Adaptive Yoga

Ingrid Yang

MD, JD, E-RYT 500, C-IAYT

Kyle Fahey

DPT, PT

HUMAN
KINETICS

Library of Congress Cataloging-in-Publication Data

Names: Yang, Ingrid, 1979- author.
Title: Adaptive Yoga / Ingrid Yang (MD, JD, E-RYT 500, C-IAYT), Kyle Fahey
  (DPT, PT).
Description: Champaign, IL : Human Kinetics, 2021. | Includes
  bibliographical references.
Identifiers: LCCN 2020017943 (print) | LCCN 2020017944 (ebook) | ISBN
  9781492596646 (paperback) | ISBN 9781492596653 (epub) | ISBN
  9781492596660 (pdf)
Subjects: LCSH: Yoga--Therapeutic use.
Classification: LCC RM727.Y64 Y36 2021 (print) | LCC RM727.Y64 (ebook) |
  DDC 613.7/046--dc23
LC record available at https://lccn.loc.gov/2020017943
LC ebook record available at https://lccn.loc.gov/2020017944

ISBN: 978-1-4925-9664-6 (print)

The web addresses cited in this text were current as of May 2020, unless otherwise noted.

Senior Acquisitions Editor: Michelle Maloney; **Developmental Editor:** Laura Pulliam; **Managing Editor:** Hannah Werner; **Copyeditor:** Rodelinde Albrecht; **Graphic Designer:** Julie L. Denzer; **Cover Designers:** Keri Evans and Racine Gruberman; **Cover Design Specialist:** Susan Rothermel Allen; **Photographs (cover):** Colin Gazley/© Human Kinetics; **Photographs (interior):** Colin Gazley/© Human Kinetics, unless otherwise noted; **Photo Production Specialist:** Amy M. Rose; **Photo Production Manager:** Jason Allen; **Senior Art Manager:** Kelly Hendren; **Illustrations:** © Human Kinetics; **Printer:** Versa Press

We thank the Prana Yoga Center in La Jolla, California, for assistance in providing the location for the photo shoot for this book.

Human Kinetics books are available at special discounts for bulk purchase. Special editions or book excerpts can also be created to specification. For details, contact the Special Sales Manager at Human Kinetics.

Printed in the United States of America   10 9 8 7 6 5 4 3 2 1

The paper in this book is certified under a sustainable forestry program.

Human Kinetics
1607 N. Market Street
Champaign, IL 61820
USA

United States and International
Website: **US.HumanKinetics.com**
Email: info@hkusa.com
Phone: 1-800-747-4457

Canada
Website: **Canada.HumanKinetics.com**
Email: info@hkcanada.com

E8019

This book is dedicated to Mom and Dad. Thank you for teaching me that we all have the potential to do something great. It is with this belief that I teach my students and patients, to help them fulfill their potential. This one's for you.

—Ingrid Yang

I dedicate this work to my patients, from whom I have learned so much. It is because of them that I am the clinician I am today. Also, to my coworkers, many of whom have provided immeasurable amounts of mentorship and support. Finally, to my parents, who taught me at a young age to strive to put others' needs before my own.

—Kyle Fahey

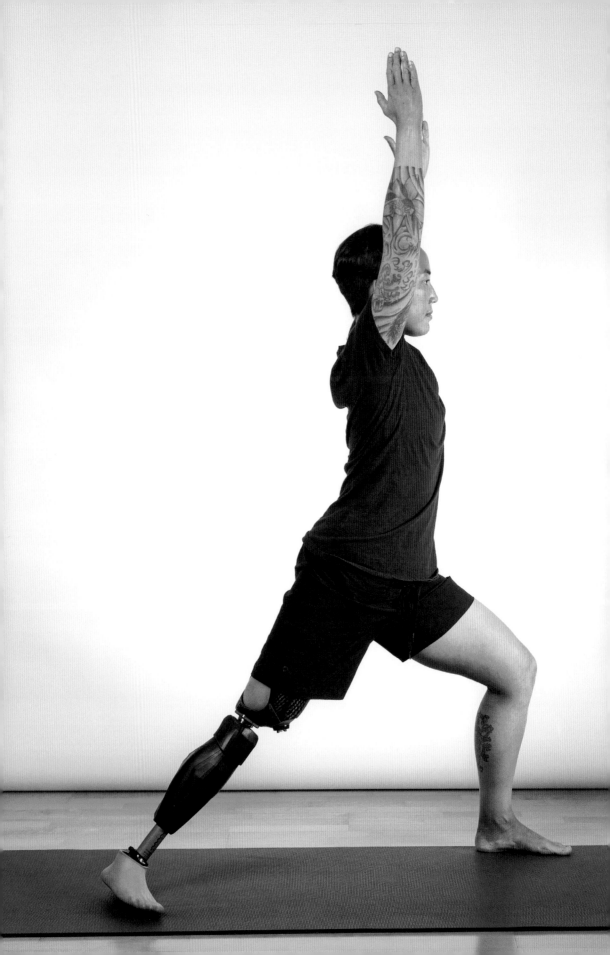

Contents

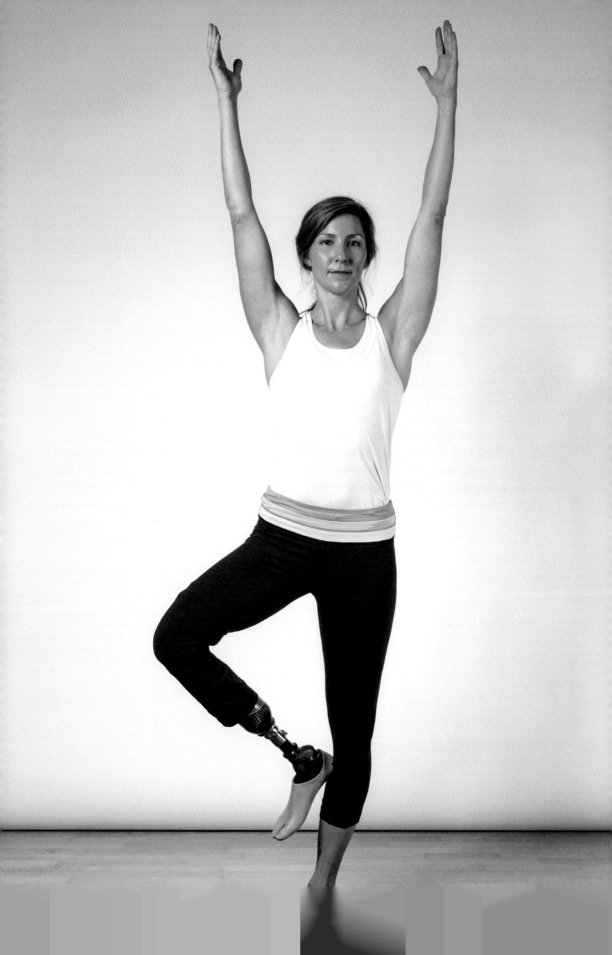

Foreword

Yoga is for every body. That's a truism that many yoga teachers, myself included, like to say. But when we say it, we're generally thinking of bodies at different sizes or different ages, not different abilities. *Adaptive Yoga* is here to expand the definition of "every body" in ways that will benefit individual practitioners as well as the field of yoga as a whole. It's a brilliant addition to the yoga and physical therapy literature, and it speaks to teachers and therapists as well as directly to yoga students.

What strikes me most about this wonderful book is that in its exquisitely specific detail of exactly how and why to use yoga to ease the symptoms of a broad range of medical conditions, it winds up pointing to the universal truths of yoga. This is fitting, because the word *yoga* itself means "union" or "connection" — a connection of the individual and mortal (the specific) with the collective and eternal (the universal). This connection is especially important when we are faced with a diagnosis or disability that defines a new way of being in our bodies and the world. It's also why most yoga practices end with *savasana*, corpse pose, as the ultimate practice of surrender and a reminder that there's more to existence than the individual ego.

If you are coming to this book to learn to adapt yoga to your own body or your students' needs, you'll pick up detailed, clearly explained, customizable ideas for how to perform yoga poses, breath exercises, and guided relaxations. But you'll also be led toward the universal truths yoga can teach us. Here are some of the main lessons that Dr. Yang and Dr. Fahey offer.

Yoga teaches its students to love and trust their bodies. It does this by allowing us to experience our strength and resilience in each moment. Yoga builds self-awareness that showcases all the things that are going right in our bodies, even when they feel less than perfect. At its most basic level, yoga teaches us to appreciate every breath.

Remember that the spine is strong and safe to move. Many yoga students — not just those suffering from low back pain — practice tentatively, in fear of doing a movement the "wrong" way, exacerbating an injury, or even drawing the teacher's attention and hence a correction. The more we can remember that bodies are made to move in all kinds of ways, the better we are able to move them and to strengthen the mind–body connection.

Promote hope, optimism, and positive expectations when practicing yoga. Metaphorically, hope and optimism are muscles. We must train them so that they become strong and capable. The more we learn to adopt positive expectations and attitudes, the easier it becomes to deploy them, even in difficult situations.

Performing the poses is not the reason to do yoga; focus on what you are trying to do for your body and find a way to do it. Amen! Know the *why* of every exercise you are doing, even if the answer is not physical but metaphysical: to learn to relax, to be in the moment, to connect to the eternal energy that animates your physical form.

I hope that by practicing the approaches you'll learn in *Adaptive Yoga*, you will have a full experience of union and connection. Dr. Yang, Dr. Fahey, and this important book are wise guides on your path toward a state of awareness and ability.

—Sage Rountree, PhD, E-RYT
Chapel Hill and Carrboro, North Carolina

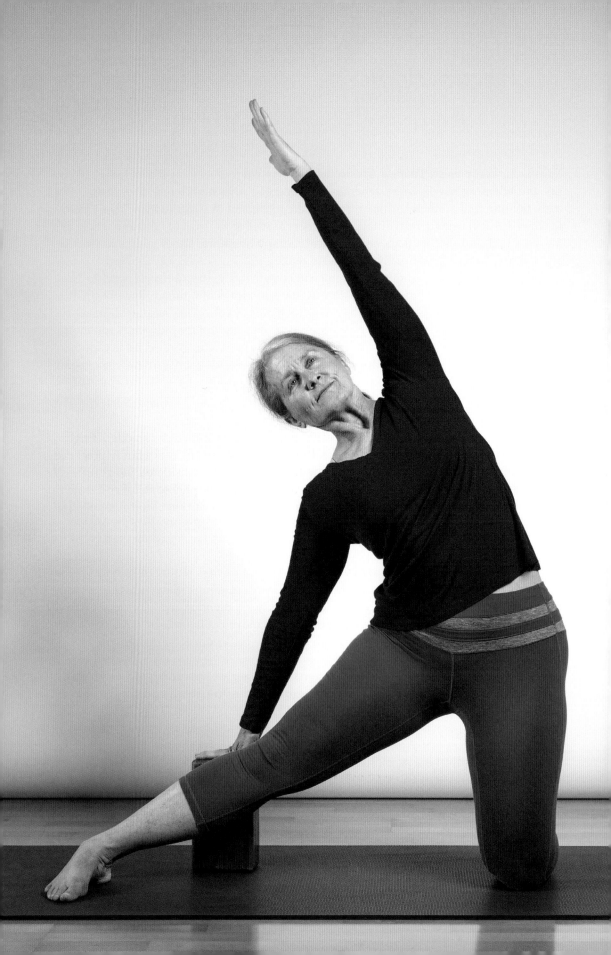

Preface

Yoga teaches us to cure what need not be endured and endure what cannot be cured.

—B.K.S. Iyengar

Yoga is for everybody. This is a saying often heard in the grand hallways of yoga conferences, in classes at yoga studio chains, and on billboards advertising stretchy yoga apparel. The pictures of that svelte 20-year-old yoga model who cranks herself into impossibly flexible positions, all while making it look easy, is indelibly embedded in our visual minds when we think about yoga. However, the normal human body does not usually bend like that, so that begs the question: Is yoga actually for everybody? Or, more specifically, for every body?

Yoga has evolved tremendously over the last century. Yoga was initially a practice created for strong young Indian men as a religious and spiritual practice. In fact, women were forced to practice yoga in secret, prohibited from practicing with a master.[1] Yoga began to gain popularity in the West at the end of the 19th century, around which time it was first formally introduced in the United States.

In the 1920s, a cleaned-up version of asana began to gain prominence as modern English language–based yoga emerged from India. Prior to this time, asana was a rarely practiced yoga tradition in India. The poses we know today were often considered the peripheral practices of yoga systems (particularly in hatha yoga). Indeed, the philosophical and esoteric frameworks of premodern hatha yoga, and the philosophy of asanas as seats for meditation and pranayama, have been sidelined in favor of systems that emphasize gymnastic movement, health and fitness, and the spiritual concerns of the modern West.

The evolution of yoga culture in the United States has taught us that we have to evolve. Yoga is a living, breathing, ever-changing phenomenon. Yoga is a practice that evolves with our bodies, communities, and lifestyles. And with this evolution, we too must adapt.

We wrote this book because it is so needed. It is beyond needed; it is necessary. Yoga is not just for robust young Indian men or willowy yoga models but for all who can benefit. (If dogs can benefit from "doga," all humans can find the rewards of a yoga practice.) This includes people whose bodies or abilities do not fit the prototype for yoga. In fact, this book proposes that people with disabilities may benefit the most from the practice of yoga.

The massive growth in popularity of yoga not only as a form of exercise but as a method of maintaining whole-body wellness has recently drawn the attention of the scientific community. Researchers have set forth countless scientific hypotheses in an attempt to quantify the health benefits of a yoga practice. Today, thousands of research studies have been published in medical and scientific journals confirming what yoga practitioners already knew: Yoga relieves stress, improves mental and emotional health, improves sleep, relieves low back and neck pain, promotes weight loss, and even enables smoking cessation. Further study has proven that yoga helps individuals with disabilities improve their mobility, experience less pain, and manage anxiety and depressive symptoms. All this study is well and good, but how do we put the science and data into practice? If yoga has been proven to help people with chronic diseases manage their symptoms and improve quality of life, what will we do with these discoveries?

This book is intended to assist the yoga community in stepping into its destined role as a healing modality for all bodies. We hope to take these studies out of the research labs and onto the yoga mat, and into therapy clinics and community centers. This book is intended to teach and empower yoga teachers, medical professionals, and individuals with chronic diseases and disabilities to utilize yoga, and its countless benefits, to maximize the potential of living and being in the spirit of yoga.

For myself, my road toward writing this book was far from straight and narrow. My journey to medicine started when I was a child (my father was a doctor and I always wanted to be just like him) but was reignited in my adulthood when I became a yoga teacher. My students would frequently approach me asking for medical advice of a biomechanical nature, and I felt ill-equipped to answer their astute and justified questions. The search for answers became purposeful, and I felt underinformed as a yoga teacher to understand the complexities that real human bodies would present to me; the level of critical thinking that was required to utilize yoga as a healing tool could not have been covered in the time frame allotted during a 200-hour teacher training. Having come from a background in academics, I poured myself into books. So, the first step in writing this book was a passion for the thing itself: books, and for giving back to the learning modality that had best assisted me in a time of need.

Eventually, I decided to follow my passion into medicine. Not only did this pursuit start to quench my thirst for all the answers to human physiology that were not covered in my initial yoga training, but it also allowed me to live the life of service that I craved. I cannot necessarily say that I entered the field of medicine because of yoga, but my study of the subject was a substantial motivator in pursuing a life in medicine. I always proudly announce that I was a yoga teacher before I was a doctor, and that's got to mean something.

My path eventually led me to work at the Shirley Ryan AbilityLab, the largest rehabilitation hospital in the United States. There, I cared for patients with all types of disabilities — spinal cord injuries (paraplegia, tetraplegia), stroke (hemiplegia, foot drops), amputations, movement disorders (Parkinson's, multiple sclerosis), osteoarthritis, and lots of low back pain. Caring for patients with disabilities is rewarding work but also presents significant challenges, because allopathic medicine can be limited in its algorithmic approach. Medicine has its own integral role, but its focus is on treating the symptoms of a specific problem and is often accompanied by an array of side effects. The allopathic algorithms can often fall short in addressing the drastic and unwelcome changes in lifestyle that accompany disabling injury or illness. Adapting to a hemiplegic lifestyle or relying on a wheelchair for mobility are some of the most difficult life transitions any human may ever experience. We have plenty of tools that assist in helping a patient get his socks on or a spoon to her mouth, but there are few tools to address the inevitable grief and loss of independence that accompany the disability. Yoga is the ultimate tool for those with chronic diseases and disabilities because it combines what the physical body needs to maintain good posture, strength, and mobility, and also emphasizes the breath, the present moment, and mindfulness. The latter aspects are the tools that actually affect quality of life. A sense of well-being, calm, and, most of all, acceptance — this is where all the healing takes place in a yoga practice.

The Shirley Ryan AbilityLab is also where I met Kyle Fahey, a young and talented physical therapist with a passion for rehabilitation and movement. When he approached me with his interest in offering yoga classes to his patients on the rehabilitation floors of the hospital, I was thrilled. Together, we set forth on a mission disseminating the good word of rehabilitative yoga with the medical structure, anatomical mastery, and deep roots in the yogic traditions that are required in an endeavor such as this.

Our experiences as practitioners in the medical field and in yoga have offered us unique insights into the gaps apparent in allopathic medicine and in the care of individuals with chronic diseases and disabilities. With our combined backgrounds of yoga, medicine, and physical therapy, we created a program integrating techniques from the ancient traditions of yoga asanas and therapeutic interventions utilized in rehabilitation hospitals and physical therapy centers. We have taken this training to physical therapy clinics and yoga centers around the world and educated people on the principles of mindfulness, breath work, and the present moment, and the response has been astounding. These cornerstones of yoga are, and will continue to be, the most important aspects of any yoga practice.

We note that yoga is not just about the physical practice but also about the eight-limbed path, which includes mental and spiritual exercises. While this book mostly focuses on the asanas (poses), it offers aids to guide the practice of breath control, Yoga Nidra, and mindfulness in the poses. These adjunctive practices can always be utilized when the physical body is unable to adapt.

The rehabilitation narrative often starts with a tragic story. Someone experiences an injury or an illness that causes a drastic change in health, mobility, and lifestyle. But the story doesn't have to have a sad ending. It can be a demonstration of the resilience of the human body and the sentient mind. It can be the triumph of a new way of living that is fulfilled and spacious in the spine and body. It can be the evolution of the spirit and the heart. It can be the path to yoga.

– Ingrid Yang

Acknowledgments

Thank you to Shoshana Clark, DPT; Lauren Rizio, OTR/L; Shari Marchbanks, DPT; Stephany Kunzweiler, DPT; and Lindsay Hoffman, DPT—expert clinicians at Shirley Ryan AbilityLab—for their guidance and education on how to make yoga focus on functional improvement.

My deepest gratitude goes to the models; our sentiments and thanks are enumerated below.

—Kyle Fahey

First, and most importantly, we want to acknowledge the models who braved the wild outside world to be photographed in a yoga studio in the middle of a pandemic: Diane Ambrosini, Nathaniel Angat, Kelly Bruno, Dani Burt, Jack Eilers, Robert Eilers, Gerhard Gessner, Sharon Houston, Diane Nelson, Steven Peace, and James Sa. Your courage and adaptability further demonstrate your resilience. To you, I offer my humblest gratitude. Your attitude, effort, and spirit will forever be part of this book of work, and I hope you acknowledge your own accomplishments every day.

Special thanks to Christina Dinh for assistance in finding models and for the world of good you are doing out there for your patients. Thank you also to the Challenged Athletes Foundation and Nico for helping identify some amazing models!

To Gerhard and Alex Gessner, owners of Prana Yoga Center in La Jolla, California, where we shot on location: Your generosity is felt not just in the community you have built but in the indelible mark you have left on the hearts you have touched. You will always be home for me in my yoga spirit. I love you both dearly.

Thank you to Rachel Krentzman, Shauna MacKay, and Jennifer Chang for being my yoga therapy guiding lights and trailblazers.

Thank you to Sage Rountree for being my mentor and confidant throughout the year. You both inspire me and embrace me with your kindness every time we talk. Thank you for being the incredible human you are.

To our photographer, Colin Gazley: You are a rock star. Your diligence, tireless dedication, charisma, kindness, attention to detail, and raw talent are unparalleled. I hope we find another project together soon because you are a true artist. The Renaissance man in you will make an indelible impression on the world and your community.

Thank you to Josh for being my biggest cheerleader, supporter, fix-it man, content editor, and lunch-delivery guy. I could not have asked for a more amazing and supportive life partner. I hope I can be the same for you.

Thank you to Racine Gruberman for lending me your amazing graphic design talents as I worked through cover options: You are an inspiration!

To my cousin, Letitia: You were always the cool cousin I looked up to for your intelligence, style, and savvy insight, all of which you still possess. Thank you for sharing your aesthetic talents with me, both for this book and because you love me. You will always have the best taste of anyone I've met, and I'm lucky to have you in my corner—and also lucky that you dress me!

My deepest gratitude to Dharma Mittra, Sarah Trelease, Cyndi Lee, David Life, Sharon Gannon, and the countless teachers I have encountered in over 20 years of practice and teaching. I have learned something from all of you that has made me more thoughtful, more open, and more flexible (in my mind, body, and heart). Yes, I'm talking about you, Brooks Rainey Pearson.

Thank you to my mentors in rehab medicine, Dr. Jason Koh, Dr. Monica Rho, Dr. Jeff Chen, Dr. Sarah Lee O'Brien, Dr. Tim Pence, Dr. Alan Anschel, Dr. Christopher Reger, and especially Dr. James Sliwa, the director of Shirley Ryan AbilityLab at the time I was employed there. Dr. Sliwa, your support meant everything to me, and I would not be where I am today if it weren't for you. And especially to Dr. Jason Ko: You are a true mentor in every sense of the word. You lead by example and have made me an exponentially better doctor with your time and care. Thank you for seeing me for my potential and allowing me to fill the role of the physician that I was meant to be.

Thank you to my mentors in internal medicine, Dr. Aashish Didwania, Dr. Tim Caprio, and the recently deceased Dr. Calvin Brown. If it were not for your encouragement and belief in me, I would not have followed the path meant for me. Because of your support, I get to serve my fellow humans with a full and hopeful heart every day. Thank you for your encouragement. To the family of Dr. Calvin Brown: I hope you remember how many hearts he touched and lives he made better. His life was spent fulfilling the worthiest of causes, in both serving patients and mentoring students and residents.

And a special thanks to the team at Human Kinetics. Michelle Maloney, we met almost a decade ago, and we are back together again—working on another book! It just goes to show that the universe has a way of bringing back people who were meant to be together. Thank you, Michelle, for believing in us and in this worthy project. I will be forever grateful. Laura Pulliam, you are not only a remarkably good editor but also an incredibly patient and kind human. Thank you for sticking through this with us! Doug Fink, the HK photo department director, made me feel like everything was going to be okay when I was stressed about all the different permutations of how to do these photos. Doug, you are both the voice of reason and the voice of sage experience. You may consider a career in radio with that million-dollar voice of yours. And to our content editors, Rodelinde Albrecht and Karla Walsh: You sure had your work cut out for you, sifting through all of our technical jargon. Thank you for your attention to detail and endurance in making our words sound pretty. And a special thanks to every individual at Human Kinetics. I could not ask for a more supportive and thoughtful publishing team. Most readers don't realize that there are so many (yet somehow, so few) individuals getting a book done. Yet, there are many hours spent on each individual piece—drafting, editing, photographing, designing, marketing, and so on. It truly takes a village of dedicated experts to do what you do. Thank you for believing in this project and the importance of this work!

And a special thanks to my coauthor, Kyle Fahey. It was quite a year-long journey writing this book, wasn't it? Your partnership has been the highlight of writing this book. Your work ethic and dedication have motivated me countless times to keep on writing, editing, and rewriting, especially when I thought I was too tired or burnt out from working in the hospital to meet our deadlines. This book would not have happened without your depth of knowledge and enthusiasm for rehab. High five, partner. We did it.

—Ingrid Yang

Introduction

How to Use This Book for Yourself

This book is divided into chapters based on specific conditions. You may have more than one of these conditions, and you will notice overlaps in some of the poses, but the instructions are different and separate based on the condition for which the chapter is written.

Depending on your condition, you may need an assistant, and it may be beneficial to work with a qualified instructor when you begin to practice yoga. Whether or not the yoga teacher is specifically trained in your condition, he or she will assist you in learning proper alignment and modifications specifically developed for your body and how to use props (blocks, straps, chairs, etc.) to gently ease into the poses. Be sure you do your research before choosing the right yoga teacher for you. The teacher should be certified, understand your goals, and resonate with you in the teacher–student relationship. You should feel safe and supported by your teacher and in the postures.

If you prefer to work on your own, be sure that you have all the props close by and available to you. Always work with your breath; if it becomes irregular and rapid, ease yourself back and out of the pose. If you feel expansive in your breath, you may be ready to advance the pose. Whatever happens, let your breath be the guide.

Your pose does not need to look exactly like the photo. In fact, we can guarantee that it will not. Your body is different, and the disease process behind your condition varies in different bodies. Read the instructions, listen to your body, use your breath, and share your experience with others. We learn the most in connection and relationship—to ourselves, our bodies, and others. And remember, what matters is how you feel and how measured your breath can be. You should always feel better after a yoga practice than when you started.

How to Use This Book If You Are a Yoga Teacher

If you teach yoga and you want to offer adaptive yoga to a student, family member, or friend: First of all, thank you. Yoga has so much healing potential, both physically and emotionally, for those you teach. This is why yoga was created and why you became a yoga teacher.

We encourage you to obtain formal training in the conditions that you seek to teach because hands-on learning is invaluable. If you are not yet ready for a live training and are seeking to use this book for ideas and references on how to help your students with these conditions, be sure that you first practice the poses in your own body using the specific instructions before teaching it to others. You will not be able to fully understand how your student is feeling if you don't have their condition, and that's okay. Your students will just be glad to be supported in their yoga journey.

Study, read the instructions, find other references, and do your research. With great privilege comes great responsibility. And if you take on this responsibility, take it with seriousness and a heartfelt desire to help. If and when you do not know what to do next or how to help your student to modify, be honest and communicate this. You can work with your student together as a team to ensure safety and progression. Enlist the help of your mentors and colleagues, and be available to hold space for your student and for yourself. You are engaging in important work. Allow there to be purpose behind your work, an unremitting sense of curiosity, and let the process open your heart in ways you never knew it could. We hope this book gives you just what you need to do the good and important work of teaching adaptive yoga.

How to Use This Book If You Are a Rehabilitation Therapist

If you do not have formal training as a yoga teacher, you can still use this book to help teach yoga poses to your patients. We spent a lot of time researching and explaining the why for each posture in the specific conditions, so that you can take these explanations in concert with your training as a professional therapist. Yoga will teach your students how to breathe within their rehabilitative journey and in each exercise and pose you teach them. If you are reading this and have acquired this book, you know the potential for yoga to help your patient in the healing practice. We hope you can use this as a reference with your formal training to enhance the rehab experience and progression of your patients.

A Note on Categorization and Sequencing

Many of the chapters are divided based on the pragmatic considerations of the specific condition. For instance, chapter 6 (Lower Limb Amputation) is split into three categories: strength and flexibility poses to be performed with a prosthetic device, strength and flexibility poses to be performed with or without a prosthetic device, and balance poses. Similarly, the chapter 7 (Spinal Cord Injury) poses are categorized as strength poses or flexibility poses. You will find this pattern for chapters in which categorization will help the reader target specific muscle groups or goals, and the categories are delineated at the bottom of each page.

Of note, the poses selected for each chapter should not necessarily be performed in sequential order. For each individual, sequencing will differ based on a variety of factors, and the poses can be tailored to the individual's needs. Therefore, there is no set order of how to practice the poses presented in this book. Instead, we encourage readers to review the poses in each chapter before practicing them so that a custom sequence can be created prior to beginning movement. Properly warming the body is integral to a safe yoga practice, particularly when seeking to dive deeper into certain poses. As always, remember to rest between postures when needed and to practice in a manner that is optimal for your body and your needs.

PART I

Principles of Adapting Yoga

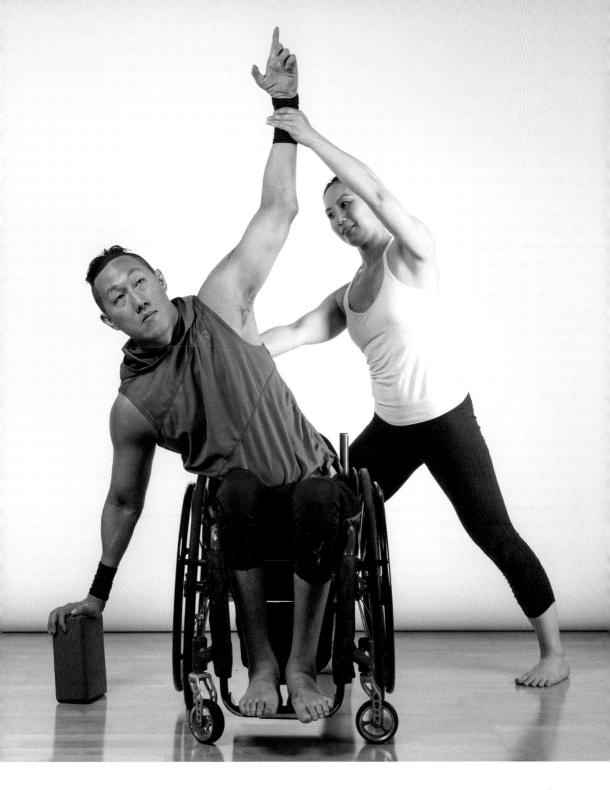

CHAPTER 1

Yoga as Rehabilitation

Disability is defined as the manifestation of a physical or psychological limitation in the context of the social environment.[17] People with disabilities (PWD) represent the world's largest minority group, with approximately 15 percent of individuals experiencing some type of disability.[18] The population of PWD includes people of all races, ethnicities, genders, and ages, and the term *disabilities* encompasses a variety of conditions.[18] For example, disabilities can be categorized by type, including physical, cognitive, emotional, and developmental disabilities; they are also often described as either congenital (present at birth) or acquired as a result of injury, aging, health condition, or other event.[16] In this book, we focus on physical disabilities, typically acquired, but we want to highlight that yoga can benefit people with any of the previously mentioned disabilities. As the global population ages, and we live longer, chronic disease increases in prevalence, causing the number of people transitioning into disability to rise. The disablement process has been described as a pathway; the transition progresses from pathology (the essential nature and origin of the disease) to impairment (the characteristics specific to that disability) to functional limitation (restrictions in basic actions) to disability (difficulty performing basic and instrumental activities of daily life).[11]

Studies have shown that PWD report higher rates of physical inactivity than those without disabilities (54.2 percent vs. 32.2 percent).[9] This pattern of low physical activity becomes more problematic across the lifespan when the effects of the natural aging process are compounded by years of sedentary living, poor nutrition, and deconditioning.[13]

Yoga is uniquely suited to be practiced by people with disabilities and chronic health conditions because each pose can be modified or adapted to meet the individual's needs. In particular, the focus on the physical poses, combined with mindfulness and breath work, not only improves flexibility, strength, balance, and stamina, but also reduces anxiety and stress, improves mental clarity, and even enhances sleep. Yoga asanas can be performed at all ability levels—while standing, lying on the floor, or seated in a chair or wheelchair. Thus, yoga is empowering because it meets individuals at their current level of function and progresses toward meeting achievable goals.

Why Yoga?

Popular yoga systems provide little guidance to those with physical disabilities, leaving many, if not most, people with disabilities minimally prepared to manage or improve their health and fitness by practicing yoga. Despite yoga's numerous potential benefits, scholars and activists have voiced that dominant media representations of yoga and its practitioners may limit how the accessibility of the practice is perceived.[13] Published analyses of mainstream yoga media contain limited visual representations of those with disabilities, and these representations have become increasingly narrow, potentially discouraging people from trying yoga despite its health benefits.[8]

Ironically, yoga is widely advertised as a practice that promotes a variety of health benefits, including lower blood pressure, increased joint mobility, improved quality of life, and reduced stress.[5] The asanas (poses) and pranayamas (breathing exercises) practiced in yoga may be especially beneficial for people with physical disabilities[5] such as arthritis, chronic pain, multiple sclerosis (MS), stroke, spinal cord injury (SCI), and Parkinson's disease.[1,6,14,15] Indeed, studies that examine yoga participation among people with MS-related disability and SCI suggest that yoga programs are safe and feasible and that participants experienced improvements in quality of life and physical and mental functioning while participating in a regular yoga practice.[3,4]

One of the keys to yoga as a rehabilitative tool is its nature as an ongoing practice rather than as an end in itself. Yoga is not simply about poses; it is a system and way of living that was created thousands of years ago to help people maintain and live a happy, healthy life. As practitioners who have worked extensively with PWD, we are most affected by how disembodied a patient feels after disability. In some ways, the body has either attacked them (such as in arthritis, Parkinson's, or MS) or failed them (such as in SCI, stroke, or low back pain). So then, why yoga? Literally translated, the word *yoga* means "union." One way to interpret this translation is that yoga is meant to unite the mind, body, and spirit. Uniting the physical poses with your breath, action with thought, and awareness with intention can be the path to peace in the body, mind, and spirit. This allows us to live again with our bodies, which we may have made an enemy of. It teaches us how to use our body again and make friends with it. This allows us to become "in-bodied" again.

Take for instance the simple practice of breathing. This is something we all do every day without conscious effort or thought. But when you become aware of what a powerful tool breathing is, and of how your breathing affects every part of your body, it becomes an object of magnificence and wonder. As you learn how to focus awareness on your breathing, you can observe how your mind can feel calmer and your body more relaxed. In this manner, mindfulness in thought can lead to actual physiologic changes in your body. This is how yoga is different from other forms of exercise: the connection to mindfulness, conscious thought and effort, and the human spirit.

And the poses themselves? Each pose is designed to stack your joints optimally and to utilize your body weight to improve your strength and flexibility. The poses support the body's joints, muscles, structure, and function, and we encourage you to modify the poses to their simplest form as you begin. As you gain confidence and ease in the poses, you can try variations and challenges. This is the beauty of yoga and why it is for everyone. It is not about lifting the most weight or hitting the ball accurately or even running the fastest; it is about modifying movement for your goals and your body's needs. You can be standing, sitting in a chair or wheelchair, or even lying on the floor or in bed—wherever you are most comfortable at that point in time. We encourage you to use the tool of visualization to combine breathing while imagining yourself performing the poses, which can help you move in the right direction when you have reduced mobility.

We also advise that you speak with your health care provider before you begin a yoga practice and discuss any questions or concerns that you or they may have. Your health care provider should be able to support you through your journey in yoga, and may even be able to educate other patients on yoga, borrowing from your experience.

The benefits of yoga can be experienced in just a few minutes of practice, whether it be through poses, pranayama, or a mindfulness practice. You should always feel better after practicing yoga than when you started. Struggling or suffering through a practice is not the purpose. The journey will present challenges; each day and each practice will be different. Some days may feel impossibly hard, other days you will feel more spacious and present. Stick with it. The answers will come and will make sense when the time is right. And at times, you will wonder whether yoga is something you can really do. It is. Be with it, and with all the emotions that arise, fully and with an open heart. There will be other moments when you wonder if yoga is too difficult. It is not. Modifications are always available, and we encourage you to take a moment to rest or simply breathe.

Every body is different—in shape, strength, flexibility, mobility, height, weight, tension, energy level, and ability. Day to day, your body will change. It will be different from the body it was yesterday, or an hour ago. And, yes, yoga is for *every* body.

What Is Adaptive Yoga?

Adaptive yoga tailors the instruction and practice of yoga to an individual's needs in a safe, comfortable, practical manner. The point is that yoga is accessible to everyone's body at every moment. Yoga asks you to start where you are, and that is different for everybody. Yoga requires you to be mindful of your body and the present moment; this mindfulness allows you to ascertain that starting point with compassion and kindness toward yourself. For example, if Locust feels impossible right now, you can adapt the pose to accommodate your body's needs and abilities. Props are encouraged, and using your breath is mandatory. Be kind to yourself and be exactly where you are. The goal is not to assume the perfect magazine cover pose; it is to do what you can and what feels right in the moment.

The beauty of exercise is that anyone, regardless of their functionality, can benefit from it. Everyone from hospital patients to professional athletes can use exercise to recover from injuries, improve general health, decrease pain, and so much more. Rehabilitation is the facilitation of exercise to optimally increase strength, flexibility, and endurance with the ultimate goal of improving function and quality of life. Rehabilitation is necessary both acutely after injury or illness and throughout life. We can always improve our musculoskeletal capabilities and function. After a life-altering injury or illness, functional improvement does not happen with prolonged rest and languishing away into muscular atrophy. Research and clinical experience have demonstrated that functional outcomes are vastly better with earlier and more frequent movement. Exercise improves and maintains function, lessens pain, and enhances quality of life for PWD. The goal of adaptive yoga is not only to modify yoga poses but to use yoga as a tool to improve mobility, function, and quality of life. The best way to build confidence and trust in your body after disability is to be mindful of and actively observe progress. In this vein, it is crucial to adapt and modify poses to your specific capabilities. Imagine being asked to perform a task or movement that you know your body can never do; the instinct is to give up. But when you are given the tools and knowledge to achieve your goals, despite the challenges, your motivation increases, and with it, your confidence.

Use Props

A key component of adaptive yoga is using all available tools to facilitate safe progression, such as the use of yoga or other exercise props (blocks, blankets, bolsters, chairs, the wall, etc.) to help support the poses. In adaptive yoga, the use of props is not just encouraged, but required; props not only increase each pose's accessibility but also offer support and a base from which to build strength and flexibility. This mirrors the use of adaptive equipment in rehabilitation. If a patient cannot stand or walk independently, a walker is used as an assistive device. For patients lacking strength in the legs to lift themselves into and out of the bed, a leg lifter is used to compensate and accomplish the goals intended. These tools provide the user with the independence and confidence to perform the tasks of daily living, and enable self-sufficient movement to improve strength, endurance, and function. Yoga props offer a similar functional purpose; if the ground seems too far out of reach, a yoga block can be used to bridge that gap. Like the assistive devices used in rehab, props enable you to perform movements and poses that will, over time, give you greater strength, flexibility, and endurance.

As you become more familiar with the yoga poses, a better understanding of your body mechanics will come naturally. Eventually the props will no longer be necessary and you will be able to rely more on your body's own strength. However, know that shedding your use of props is no badge of honor or measure of your skill. Props can and should always be used for support when needed, and if you hope to progress with your use of them, you can change their size and height at any time.

Adapt Poses

In this book, we recommend various methods of adapting poses. Whether the limitation is decreased balance, strength, or pain, therapeutic yoga can still be used to strengthen targeted muscle groups. Poses can be modified to meet specific needs and can be selected to facilitate progress to improve function and mobility.

The primary adaptation is the use of props as discussed in the previous section. Props enable you to place and keep your body in a position that it may not otherwise be able to achieve. The secondary method of adapting is through the selection of poses. Our recommended poses in each chapter are based on current research and rehabilitation practices. The purpose of choosing these specific poses for each condition is to facilitate targeted strengthening and stretching to the muscle groups that will create the most improvement for each medical condition. Our third method of yoga adaptation is through pose modification. Within each pose instruction, we provide a list of ways you can modify traditional yoga poses to increase their accessibility. Every body is different, just as every disease process is different. Modifications are integral to any yoga practice, whether or not you have a disability. Pay attention to the ways your body wants to modify and allow yourself to move in ways that make each pose approachable and accessible.

Our goal for this book is not to target yoga for specific conditions only. We don't want to hand you a narrow version of yoga; we want to teach you how to adapt yoga to the unique needs of your body. That is why we have set out to teach you the tools needed for each specific adaptation. This encompasses the mechanics and pathology of the diseases, the consequent mobility deficits, how to use props and other modifications, and how to select poses to perform targeted muscle strengthening or stretching. With these tools you will be able to create practices to meet the abilities for every body.

A NOTE ABOUT THE PHOTOGRAPHS

You may notice that the photographs sometimes look different from their corresponding instructions, or that you are able to perform more (or less) of the pose than depicted in the selected images. Please don't worry. We wrote this book on the premise that each individual's body is different. Your pose will look different than the model's demonstration, and also different from the ones you may discover on the internet. If the instructions recommend that you point the toes, point them with all your might, even if the model doesn't have the perfect ballerina point. We selected models with the exact conditions discussed in their respective chapters because we value integrity and authenticity, which are essential to your confidence when performing the poses. Know that the conditions' manifestations may present differently in the pictured individuals for an infinite number of reasons. Do what works in your body, not someone else's. We promise you that perfect is not better. You are all you need to be in this moment to perform the poses as they were meant to be practiced in your body. We encourage you to summon your courage and confidence, and know that you are capable of putting these techniques into practice.

Incorporate Open and Closed Chain Exercises

Open chain exercises are an excellent starting point for exercise, whether in yoga, strength training, or rehabilitation. An open chain exercise is an exercise in which the distal segment of a limb (the foot or hand) is free to move in space. For example, in strengthening the arm, the hand remains free, and in strengthening the leg, the foot remains free. Boat is an example of an open chain exercise that strengthens the hip flexors—the feet are free as the hip flexors contract to elevate the legs. Gate is another open chain exercise—the hand is free while the shoulder abductors contract to elevate the arm overhead. Open chain movements permit isolated muscle activation, allowing for targeted muscle strengthening.[10] Because these exercises are not weight-bearing on the specific targeted muscle, there is minimal load through the joints of the extremities, and therefore more ease of movement in otherwise painful limbs. Open chain movements are incredibly accessible because they can be performed in any position and can be assisted by a yoga strap to gain full range of motion.

From open chain, exercises can progress to closed chain. In closed chain exercise, the distal portion of the limb is fixed against the floor, the wall, or a yoga block. A good example of a closed chain pose is Plank, which strengthens the shoulders with the feet and hands fixed on the floor. Warrior I is another closed chain pose that strengthens the knee extensors (quadriceps) of the front leg with the feet fixed on the floor. In closed chain exercises, movements occur at multiple joints simultaneously. For instance, in Chair, hip flexion, knee flexion, and ankle dorsiflexion occur simultaneously to achieve the squatted pose. The multijoint movements generate multiple points of muscle activation, promoting greater strength gains because they require stability and control while the feet are fixed. Many of these movements closely mimic movements that are used in daily life (moving from Chair to Mountain simulates standing up from a seated position) and are practiced conceptually to improve function in daily life.[10]

Introduce Unstable Surfaces

Exercising on unstable surfaces has been shown to produce greater muscle activation.[7] In the gym, this might be done on a stability ball or a foam pad. For the purposes of this book and working with the disabled population, we recommend making a surface unstable by decreasing the surface area of its base (narrowing the base of support or switching to one-legged postures). This is one of the ways we challenge the practitioner and create an unstable surface on which to build strength. In any position, strength and muscle control are used to stabilize the body's center of mass (COM). In yoga, typically the torso is positioned over the feet (acting as the base of support, or BOS). A greater challenge can be created by narrowing the BOS (think Warrior I vs. Chair vs. Tree), creating opportunity for larger increases in strength, control, and balance.

Poses can also be simplified by broadening the BOS or lowering the COM closer to the BOS to facilitate accessibility. Broadening the BOS can be as simple as repositioning the feet (e.g., widening the feet in Warrior I). For some, holding onto a chair or a block may be necessary, and this actually widens the BOS by giving the body another point of contact, and increases the base between the feet and the additional support mechanism. To lower the COM closer to the BOS, you can bring your arms alongside your body or to heart center (e.g., modifications in Chair).

Use the Breath

A crucial component of your adaptive yoga practice is to use the breath with the poses. Your breath keeps you grounded and mindful of where you are in each pose and movement. When you are breathing too rapidly, it is a signal to your body to ease back on a pose, or perhaps to exit the pose altogether. If you notice a yawn (which is also a method of breathing), perhaps it is time to push your body and try a challenge modification of the pose.

Practice Mindfully

Yoga is distinct and unique from other forms of rehabilitation and exercise because you must practice it mindfully. Psychosocial factors play important roles in pain and associated physical and psychosocial disability.[12] If yoga will give you anything, it is a sense of peace and wellness. But this idea is neither new nor novel. In fact, four of the eight nonpharmacologic treatments recommended for persistent back pain by the American College of Physicians include mind–body practices.[2] Mindfulness practice in yoga calls upon a mind–body approach to increase awareness and acceptance of moment-to-moment experiences, including physical discomfort and difficult emotions, which inevitably arise whether or not you have a societally defined disability. Yoga cannot be practiced properly without an emphasis on mindful action to enter, exit, and exist in each pose. This is yet another reason why hatha yoga (the branch of yoga that studies the physical postures) is such an ideal physical activity for those with specific medical conditions and within the rehabilitative journey; when we move our bodies mindfully, we have less risk of injury and greater opportunity to activate the relaxation response. And what better way to feel good within our bodies than to be able to master our ability to relax the nervous system.

We do encourage a formal meditation practice, not just mindfulness during the poses. Start with just five minutes a day of paying attention to your breath, without distraction or movement. You can sit, stand, or lie down during this time. The key is to follow the breath and be in the present moment. When thoughts arise, bring your attention back to the breath, and let go of following the trail of your thoughts. It will be challenging at first. You will have to fight every urge to disturb the process of meditation and the desire to distract your mind. But if you can be with it, truly sit with it, you will notice transformations in your body and mind that will change your life. You can build up the minutes each day or each week to eventually form a dedicated and sustained practice. Yoga and mindfulness are inextricably linked. Without mindfulness, you are simply stretching, not practicing yoga. Yoga is your entrée into mindfulness, and mindfulness is your key to unlocking the door to a happy and fulfilled life. Practice—often and well. You will notice changes in your mind, body, and heart that you never anticipated, but they will be your springboard to soar through your life with joy and triumph.

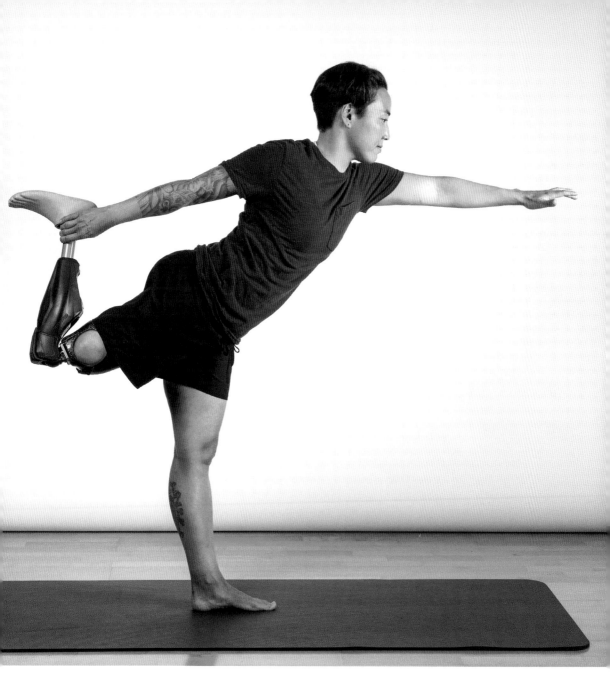

CHAPTER 2

How the Body Moves

Anatomy is the study of the basic structures of the body. It includes knowledge of the bones, muscles, joints, blood vessels, nerves, and organs of the body. Familiarity with the anatomy of the human body is integral for any yogi seeking to teach adaptive yoga, and helpful for any student practicing it. Knowing the muscles and how they move the body is integral to the practice of adaptive yoga, particularly in deciphering which poses target the strength and flexibility of specific muscle groups to facilitate healing and functional improvements. Our musculoskeletal system is brilliant and sophisticated. It provides our bodies with tremendous support and stability while enabling us to perform a countless number of movements. This book focuses primarily on how yoga affects the musculoskeletal system, and more specifically on how yoga can be used to improve this system to enhance quality of life and physical function.

Anatomy Basics

For decades, the scientific community has been studying the medical conditions included in this book. In an effort to improve how we rehabilitate our bodies after injury or illness, we have focused a large segment of our research on the effects these conditions exert on the strength, endurance, flexibility, and power of the muscles. For each specific condition, we know which muscle groups are most commonly weak and which are most commonly tight. If you are able to learn how to address these muscle deficits, you will be able to perform a variety of poses and modifications.

There are 206 bones in an adult human body that comprise the skeletal system. Bones are remarkable structures that are strong enough to withstand the forces we demand from them day after day, yet light enough to allow us to move through our world to perform our daily activities with ease and elegance. The skeletal system gives structure and support to our body by providing attachment sites for muscles and pathways for nerves and arteries. Our bones protect our vital organs: The skull encases the brain while the sternum and ribs shield the heart and lungs. The skeletal system allows for movement where there is a relationship between two or more bones; this connection is defined as a joint.

Bones connect at the joints and are supported by ligaments and other connective tissue to provide stability while allowing considerable mobility. The bones themselves are brilliantly shaped in specific configurations to promote stability and mobility. For example, the hip and shoulder joints are known as ball-and-socket joints because the ball-shaped head of the thigh and upper arm bones sit inside the concave hip and shoulder sockets. However, joints only enable movement where muscles create movement. Without the muscular system these bones and joints would only be able to respond to forces from outside the body.

The muscles and bones work together to allow us to control our relationship to gravity, provide an upright posture, and let us move through and interact with our environment. Simply put, the muscles act to move the bones into a desired position or maintain them there. An example of when the muscles and bones do not work optimally is in Parkinson's disease (PD). In PD, the postural muscles tend to become weak and stiff, which can result in a forward-bent posture at the waist when standing and walking. Consequently, many of the poses recommended for PD focus on improving the strength and flexibility of these postural muscles to enable a more upright posture, thus allowing the bones to better stack against gravity and decrease the effort required to maintain optimal posture.

Muscles are made up of multiple bundles of muscle cells known as muscle fibers. Generally, these fibers run parallel to one another. When a muscle is contracted, the muscle fibers shorten to create movement at the joints they cross. For example, your biceps muscle (biceps brachii) attaches to the upper arm and forearm bones and crosses in front of the elbow joint. In order to bend the elbow, the muscle fibers of the biceps contract and shorten, decreasing the angle between the upper arm and forearm.

Keep in mind that not every muscle contraction is the same. In fact, our musculoskeletal system produces various types of contractions as we move throughout the day, such as the following.

- *Concentric contraction* occurs when muscle fibers contract and **shorten** as a joint moves. This requires the muscle to produce more force to overcome the resistance at the joint, thus shortening the length of the muscle while it produces tension. For example, lifting the torso up from a Standing Forward Bend requires the hamstrings, glutes, and muscles in the back to shorten, concentrically contracting.

- *Eccentric contraction* occurs when muscle fibers contract and **lengthen** as a joint moves. In eccentric contraction, the resistance at a joint is greater than the force produced by the muscles, therefore the muscle elongates while under tension due to the opposing force of the joint. A good example is while moving from Plank to bent elbows, the pectoralis and triceps muscles contract while lengthening to lower slowly and with control.

- *Isometric contraction* occurs when muscle fibers contract, but without joint motion or a change in muscle length. To maintain Plank, the pectoralis and triceps muscles must isometrically contract (without actual visible movement) to keep the shoulders and elbows from collapsing under gravity.

Each of these contractions (concentric, eccentric, and isometric) is repeatedly performed during yoga and can improve strength in the muscles involved. Regular exercise causes muscles to contract against resistance, producing greater force in contraction of the muscle fibers, which results in increased strength. This increase in muscle strength occurs in two major ways.

- *Changes in the nervous system:* Initial gains in strength occur due to an enhanced nerve–muscle connection. The nerves that stimulate a muscle causing that contraction connect to a greater number of muscle fibers. Therefore, recruiting more muscle cells at a time generates more force. This accounts for much of the strength increases in the initial stages of strength training and can allow for weak muscles to become stronger through activation alone, even without the addition of resistance (weights and pulleys). As an example, the presence of knee pain may cause difficulty in knee extensor contraction. A principle of rehabilitation in knee osteoarthritis is performing exercises to increase control of the knee extensors. This often includes simply practicing activation of this muscle group, as demonstrated in Staff.

- *Increased size of muscle fibers:* Enlargement of the muscle fibers is called *hypertrophy*, causing muscle cells to perform greater protein synthesis. Contrary to common belief, the number of muscle cells does not increase during this process of protein synthesis; the muscle cells themselves become larger. This increased muscle volume produces greater amounts of force, yielding more strength potential during functional use. Note that hypertrophy does not occur until after several weeks of exercise, so practice, practice, practice. For example, weakness or paralysis of the legs may result from spinal cord injury. As a compensatory measure, the upper body is utilized to shift body weight and perform activities of daily living. A notable hypertrophy of the shoulder muscles is typically observed and is crucial to enable the use of the arms to compensate.

Flexibility is another functional characteristic that is improved with a regular yoga practice. Muscle flexibility is the ability of a muscle to be passively lengthened. This happens constantly and unintentionally as we move. During any joint movement, some muscles are shortening and others are lengthening. As the elbow straightens, the triceps muscle shortens and its antagonist muscle (the biceps) lengthens. Deficits in a muscle's ability to lengthen limits mobility and can lead to pain or decreased function. Loss of muscle flexibility can occur through muscle injury, pain, disuse over time, the normal physiologic effects of aging, or changes in the nervous system. For instance, individuals with cerebral palsy (CP) and multiple sclerosis (MS) often have significant loss of flexibility in the legs due to the lack of use and inefficient body mechanics. This in turn can lead to changes in gait and posture. Therefore, increasing flexibility is not as simple as stretching a tight muscle but also includes the process of retraining the nervous system to allow the muscle to relax and lengthen. It should be noted that joints can become stiff themselves, limiting movement. Joint stiffness is often mistaken for a loss of muscle flexibility.

In the chapters ahead, we will recommend yoga poses that can be utilized to improve the strength or flexibility of muscles for specific medical diagnoses. In each chapter, we target muscle groups rather than individual muscles. Muscle groups are muscles that are located in close proximity to one another and which, when they contract, perform the same action. For example, there are four muscles located on the front of the thigh (commonly known as the quadriceps): vastus medialis, vastus lateralis, vastus intermedius, and rectus femoris. These muscles all act to straighten or extend the knee. Therefore, they are referred to as the *knee extensors*. It is important to understand the names of muscle groups, and the specific terms that are used to describe muscle and joint actions:

- *Flexion:* Generally, replaces the term *bending*. For example, bending the knee to bring the heel toward the buttocks is known as knee flexion.
- *Extension:* Generally, replaces the term *straightening*. For example, straightening the knee to kick a ball is knee extension.

- *Rotation:* Movement around the axis of a limb. In the hips and shoulders this occurs as internal (toward the midline of the body) or external (away from the midline). For example, when a pitcher brings the hand back during windup the shoulder is externally rotated, and with the action of throwing the ball the shoulder is internally rotated.
- *Abduction:* Movement of the limb away from the midline. For example, in a jumping jack, the hands lift overhead, and the shoulders abduct.
- *Adduction:* Movement of the limb toward the midline. When the hands come back alongside the body during a jumping jack, the shoulders adduct.

It is important to note that this terminology can present an initial challenge when differentiating between strength and flexibility training. Bending your elbow to bring your hand toward your shoulder can be used to strengthen the elbow flexors. However, that same movement can be used to stretch (increasing flexibility of) the elbow extensors. With time, you will develop a firm grasp on these concepts from kinesthetic muscle memory. And, with practice, you will understand how to utilize poses to strengthen weakened muscles and lengthen tight muscles.

Muscle Anatomy Reference Guide

Tables 2.1 to 2.3 show the most commonly targeted muscle groups in this book. In the chapters ahead, we will be recommending poses for each medical condition. These poses have been selected to strengthen or stretch targeted muscle groups. For example, Bound Angle stretches the hip adductor muscle group and Bridge strengthens the hip extensors. This section is provided as a guide and reference for the location or action of these muscle groups. As you read through this book and learn the yoga poses, there may be terms that are unfamiliar to you. We encourage you to review this section alongside each condition chapter to obtain a solid grasp of the anatomical benefits of the yoga poses chosen for each condition.

Lower Extremity Muscle Groups

The muscles of the legs are generally the longest and the strongest of the body, but their key function is locomotion. Locomotion is the ability to move from one place to another. Whether it consists of walking up a flight of stairs, running a mile, or walking from one room to another, locomotion is a key component of quality of life. All of the conditions discussed in this book have strength and flexibility deficits in the lower extremity muscles. These deficits result in challenges, such as pain and inefficiency in locomotion. See table 2.1 for an explanation of the muscles included in the lower extremity muscle groups.

Table 2.1 Lower Extremity Muscle Groups

Muscle group name	Components of muscle group	Muscle action
Hip flexors	*Prime mover:* iliopsoas *Accessory muscles:* rectus femoris, tensor fasciae latae, sartorius	Moves the thigh forward to flex the hip (up toward the chest)
Muscles of the iliopsoas: Psoas major Iliacus Tensor fasciae latae Sartorius Rectus femoris		
Hip extensors	*Prime mover:* gluteus maximus *Accessory muscles:* biceps femoris, semimembranosus, semitendinosus	Straightens the hip joint, moving the thigh backwards and the foot back behind you
Gluteus maximus Gluteus maximus (cut) Biceps femoris (long head) Semimembranosus Semitendinosus Biceps femoris (short head)		
Hip adductors	*Prime movers:* adductor magnus, adductor longus, adductor brevis *Accessory muscles:* gracilis, pectineus	Moves the thigh inward, toward the midline of the body
Pectineus Gracilis Adductor brevis Adductor longus Adductor magnus		

Muscle group name	Components of muscle group	Muscle action
Hip abductors 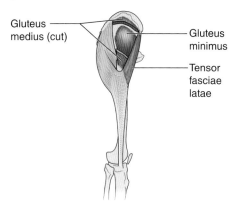 Gluteus medius (cut), Gluteus minimus, Tensor fasciae latae	*Prime mover:* gluteus medius *Accessory muscles:* gluteus minimus, tensor fasciae latae	Moves the thigh outward, away from the midline of the body
Hip internal rotators 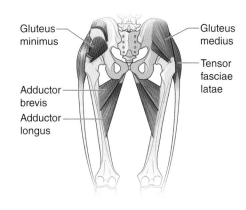 Gluteus minimus, Adductor brevis, Adductor longus, Gluteus medius, Tensor fasciae latae	*Prime mover:* gluteus medius *Accessory muscles:* gluteus minimus, tensor fasciae latae, adductor longus, adductor brevis	Rotates the thigh toward the midline, bringing the foot inward
Hip external rotators 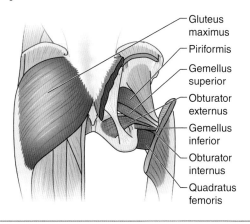 Gluteus maximus, Piriformis, Gemellus superior, Obturator externus, Gemellus inferior, Obturator internus, Quadratus femoris	*Prime mover:* gluteus maximus *Accessory muscles:* obturator internus, obturator externus, gemellus superior, gemellus inferior, piriformis, quadratus femoris	Rotates the thigh away from the midline, bringing the foot outward

(continued)

Table 2.1 (continued)

Muscle group name	Components of muscle group	Muscle action
Knee flexors Biceps femoris (long head) Biceps femoris (short head) Semimembranosus Semitendinosus Gastrocnemius	*Prime mover:* biceps femoris *Accessory muscles:* semitendinosus, semimembranosus, gastrocnemius	Flexes the knee, and assists with hip extension (see *hip extensors* in this table)
Knee extensors Rectus femoris Vastus lateralis Vastus medialis Vastus intermedius (under rectus femoris)	*Prime mover:* rectus femoris *Accessory muscles:* vastus lateralis, vastus medialis, vastus intermedius	Straightens the knee, and assists with hip flexion (see *hip flexors* in this table)
Ankle dorsiflexors Tibialis anterior Extensor digitorum longus Extensor hallucis longus	*Prime mover:* tibialis anterior *Accessory muscles:* extensor digitorum longus, extensor hallucis longus	Flexes the ankle to lift the foot, causing the angle between the top of the foot and the lower leg to decrease

Muscle group name	Components of muscle group	Muscle action
Ankle plantar flexors Gastrocnemius, Soleus, Peroneus longus, Peroneus brevis	*Prime movers:* gastrocnemius, soleus *Accessory muscles:* peroneus longus, peroneus brevis	Straightens the ankle to point the toes, causing the angle between the top of the foot and the lower leg to increase

Upper Extremity Muscle Groups

In conditions in which the function of the lower extremity muscles does not return, the upper extremity muscles are used to compensate. For example, the upper extremities are heavily relied upon to propel a wheelchair in spinal cord injury. A walker is often required for ambulation in CP. In these cases, upper extremity strength is integral, and range of motion must be maintained to reduce the risk of injury.

While locomotion is the key function of the lower extremity muscles, object manipulation is the key function of the upper extremity muscles. We use our shoulder and elbow muscles to bring our hand to an object and our fingers to grasp and use objects. This function is crucial for self-care. Specific yoga poses are recommended to maintain the strength and flexibility of the upper extremity muscle groups to promote optimal function of the upper body. See table 2.2 for an explanation of the muscles included in the upper extremity muscle groups.

Table 2.2 Upper Extremity Muscle Groups

Muscle group name	Components of muscle group	Muscle action
Scapular retractors Trapezius Upper Upper middle Lower middle Lower Levator scapulae Rhomboids	*Prime mover:* trapezius *Accessory muscles:* rhomboids, levator scapulae	Moves the shoulder blade in the horizontal plane toward the spine
Scapular protractors Pectoralis minor Serratus anterior	*Prime mover:* serratus anterior *Accessory muscle:* pectoralis minor	Moves the shoulder blade in the horizontal plane away from the spine
Scapular depressors Pectoralis minor Serratus anterior Lower trapezius Anterior Posterior	*Prime mover:* lower trapezius *Accessory muscles:* pectoralis minor, serratus anterior	Moves the shoulder blade downward in the vertical plane

Muscle group name	Components of muscle group	Muscle action
Scapular elevators 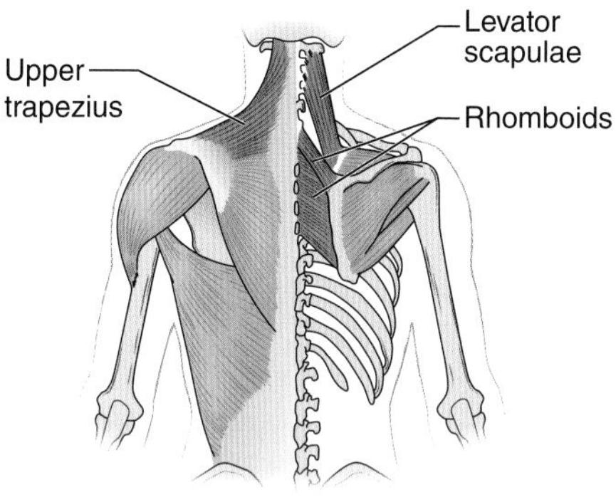 Upper trapezius, Levator scapulae, Rhomboids	*Prime mover:* upper trapezius *Accessory muscles:* rhomboids, levator scapulae	Moves the shoulder blade upward in the vertical plane
Scapular upward rotators 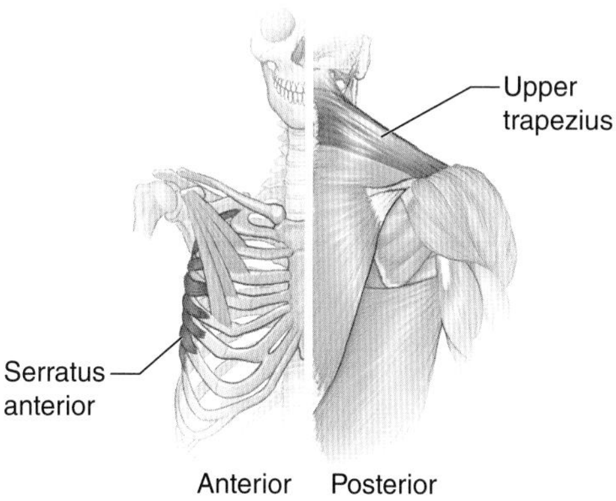 Upper trapezius, Serratus anterior, Anterior, Posterior	*Prime mover:* serratus anterior *Accessory muscle:* upper trapezius	Rotates the shoulder blade in the vertical plane in such a way that the inferior angle points away from the spine
Scapular downward rotators 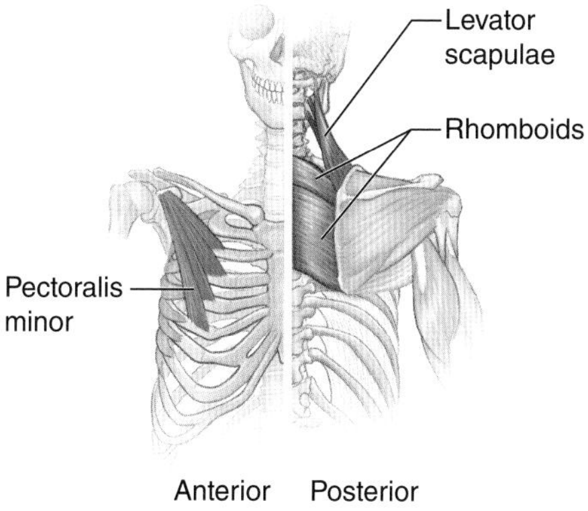 Levator scapulae, Rhomboids, Pectoralis minor, Anterior, Posterior	*Prime mover:* rhomboids *Accessory muscles:* levator scapulae, pectoralis minor	Rotates the shoulder blade in the vertical plane in such a way that the inferior angle points toward the spine

(continued)

21

Table 2.2 (continued)

Muscle group name	Components of muscle group	Muscle action
Shoulder flexors 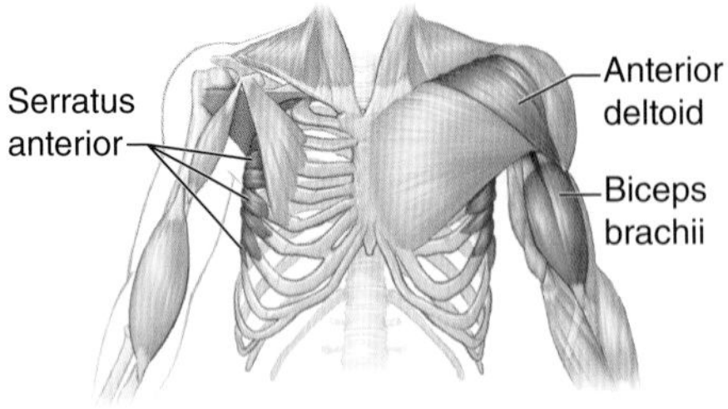	*Prime mover:* anterior deltoid *Accessory muscles:* serratus anterior, biceps brachii	Moves the upper arm forward
Shoulder adductors 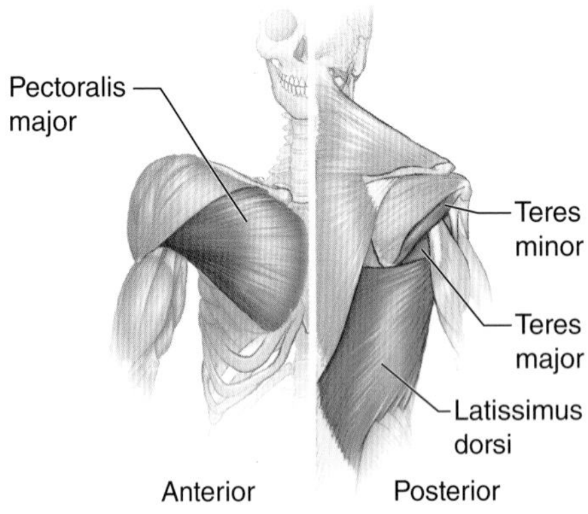	*Prime movers:* pectoralis major, latissimus dorsi *Accessory muscles:* teres major, teres minor	Moves the upper arm out to the side, away from the body
Shoulder extensors 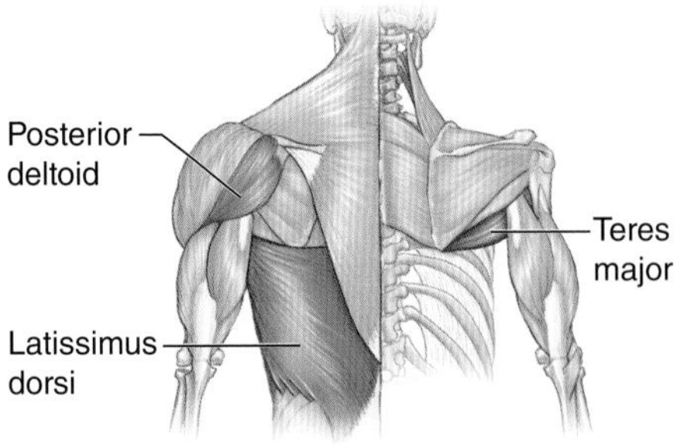	*Prime movers:* posterior deltoid, latissimus dorsi *Accessory muscle:* teres major	Moves the upper arm backward

Shoulder flexors figure labels: Serratus anterior, Anterior deltoid, Biceps brachii

Shoulder adductors figure labels: Pectoralis major, Teres minor, Teres major, Latissimus dorsi, Anterior, Posterior

Shoulder extensors figure labels: Posterior deltoid, Teres major, Latissimus dorsi

Muscle group name	Components of muscle group	Muscle action
Elbow extensors 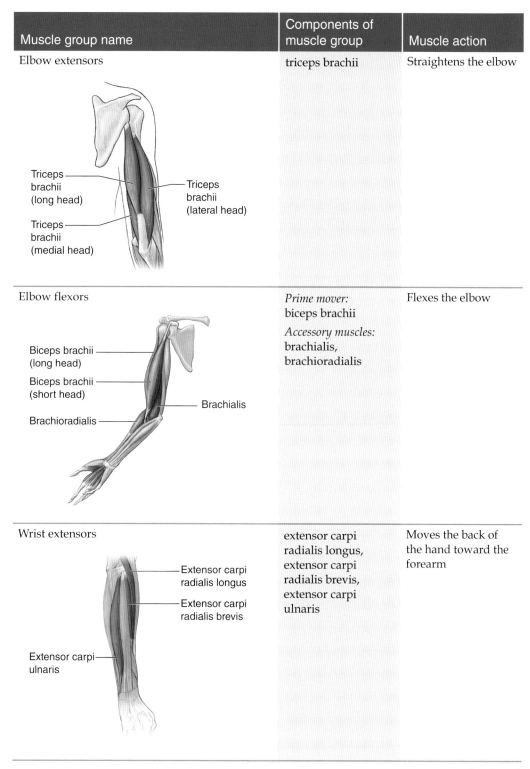 Triceps brachii (long head) — Triceps brachii (lateral head) — Triceps brachii (medial head)	triceps brachii	Straightens the elbow
Elbow flexors Biceps brachii (long head) — Biceps brachii (short head) — Brachialis — Brachioradialis	*Prime mover:* biceps brachii *Accessory muscles:* brachialis, brachioradialis	Flexes the elbow
Wrist extensors Extensor carpi radialis longus — Extensor carpi radialis brevis — Extensor carpi ulnaris	extensor carpi radialis longus, extensor carpi radialis brevis, extensor carpi ulnaris	Moves the back of the hand toward the forearm

(continued)

Table 2.2 (continued)

Muscle group name	Components of muscle group	Muscle action
Wrist flexors	flexor carpi radialis, flexor carpi ulnaris	Moves the palm of the hand toward the forearm

—Flexor carpi radialis

—Flexor carpi ulnaris

Core Muscle Group

As the name insinuates, *core* refers to the center of your body, lumbar spine, and pelvis. *Core stability* refers to the active component of the stabilizing system of this area, the deep and superficial muscles. The deep muscles (e.g., multifidus and transversus abdominis) attach directly to the spine and the pelvis. When these muscles are contracted, they do not produce movement in the spine, but rather create stability. The superficial core muscles (e.g., rectus abdominis and paraspinals) produce movement in the spine, but also assist with stability during physically demanding tasks. This is why core-strengthening yoga poses are recommended in low back pain, to provide both stability for weight-bearing activity, as well as flexibility for pain-free movement.

Stabilization is achieved through strength and control of core muscles. Back pain and a sedentary lifestyle can cause weakness and challenges in activating the core muscles, especially the deep stabilizers.[1] Therefore, a key component to increasing core stability is to learn to turn on the core muscles. In later chapters, we will discuss several yoga poses that strengthen the core, and offer instructions for promoting core muscle activation and control.

Core strength and stability are needed for movement, carrying loads, and spinal protection. Stability creates a strong base from which all movements in your body arise. For example, several muscles of the upper leg that control movement of the hip and knee attach to the pelvis. These leg muscles work much more effectively if the pelvis is stabilized by the core muscles. In contrast, if the pelvis moves excessively (is *hypermobile*) due to weakness or poor control of the core muscles, the leg muscles will work less efficiently. See table 2.3 for an explanation of the muscles included in the core muscle group.

Table 2.3 Core Muscle Group

Muscle group name	Components of muscle group	Muscle action
Stabilizers	multifidus, transversus abdominis	Produces a stabilizing or stiffening effect of the lumbar spine
Spinal extensors	paraspinals, quadratus lumborum	Flexes the spine backward or to neutral from a bent forward position
Obliques	internal and external obliques	Produces rotation and sideways flexing of the low back

(continued)

Table 2.3 (continued)

Muscle group name	Components of muscle group	Muscle action
Spinal flexors External oblique Internal oblique Rectus abdominis	*Prime mover:* rectus abdominis *Accessory muscles:* internal obliques, external obliques	Flexes the spine forward
Diaphragm Diaphragm	diaphragm	Primary muscle of inhalation, assists in increasing intra-abdominal pressure

PART II

Adapting Yoga for Specific Disabilities

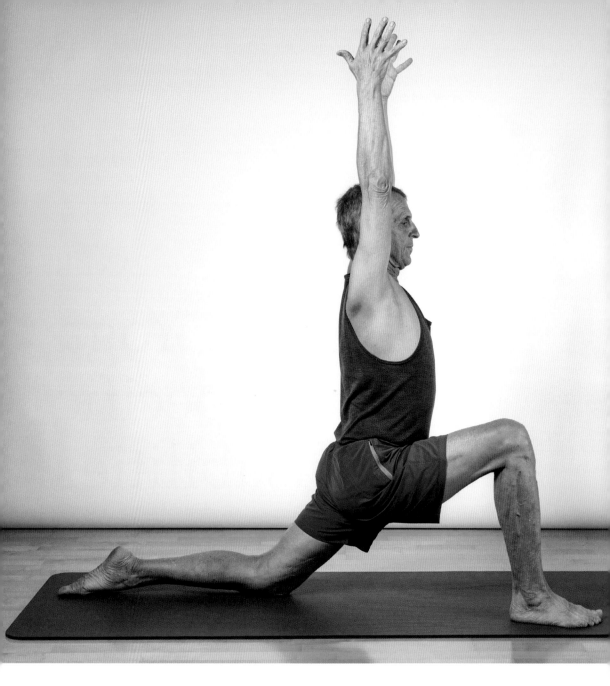

CHAPTER 3

Low Back Pain

It is important that we introduce low back pain (LBP) early on because the principles of LBP set a groundwork for treating all disabilities. Chronic LBP is considered a disability because it causes a decrease in functional status, quality of life, and social life.[4] We would venture to guess that anyone reading this has experienced it themselves, or has a loved one who has suffered from LBP. With up to 84 percent of adults in the United States having reported LBP, it is one of the most commonly experienced medical conditions.[3] It is the number one cause of activity modification[13] and missed work[12] throughout much of the world. LBP is responsible for an enormous economic burden. In a study of U.S. health care costs in 2013,[5] the estimated spending related to LBP and neck pain was $87.6 billion.

LBP causes such a high economic burden and is so common due to its high rate of recurrence (repeatedly afflicting the same person) and the propensity to progress to a chronic (long-standing) condition. LBP can be categorized as acute (pain up to 4 weeks), subacute (4 to 12 weeks), or chronic (more than 12 weeks). A seminal study on LBP found that among patients with one episode of acute LBP, 65 percent experienced additional incidences of LBP with a second episode occurring within two months.[1]

Modern medical practice is moving away from the use of opioid medications and invasive procedures such as spinal injections and surgeries in the treatment of LBP. Instead, we are now trending toward treatments such as physical therapy, yoga, and mindfulness. Yoga has recently been proven to be an effective tool to help prevent recurrences of LBP, stop the progression from acute to chronic LBP, and improve function and quality of life in individuals with chronic LBP.[2]

The United States Department of Defense (DOD) recommends that patients with LBP remain active in "an exercise program, which may include Pilates, yoga, and tai chi."[2] A study published in 2019 found that after just six weeks of yoga, individuals can achieve significant improvements in back pain at rest, back pain during activity, spinal performance, and quality of life. In fact, the functional hypothesis for utilizing yoga in LBP proposes that by improving balance and body awareness to correct alignment, yoga reduces muscle spasms in the spine by decreasing spinal stress and loading.[4]

LBP is also complicated by a strong mental and emotional component. Studies have found that emotional distress or depression increases the risk of developing chronic LBP[11] as well as fear of pain, movement, and reinjury.[6] The DOD recommends the use of mindfulness-based stress reduction (MBSR) for patients with LBP. Yoga consists of breathing and relaxation exercises that have been proven to reduce stress, anxiety, and depression by mechanisms and techniques in line with cognitive behavior therapy.[9] In short, yoga teaches its students to love and trust their bodies.

We know that, generally, yoga can help patients with LBP, but how do we select which poses are best? A multitude of yoga asanas coincide with the treatments recommended by current medical guidelines. The American Physical Therapy Association's practice guidelines on LBP recommend physical therapists (PTs) use trunk exercises *to improve core coordination, strength, and endurance* to reduce LBP and its consequential disability. A key principle of yoga is to engage and strengthen the trunk and core muscles. We also recommend the use of spinal extension–based exercises to increase spinal flexibility. There are countless poses that incorporate spinal extension. In some cases, it is recommended that PTs use spinal traction techniques. In this chapter, we will teach you how to perform self-traction with two yoga straps. It is well established that sitting with slouched posture increases the risk of developing LBP[10] and yoga can help to prevent or mitigate LBP through its emphasis on upright posture and body awareness.

The poses and exercises in this chapter have been chosen to combine the principles of yoga and modern medicine to decrease pain and disability and to improve function and quality of life in those suffering from LBP. In utilizing the poses in this book to alleviate and prevent LBP, please do so after physician assessment regarding the origin of the LBP to ensure the symptoms are truly musculoskeletal in nature, and not a more sinister pathology (tumor, fracture, etc.) that may require medical or surgical intervention.

GENERAL GUIDELINES

- End range positions of the spine (flexion, extension, rotation) should initially be avoided. However, make it a goal to progress into the full expression of the poses as tolerated.
- Avoid standing flexion (deep forward bends) without support (wall, block, chair) because the extreme forward-flexed position places the most load on the intervertebral discs.[7]
- You do not need to avoid flexion movements but should incorporate more extension compared to flexion in your yoga practice for LBP.
- Incorporate flowing movements through a middle range of motion of the spine.
- Always include core activation.
- Remember that the spine is strong and safe to move.

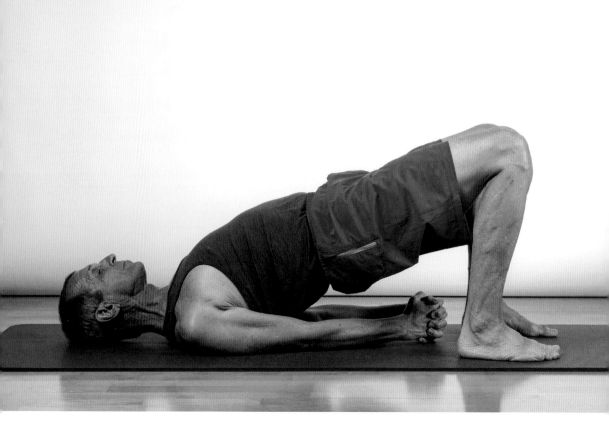

BRIDGE Setu Bandha Sarvangasana

Bridge is a great starter pose for individuals with LBP because fear of movement (especially of the spine) is a common emotion for those experiencing LBP. The purpose of the pose is to extend the spine, with the benefit of doing so in an unloaded position, thus decreasing pain and extending the spine through a controlled range of motion.

More specifically, when you are lying flat on the mat, the lumbar (low back) spine is considered to be unloaded from the forces of weight and gravity because it is not experiencing the compressive forces of the head and torso. In Bridge, there is relative spinal extension. Because the hips elevate with the spine, the force on the spine is minimal. In addition to achieving the benefits of spinal extension in this pose, the spinal extensors (paraspinals) and hip extensors (glutes) are also strengthened. Furthermore, hip flexors are also stretched because the hips are elevated with the feet planted on the floor.

Benefits

- Improves mobility in spinal extension.
- Strengthens the spinal extensors.
- Strengthens the hip extensors.
- Stretches the hip flexors.

Precautions

Avoid this pose if you have a history of neck injury.

Before You Begin

Have a strap or a block handy for variations.

How To

1. Start lying on your back with your knees bent, feet flat on the floor, and arms alongside your body with palms facing down.
2. Press your feet and shoulders into the mat as you lift your hips.
3. As you rise, walk the feet closer to your buttocks and scoot your shoulders into midline and underneath you so they act like a slight shelf with the upper arms, to further elevate the hips and lengthen the tailbone.
4. Keep your knees parallel as you engage the inner thighs.
5. Interlace the fingers or hold on to a strap with each hand.
6. Relax your chin away from your chest to preserve the natural curve of your cervical spine.
7. Your shoulders, feet, and back of the head support the lift of your pelvis comfortably on the mat as you use the muscles of your buttocks and back to lengthen your hips.
8. Hold for 5 to 10 breath cycles.
9. To exit the pose, release the interlace of the hands and slowly roll down your spine.

Modifications

Wrap a strap around the upper thighs to relax the hip adductors (groin) and keep the knees in line with the hips to focus on spinal extension.

Variations

- *Challenge variations:* Bend one knee into the belly, *or* for a further challenge, you can extend the leg straight up.
- *Restorative variation:* Place a block or bolster directly under your sacrum and allow the prop to take the weight of your body. Be sure that you continue to lengthen your neck by resting the head's weight on the back of the head and not on the neck. Lift the chest toward your chin, and your chin slightly away from your chest.

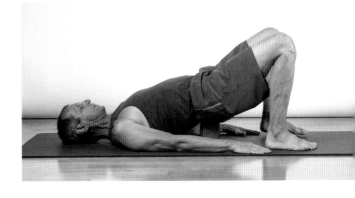

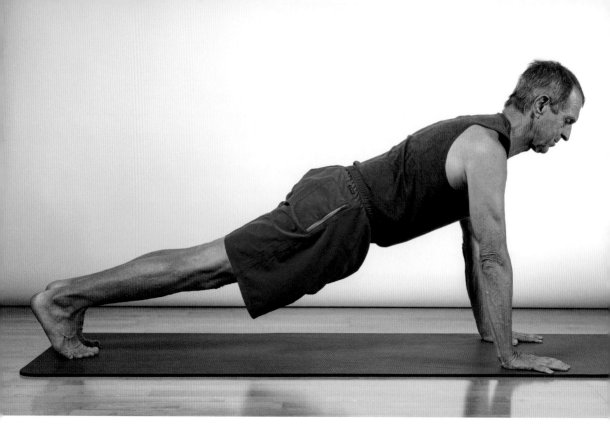

PLANK

Phalakasana

A muscle can have one of two roles: a mobilizer or a stabilizer. A mobilizer contracts to *cause movement* of a joint (think of the biceps bending your elbow), while a stabilizer contracts to *prevent movement* of its corresponding joint. Therefore, core stabilization refers to strengthening of the muscles that attach to the spine and pelvis that stabilize the spine by preventing movement. Because Plank strengthens the spinal muscles in a neutral position, this is the perfect pose to initiate core stability. With the ability to progress from Plank on elbows to Plank on hands, there is a form of Plank for everybody.

Benefits

- Stabilizes the core.
- Strengthens the hip extensors.

Precautions

If you have a wrist injury, use your forearms.

How To

1. Start in Downward-Facing Dog (pages 90-91).
2. Inhale as you extend your chest forward and heels back and bring the shoulders over the wrists.

3. Align your body in a straight line from your head to your heels.

4. Engage the abdominal muscles in and up, firming your outer arms in toward midline.

5. Press into the hands, separating your shoulder blades, drawing your sternum in the direction of your spine, and filling out your thoracic spine.

6. Energize the inner thighs toward each other and up as you press back into your heels and forward with your chest, lengthening the spine and neck.

7. Your gaze should be two feet in front of the hands on the floor for a long neck.

8. Be sure the hips do not sag and are in alignment with the chest and legs.

9. Hold for 5 to 8 breath cycles.

10. Come down to rest in Child's Pose (pages 38-39).

Modifications

- Another way to get into the pose is to start in Table Top (pages 250-251) with the shoulders over the wrists, engage the core, and extend one leg back, and then the other.

- *Standing Plank:* Face the wall and extend your arms to place your hands on the wall at chest height. Walk the feet back until the hands are at shoulder height and the abdomen engages. You can walk the feet back further until you feel the upper arm muscles engage. Be sure you are tucking the tailbone, so the hips stay in line with the diagonal of the body.

- *Supported by the knees*: Start with steps 1 to 5 above. In Plank, lower the knees directly to the floor, without moving your hands and chest. Continue engaging the abdominal muscles and hugging the outer arms into midline. Hold for 10 breaths and come down to rest in Child's Pose.

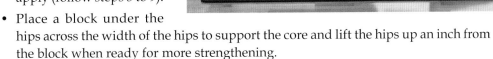

- *Forearm Plank:* Simply place the forearms instead of setting the weight on the hands. The remaining principles of spinal alignment as described earlier apply (follow steps 3 to 9).

- Place a block under the hips across the width of the hips to support the core and lift the hips up an inch from the block when ready for more strengthening.

Variations

To challenge yourself, lift one foot off the floor, maintaining a neutral position in the hips. Hold for a few breaths, then release the foot down and switch to the other foot, holding for the same amount of breaths.

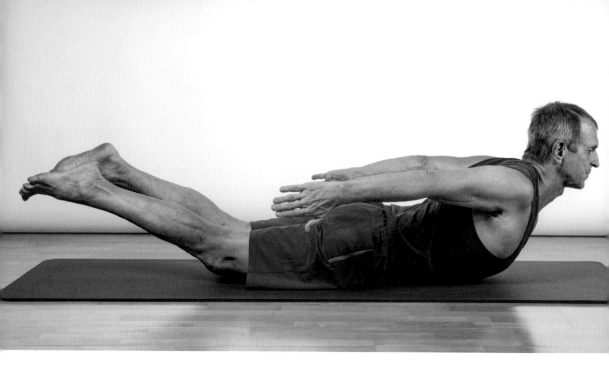

LOCUST

Salabhasana

We live in a world of spinal flexion: sitting at work, looking down at our phones, lounging on the couch while binge-watching TV, even putting on our socks in the morning. Gone are the days of running to hunt for food and climbing trees to escape from predators. Extending the spine in Locust counteracts the repeated spinal flexion of modern life. Locust is a great way to initiate spinal extension because this pose actively utilizes the spinal muscles to protect the joints of the low back.

Benefits

- Improves mobility in spinal extension.
- Strengthens the hip extensors.
- Strengthens the spinal extensors.
- Stretches the hip flexors.

Precautions

- Do not rest your weight on the abdomen if you are pregnant.
- Be cautious with spinal extension if your medical history includes severe stenosis of the lumbar spine.

How To

1. Start by lying face down with your forehead on the mat, and hands alongside your hips, palms alongside the hips.
2. Inhale, and with the action of dragging your shoulder blades down your back, extend your head, chest, and arms up and off the mat.
3. Lift the belly button up and in and start to lift your legs off the mat with the action of reaching the feet behind you and slightly toward each other while keeping the knees straight.
4. Firm and strengthen the legs and buttocks as you extend your arms further back toward your feet, and your legs higher.
5. Interlace the fingers or bring your hands closer alongside the body as you squeeze the shoulder blades closer toward each other.
6. Allow the gaze to extend forward on the ground or to the space in front of you; you can also look down if that's more comfortable for your neck.
7. You should be balancing on your belly and pelvis.
8. Hold for 5 to 8 breath cycles.
9. Rest for a few breaths by releasing the body down and turning one cheek to the mat, then repeat three more times.

Modifications

- Rest the forehead on the mat to avoid neck strain.
- Place the hands on the ground alongside the body and just lift the legs, or keep the legs on the mat and extend the arms only for a chest lift. This is especially helpful if this feels uncomfortable in your low back or if you are just beginning to learn this pose.
- Unlock hands and extend the arms alongside the torso and hips.

Variations

- *Challenge variations:* Interlace the fingers behind your back and draw the biceps toward each other for increased lift in the chest, *or* reach the arms forward like Superman flying and lift the hands and feet up and away from the mat.
- *Restorative variation:* Place a bolster under the chest and rest the chest on the bolster. This still allows you to experience spinal extension.

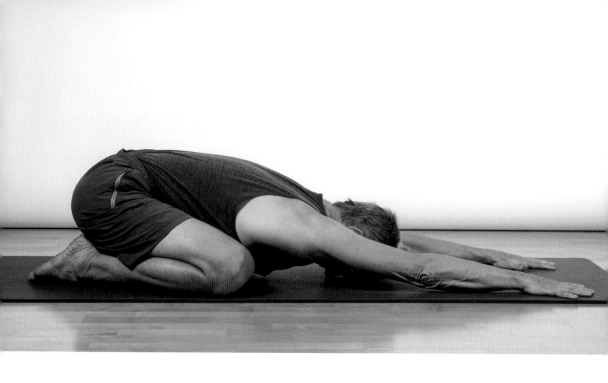

CHILD'S POSE Balasana

Child's Pose is a great way to decompress the spine. By placing the spine in gentle flexion without the weight of gravity compressing the spine, Child's Pose creates a slight traction force (creating more space between each of the vertebrae) through the spine. Additionally, this pose lengthens and relaxes several muscle groups: spinal extensors, hip extensors, and hip external rotators. Another way to keep the spine neutral is to widen the knees if the low back is easily irritated with spinal flexion.

Benefits

- Fosters spinal traction or decompression.
- Stretches the spinal extensors.
- Stretches the hip extensors.
- Stretches the hip external rotators.

Precautions

- Avoid this pose if you have a current or recent knee injury, or if extreme knee flexion causes pain.
- Avoid this pose if you have a history of ankle injury, or if end range plantar flexion causes pain.

How To

1. Place your shins on the floor, knees hip width apart, with sitting bones resting on the heels.
2. Hinge forward from the pelvis and walk your hands in front of you to straighten the arms.
3. Lower your torso to the thighs and rest your forehead on the floor.
4. Rest your elbows, forearms, and palms on the floor in front of you. (You can also stack the hands under the forehead or place a block under the forehead to ensure your neck is comfortable.)
5. Direct your breath to your lower back and side ribs, expanding the back of your body when you inhale and release into the mat on your exhale.
6. Hold for 10 breath cycles.

Modifications

- If Child's Pose causes knee or chest discomfort, perform it on your back with your knees drawn into your chest.
- Can bring arms alongside the body if the shoulders are tight.
- *Wide-knee Child's Pose*: If keeping the knees together causes pain in your back due to spinal flexion, you can draw the knees wide apart and lay the belly between the thighs to obtain a more neutral position.
- If resting on the tops of the feet elicits pain in the ankles, keep the toes tucked.
- If the weight on your knees elicits pain in the knees, fold a blanket behind the knee creases.
- If the neck is uncomfortable, rest the forehead on a block, bolster, or folded blanket.

Variations

- *Challenge variation:* Child's Pose is meant to be a restful pose; we do not recommend creating challenge out of this pose.
- *Restorative variation:* From a wide-knee Child's Pose, place a bolster far up into the thighs and under the belly to completely support the weight of your torso.

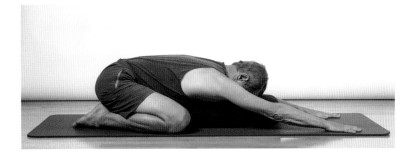

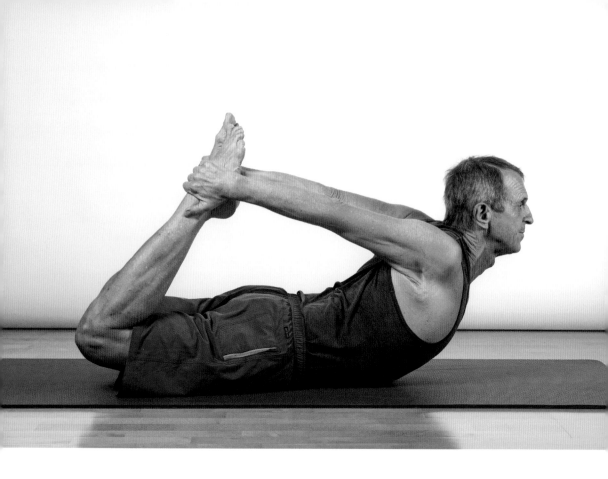

BOW

Dhanurasana

If Bow seems intimidating for someone with LBP, think of the pose as a progression to work toward. Bow extends the spine actively via use of the spinal extensors, with gentle pressure provided by the arms to improve spinal mobility. Daily life requires repeated forward bending, and this pose moves our spine in the opposite direction with spinal extension, relieving the pressures of the persistent modern-day slouching. Additionally, Bow requires you to engage the abdominal muscles to prevent overextension of the low back, thus providing core strengthening. Keep in mind this is an advanced pose, so allow this to be an aspiration, and consider starting with Locust (pages 36-37) and working toward Bow.

Benefits

- Improves mobility in spinal extension.
- Strengthens the spinal extensors.
- Stretches the hip flexors.
- Stabilizes the core.

Precautions

Avoid this pose if you have high blood pressure or headaches because bearing down can further increase your blood pressure.

How To

1. Start by lying face down with your arms alongside your body and palms facing up.
2. Bend the knees while lifting your chest and head to reach back for your ankles.
3. Wrap your hands around your ankles and kick the ankles back to lift your chest.
4. Keep your knees no more than hip width apart as you continue to kick the feet back and draw your shoulder blades down your back to enhance the opening of your chest.
5. Engage the belly button up toward the spine to support the low back.
6. Hold for 5 breath cycles.
7. Exhale to release, turn one cheek to the mat, and bring your arms down by your sides to rest.

Modifications

- Place a bolster under the chest and front ribs to support the backbend.
- If you cannot reach your feet, wrap a yoga strap around each ankle and reach for the straps with the hands.

Variations

To challenge yourself, ground the knees on the floor while strongly kicking the feet against the resistance of your hands; this further opens the chest and strengthens the quadriceps.

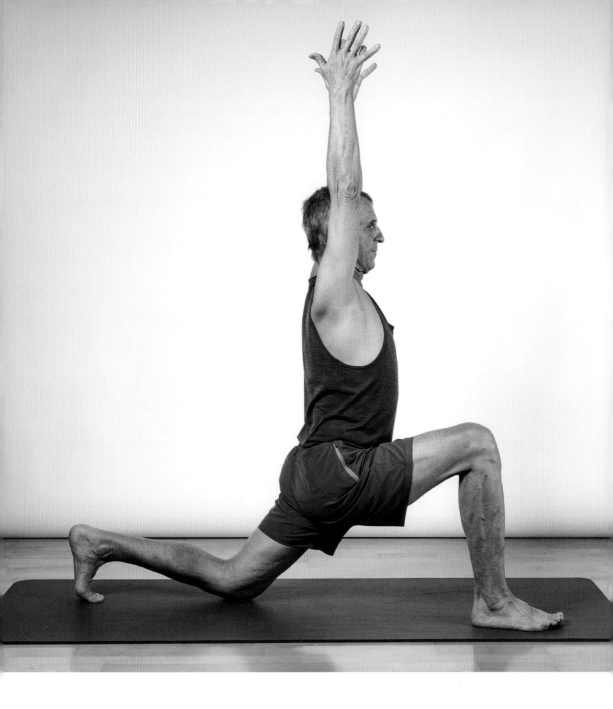

CRESCENT LUNGE Anjaneyasana

Prolonged sitting, which is common in our daily modern lives, shortens the length of the hip flexor muscles. Because these muscles attach to the pelvis and the thigh, shortened hip flexors can cause poor mobility of the pelvis. This, in turn, requires more movement of the lumbar spine, which can increase LBP. Crescent Lunge stretches the hip flexors of the back leg while also strengthening the hip extensors and abductors of that same leg. This pose also places the spine in mild extension and rotation toward the front leg, which strengthens the spinal extensors and the obliques, thus stabilizing the spine.

Benefits

- Improves mobility in spinal extension.
- Strengthens the spinal extensors.
- Stabilizes the core.
- Stretches the hip flexors.
- Strengthens the hip extensors.
- Strengthens the hip abductors.

How To

1. From Downward-Facing Dog (pages 90-91), raise your right leg up and back to extend it.
2. Step the right foot forward in between your hands. If it doesn't make it all the way between the hands with your step, catch the ankle with your hand and assist it forward so it aligns with your hands.
3. Bring your torso and chest upright and bend the front knee.
4. Make sure that your knee is above your ankle, not forward of the ankle.
5. Lower the back (left) knee to rest on the ground; you can place a blanket or towel under the knee for cushioning. Your back toes can be tucked or extended, whichever is best for your balance.
6. Extend your arms up with the palms facing each other.
7. Expand your chest to the sky as you draw your arms further behind your ears, and lift the chest up to deepen the stretch of your left knee.
8. Gaze directly in front of you or slightly up to where the wall meets the ceiling, with the goal of extending the back of your neck.
9. Hold for 5 breath cycles.
10. To exit the pose, release your hands down to the mat to frame the foot and step the right foot back to Downward-Facing Dog.
11. Repeat on the left side.

Modifications

Your hands can be on blocks, on your hips, or in prayer, depending on the support you need.

Variations

- *Challenge variation:* You can also practice this pose with the back knee off the mat for increased leg strengthening. Note that this tilts the pelvis forward, so you can add a slight bend in the back knee to neutralize the pelvis.
- *Restorative variation:* Place a bolster in front of the back knee and rest the quadriceps on the bolster.

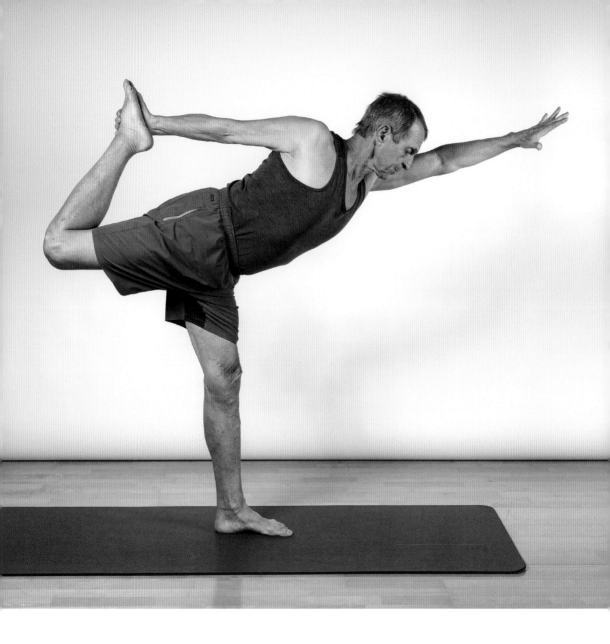

DANCER

Natarajasana

An important aspect of managing LBP is learning to trust that it's safe to move the spine and that it can be challenged. A significant part of that process is attempting (and often failing) new movements. Dancer requires the ability to balance on one leg and the flexibility to extend the spine, which is why this pose can feel especially challenging for those with LBP. Thus, attempting a challenging pose such as Dancer and being none the worse for wear can teach us that it is safe to move our bodies in new ways. This pose positions the spine into extension while activating the spinal extensors, hip extensors, and core muscles, which ultimately protects and stabilizes the spine. It also facilitates strengthening of the hip abductors on the standing leg.

Benefits

- Improves mobility in spinal extension.
- Strengthens the spinal extensors.
- Stabilizes the core.
- Strengthens the hip abductors.
- Strengthens the hip extensors.

How To

1. Start standing at the front of your mat in Mountain (pages 150-151).
2. Focus the weight of your body on the left leg as you bend your right knee to lift the right foot toward your right buttock.
3. Hold onto the inner right ankle with the right hand to bend the knee more deeply so you feel a stretch in your quadriceps.
4. Make sure you feel balanced on your left leg as you begin to kick the right foot back and away from the buttocks, maintaining a steady grip of the right ankle in your hand.
5. Continue extending the right leg back, aiming to lift the upper thigh parallel to the floor.
6. Extend your chest forward and slightly up to arch your back as you kick your foot back farther away from the body; you will also feel a stretch in your right pectoralis (chest) muscles.
7. Hold for 5 breath cycles.
8. To release, inhale to lift your chest and bring the right foot back toward your buttocks.
9. Stand in Mountain for a few breaths before switching to the other side.

Modifications

Place your hand on a wall or chair in front of you for more support.

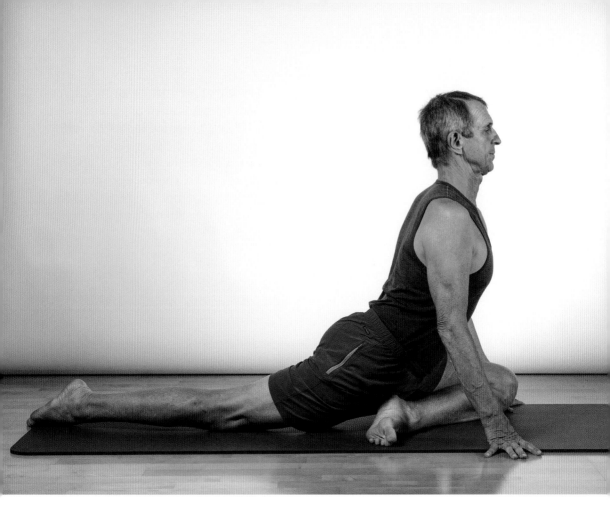

PIGEON Eka Pada Rajakapotasana

We have discussed that prolonged sitting in a slouched position can lead to low back pain by decreasing mobility of the spine, but it also affects the hips. Pigeon checks every box for improving hip mobility and encouraging an upright position. This pose places the spine into spinal extension, unloads the intervertebral discs, and actively engages the spinal extensor muscles, which protects the joints of the spine. Additionally, core muscles are engaged; the obliques activate to lift the spine upright because of the asymmetry of this pose.

Pigeon also lengthens the hip flexors of the back leg to improve lumbopelvic mobility while strengthening the gluteal hip extensors, which aids in spinal stabilization and motor control.

Benefits

- Improves mobility in spinal extension.
- Stabilizes the core.
- Strengthens the spinal extensors.
- Stretches the hip flexors.
- Strengthens the hip extensors.

Precautions

- Be careful if you have a history of or an active knee injury because this pose places force on the lateral aspect of the front knee.
- Be cautious if you have sacroiliac joint issues, especially during pregnancy, because the pose places asymmetrical forces on the pelvis, which can cause sacral pain.

How To

1. Start in Downward-Facing Dog (pages 90-91).
2. Shift halfway forward with your hips and bend your left knee while rotating your hip out so that the left ankle slides behind your right wrist.
3. Your left lateral shin will relax onto the floor and the left knee will rest just outside the alignment of the hip.
4. Extend your right leg back with a straight knee, hip rotated slightly inward, and right upper thigh resting on the floor.
5. With the support of your arms, lower the left buttock to the floor or onto a block and dorsiflex the left foot.
6. With the hands still supporting you, settle into the hip stretch: Walk the hands back alongside the hips, or place the hands on blocks next to the hips.
7. The torso lifts up and the lower back lengthens with core engagement.
8. If this feels uncomfortable, scoot your left foot closer to the body. To make the pose more challenging, walk the foot closer to the right wrist to bring the left shin parallel to the front of the mat.
9. Hold for 5 to 10 breath cycles.
10. To exit the pose, tuck the right toes under to straighten the leg, press into the hands to lift the left leg up and back again into Downward-Facing Dog.
11. Switch to the right side.

Variations

- Place a block or blanket under the front hip to support your pelvis and achieve a leveling of the hips.
- *Challenge variation:* Bend your back knee and use the hand on the same side to catch hold of the foot or ankle to deeply stretch the quadriceps and hip flexor.
- *Restorative variation:* From the upright position, walk the hands forward to lie over the front leg or over a bolster, or, optionally, you can rest your forehead on stacked hands, a folded blanket, or a block.

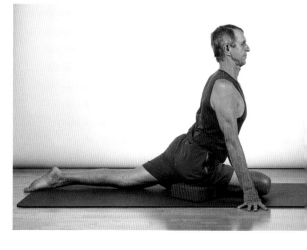

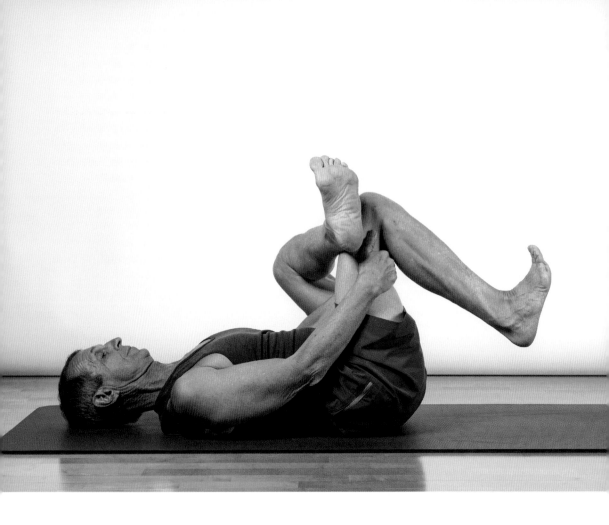

RECLINING PIGEON Supta Eka Pada Rajakapotasana

This pose offers a modification for those with knee pain or low back discomfort in the seated Pigeon. The same benefits apply in the hips, while keeping the spine in a neutral position—stretching the hip external rotators and extensors, which can sometimes be the cause of low back pain (the tightness of these muscles flattens our natural lordotic curve, which changes the distribution of forces in the spine).

Benefits

- Strengthens the hip flexors.
- Stretches the hip extensors.
- Stretches the hip external rotators.

Precautions

Be cautious if you have sacroiliac joint issues, especially during pregnancy, because the pose places asymmetrical forces on the pelvis, which can cause sacral pain.

How To

1. Starting on your back, bend the knees and place the feet on the floor, walking them under the knees, hip width apart.
2. Bend the left knee into the chest and cross your left ankle above your right knee. In this manner, you will create a figure 4 with your legs.
3. Draw your right knee into your chest and thread your left arm through the triangle created by your ankle and knee.
4. Interlace your fingers around the right shin or the back of your right thigh and draw your knees close to your chest.
5. Your head and shoulders should be resting on the ground. If they need to come off the floor to catch hold of the shin or thigh, you can use a strap to draw your legs into the body.
6. Bonus: You can push your left knee away with your left arm while simultaneously drawing the right knee in for increased stretch.
7. Relax your sacrum, head, and shoulders on the ground while you draw the knees in.
8. Hold for 5 to 10 breath cycles.
9. To exit the pose, uncross and extend the legs.
10. Switch sides.

Modifications

Push your left knee away with your left arm while simultaneously drawing the right knee in for an increased stretch.

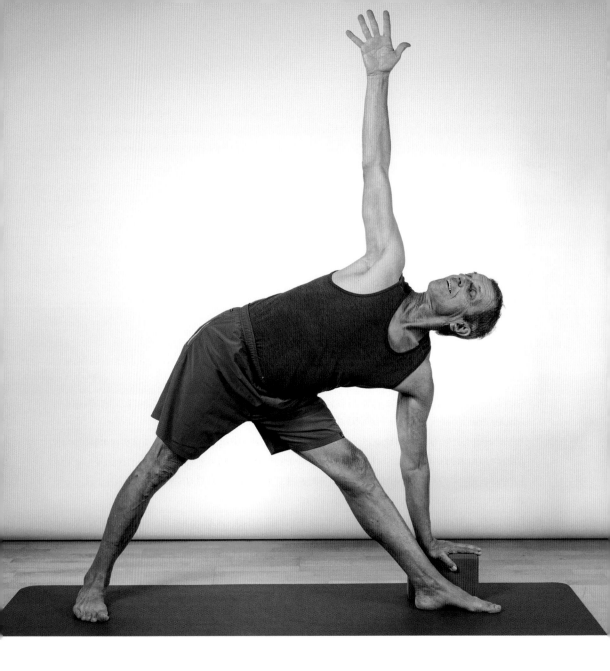

EXTENDED TRIANGLE   Utthita Trikonasana

This pose is a great core stabilizer, but the real benefit is to help you differentiate movements of the spine and hips. The spine should remain in a relatively neutral (slight rotation) position in reference to the legs; to achieve this, the pelvis rotates at the hip joints to avoid side bending the spine. Learning to move the trunk at the hip joint rather than through the low back is a valuable skill to reduce stressful, injury-causing forces through the low back.

In Extended Triangle, there is a co-contraction of the spinal extensors, flexors, and obliques, which keeps the spine neutral. Furthermore, the back leg's abductors activate to control the amount of lateral pelvic tilt: too little and the spine will side bend, too much and the weight of the torso will be incorrectly distributed over the front arm and leg.

Benefits

- Increases body awareness and control.
- Strengthens the hip abductors.
- Stabilizes the core.

Precautions

Avoid looking up if you have a neck injury; you can perform this pose with your gaze down toward the floor.

How To

1. Start in Warrior II (pages 104-105), with the left foot forward (left foot pointing forward, right foot parallel to the short edge of the mat).
2. Keep the arms extended.
3. Straighten the left leg and extend the left fingertips forward, lengthening both sides of your waist.
4. Continue to extend your torso forward in line with your left leg, grounding through the right foot and leg to anchor your movement.
5. Rotate the torso, hinging at the left hip and extending both sides of the waist.
6. Your right hip will roll slightly down, which is okay. Make sure that both sides of the torso extend equally long and you are not rounding the right side waist.
7. Rest your hand on a block or your shin.
8. Lengthen through your tailbone and engage your abdominal muscles to support your spine.
9. Point the right arm to the sky, in line with your shoulder and your palm facing forward.
10. Maintain extension of your neck in line with your spine and look up or forward (or down if looking up strains your neck).
11. Hold for 5 breath cycles.
12. To exit the pose, bend the left knee slightly and press firmly into the feet to lift your torso upright again.
13. Switch sides by pivoting your heels or resetting in Downward-Facing Dog (pages 90-91).

Modifications

Practice with a wall behind you for additional support and a block under the hand.

Variations

To challenge yourself, hover the bottom hand in front of the shin, rather than on the shin, to engage the abdominal muscles and increase core strength.

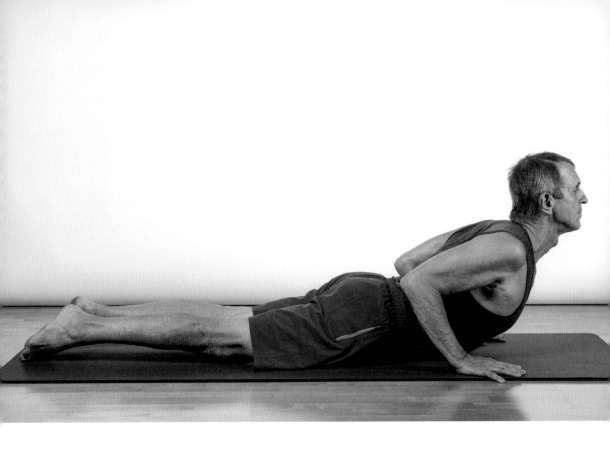

COBRA

Bhujangasana

Cobra is similar to the "press-up" exercise that physical therapists commonly use to treat low back pain. This pose can be used to progressively increase extension of the lumbar spine, which is facilitated by activation of the arm muscles. Without use of the spinal extensor muscles, the movement of the spine is passive, thus isolating the joints of the low back. Moving the lumbar vertebrae into extension is thought to decrease force on the intervertebral discs, allowing them to move forward and out of the joint space and away from the nerves. This increases mobility and decreases pain.

Benefits

- Improves mobility in spinal extension.
- Stretches the hip flexors.

Precautions

- If you are pregnant, be mindful of not putting weight on the belly, or skip this pose altogether.
- Be cautious if you have an active wrist injury.

How To

1. Start by lying face down with the forehead to the ground, legs extended, and hands directly under the shoulders.
2. Scoop the elbows in toward your body and spread the fingers wide to create a firm foundation with the hands.
3. Press into the hands to lift the chest as you engage the abdominal muscles.
4. Draw the shoulders down your back as you begin to straighten the arms (it's okay to maintain a bend in your arms for the comfort of your back).
5. Make sure that you continue to engage your abdominal muscles to protect the spine as you lift your heart up and draw the scapulae down your back.
6. The head balances comfortably in line with the curve of the spine.
7. The pubic bone rests on the mat, in conjunction with the action of lifting slightly up toward the chest to lengthen the lumbar spine.
8. Hold for 5 to 8 breath cycles.

Modifications

Place a bolster under the belly to take the weight off of the arms and shoulders.

Variations

- *Challenge variation:* Walk the hands farther in toward the body to lift the chest higher and move toward a more upright spine. Make sure the shoulders continue to draw down the back and away from the ears, and the abdomen remains engaged.
- *Restorative variation:* Place a bolster under the low belly to support the spine.

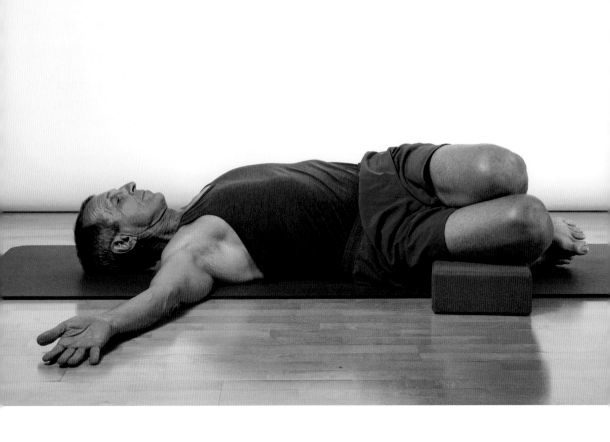

BELLY TWIST

Jathara Parivrtti

When it comes to back pain, movement is far superior to maintaining a fixed position. This lying spinal twist increases rotational mobility of the spine while reinforcing the fundamental principle that moving the back is safe. Using the legs to create rotational movement encourages flexibility in the lumbar spine and allows for control over the degree of the twist.

Benefits

Improves rotational mobility of the spine.

Precautions

Be mindful of disc herniation because the pose can exacerbate radiculopathy (sciatica).

How To

1. Start lying on your back.
2. Draw the knees into your chest and hold here for a few breaths to feel the spine lengthen.
3. Extend your arms straight out to the sides, with your palms up.
4. Roll your knees to the right, keeping them stacked.
5. If the knees do not reach the floor, place a bolster or blanket under them.
6. Ground the opposite (left) shoulder as best you can (it's okay if the shoulder comes off the ground a bit to maintain comfort in your low back).
7. Hold for 5 breath cycles.
8. Bring the knees back to center and hold for a few breaths before shifting the knees to the left.
9. To exit the pose, draw the knees back into the chest and extend the legs out to neutralize the spine from the twist.
10. Repeat on the other side.

Modifications

- Place a bolster or block between the knees to decrease the force on the spine and sacrum.
- Place a block or bolster to the side under both knees if the knees do not reach the floor.

Variations

- *Challenge variation:* Straighten both legs or just the top leg and catch hold of the foot with the opposite hand.
- *Restorative variation:* Place a folded blanket or bolster between the knees to neutralize the pelvis. As noted, a bolster or folded blanket can be placed under the knees if the knees do not reach the floor.

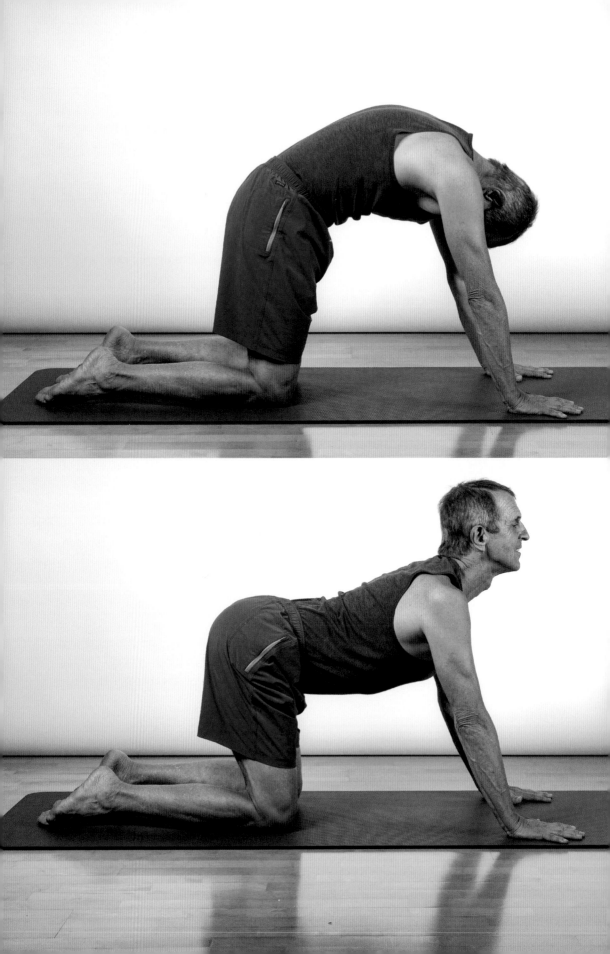

CAT COW Marjaryasana Bitilasana

We are about half an inch shorter at the end of the day than we are when we first wake up in the morning.[10] This is because the height of our intervertebral discs decreases throughout the day. The more we sit during the day, the shorter our discs become. Alternating flexing and extending the spine in Cat Cow rehydrates the discs and revives a healthy disc shape with movement, and in so doing, decreases pain and increases spinal mobility. Additionally, the pose helps you gain postural control and improve the kinesthetic connection between the pelvis and the spine.

Benefits

- Stabilizes the core.
- Improves spine and pelvis motor control.
- Improves spinal mobility.

Precautions

- Be gentle in the rounded spinal pose if you have a herniated disc.
- If you have wrist pain, be careful not to place too much weight on the hands.

How To

1. Start in Table Top (pages 250-251), making sure your hips are aligned over your knees and your shoulders over your wrists.
2. Inhale and start to tilt the pelvis back as you arch the spine to drop your belly and lift the chest into Cow.
3. Press your hands into the mat as you broaden the collarbones and lift the heart to counter the extension of the belly to the floor.
4. Transition with your exhale and initiate the spinal movement from the hips to tuck the pelvis underneath you as you start to curve into a rounded spine for Cat.
5. In the full expression of Cat, tuck your chin into your chest and tuck your pelvis toward your nose while pressing the hands strongly into the floor.
6. Cycle through 5 to 10 rounds of Cat Cow with the breath. Finish by pressing the hips back over the heels into Child's Pose (pages 38-39).

Variations

Practice against a wall by standing at arm's length from the wall with the hands at the height of your chest. Inhale to lift the chest and arch your back (Cow) and round your spine (Cat).

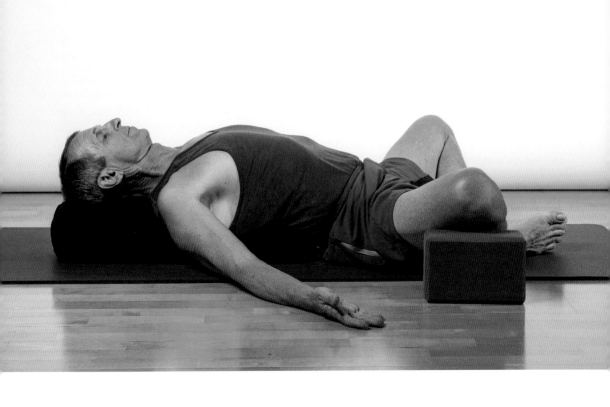

RECLINING SUPPORTED BOUND ANGLE

Supta Baddha Konasana

This pose is an excellent way to start or end a yoga session. This passive position of lumbar extension and hip external rotation decompresses the spine and relaxes the spinal muscles. It's a great pose in which to incorporate breathing techniques and to realize the need and the safety of doing so.

Benefits

- Relaxes the spinal muscles.
- Stretches the hip adductors and internal rotators.
- Extends the spine gently.
- Emphasizes breath control.

How To

1. Start by sitting up with your feet on the mat and knees bent.
2. Place a bolster lengthwise behind you on the mat and wiggle it to lie flush against your lower back.
3. Let the knees roll out into Bound Angle (pages 186-187) with the bottoms of the feet together.
4. Hold the bolster in place behind your low back as you lower your back toward the bolster.
5. Lay your arms on the floor, angled at about 45 degrees from the sides of your torso, palms up.
6. The key here is to relax. You can place blocks under the knees to soften the tension on your hip abductors.
7. Hold the pose for up to 3 to 5 minutes while taking deep breaths.
8. To exit the pose, draw the knees together with the hands and roll onto one side.

Variations

- You can start with a looped strap around your waist and hook the strap around the outsides of the feet before you lie back. This allows for traction between your feet and back and helps to lengthen the lumbar spine while holding your feet in place, removing tension from your hips.
- *Restorative variation:* Place blocks under the knees to support the hip flexors if the hips feel strained.

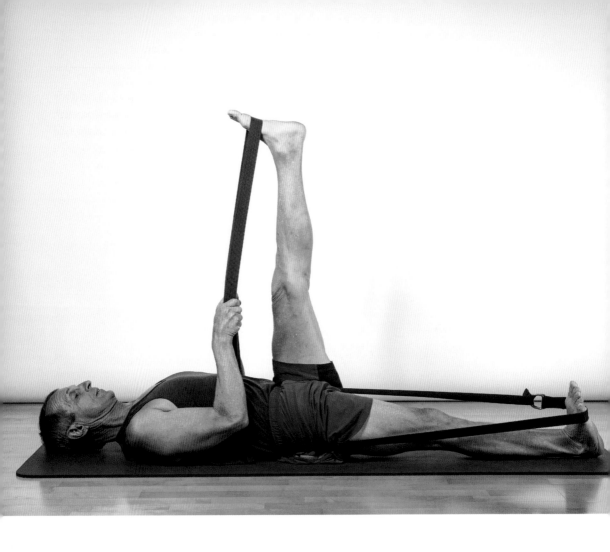

RECLINING HAND-TO-TOE WITH STRAPS
Supta Utthita Hasta Padangusthasana

Traction has been used in the management of low back pain for decades. Traction increases space between the vertebrae, allowing for increased room for nerves to travel and restoring proper disc position. Luckily, in this pose there is no need for a traction or inversion table because traction can be achieved with the use of yoga straps.

Benefits

- Increases spinal mobility.
- Relaxes the spinal muscles.
- Decreases pressure on the intervertebral discs.

How To

1. Measure the length from your hip to your foot with a strap and loop the strap to that length.
2. Have another, unlooped strap next to you.
3. Put the looped strap over your head and around your waist and hook it over the ball of your right foot. Straighten your right leg.
4. Lie on your back with the strap hooked on your right foot and bend the left knee into your chest; you may need to readjust your strap for comfort to attain a straight right leg.
5. Take the other strap and step your left foot into it, with one hand on each side of the strap.
6. Keep your elbows bent as you draw the left knee in to your chest with the strap of the left foot.
7. Move toward straightening your left leg, or keep the left knee bent if the hamstring does not feel comfortable straightening.
8. Hold for 5 breath cycles.
9. Switch sides.

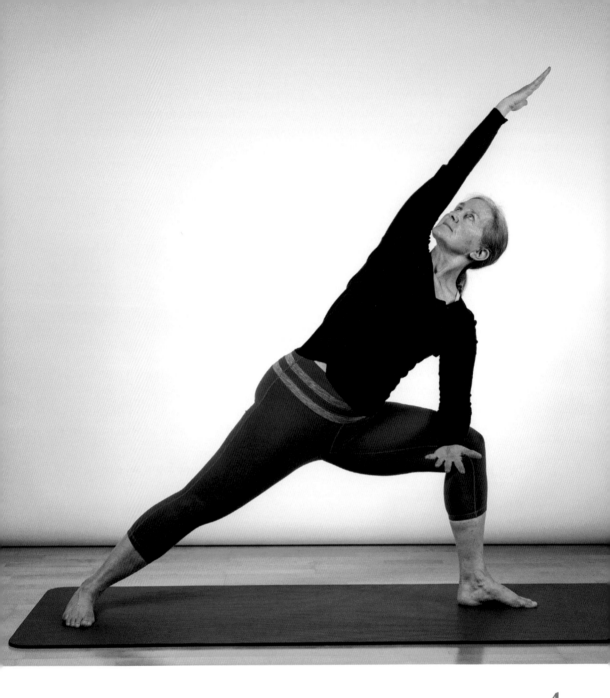

Osteoarthritis of the Hip and Knee

Osteoarthritis (OA), typically referred to in its truncated term simply as *arthritis*, is the most common condition affecting the musculoskeletal system, with the knee and the hip being the two most commonly affected joints.[14] Approximately 21 percent of adults in the United States live with OA.[22] In fact, OA is the leading cause of lower extremity disability in older adults.

OA is characterized by the slow and sometimes progressive loss of cartilage that covers the bones of a joint. Those with OA of the hip or knee often experience pain when performing daily tasks, such as walking and climbing stairs, resulting in loss of mobility, stiffness, or instability. OA diagnoses are often associated with reduced participation in various activities such as work, recreation, and sports.[14]

It is important to understand that when considering pain and function, the problem with OA is not the evidence or severity of OA that is seen on X-ray. In fact, many people with evidence of arthritic changes on X-ray actually experience no pain at all.[15] It is reasonable to think that after an OA diagnosis, pain will be a ubiquitous part of life, and the only solutions may be medication or joint replacement surgery. However, recent studies demonstrate that pain and function in OA can significantly improve with exercise and activity modification.[2]

So, if the problem does not rely on the amount of arthritis present, then what is the actual issue? It turns out that muscular weakness is the leading cause of pain and disability in individuals with OA.[22] Increasing evidence has demonstrated that conservative treatment (i.e., targeted exercise and strength training) can actually delay or, in certain circumstances, prevent the need for surgery in younger patients.[6] The guidelines set forth by both the Centers for Disease Control and Prevention (CDC) and the Arthritis Foundation recommend exercise programs for hip and knee OA that include flexibility, strengthening, endurance, and balance. Because yoga has all four components, we highly recommend yoga as a therapeutic method for reducing pain and disability in those diagnosed with OA.

The loss of strength and range of motion (ROM) in a joint directly correlate to the progression of OA.[5,16] A 2018 retrospective cohort study found that individuals with hip OA had decreased strength in their knee flexors (hamstrings), knee extensors (quadriceps), hip extensors (glutes), and hip abductors (outer thighs).[16] Keep these muscle groups in mind; these are important concepts to understand when learning yoga targeted specifically for OA.

Furthermore, decreased joint ROM is correlated with the presence of OA.[5] Studies have shown that joint impairment is a predictor of disability, particularly due to decreased ROM.[7] We also know that maintaining physical activity through midlife improves flexibility and has measurable benefits on knee function and joint mechanics in osteoarthritis. All this being said, flexibility can translate to a more stable loading environment in the knee and can thus reduce the risk of knee OA in the long term.[12]

The 2019 guidelines from the Osteoarthritis Research Society International specifically recommend yoga for individuals with hip or knee OA, as being "effective and safe."[2] Goh and colleagues[11] state that "aerobic and mind-body exercises [yoga] were found to be the best for pain and function" in OA. The poses in this chapter will target improving strength and flexibility in the muscle groups that have been found most effective in improving pain and function in hip or knee OA. Additionally, select poses will address how to safely progress balance training to improve function and pain in OA. When we focus on the body as a whole and not just on the arthritic joint, we can facilitate great changes.

GENERAL GUIDELINES

- Hip strengthening is beneficial for both hip and knee OA.
- Knee extensor activation and strength are particularly important with knee OA.
- Focus on activating the intended muscle group.
- Progress strengthening exercises from nonweight-bearing to partial weight-bearing to full weight-bearing poses.
- Progressively work *toward* end range positions of the affected joints; do not start at the end ranges.
- Repeated, mindful movements assist in improving joint mobility.
- Promote hope, optimism, and positive expectations when practicing yoga.
- Increase hip mobility in all directions to obtain the highest benefits in yoga for OA.

When considering arthritic joints, the degree of strength in the muscles surrounding the corresponding joint directly correlates to the degree of pain and function. This is because strength equates to stability. Stability can be defined as "the ability to maintain the position of a joint or to control movements affected by external forces."[14] In hip OA, the passive support structures of a joint such as the cartilage and the capsule can be compromised, decreasing joint stability. Therefore, it is critical to focus on increasing muscle strength and proprioception (your sense of where you are in space) to provide active support for the joint. Strength and proprioception combine to reduce forces on the arthritic structures of a joint, reducing pain and inflammation.[22]

The principles of strengthening muscles around an arthritic joint in the hip also apply to knee OA. More strength around an arthritic joint will decrease stress and suboptimal joint loading. With reduced joint stress and improved strength, pain and function improve. Thus, we emphasize strengthening the knee extensor muscles in knee OA to stabilize the knee joint and decrease joint loading. There is an insightful saying that "the knee is the victim of a weak hip and a tight ankle." This principle best explains that weakness at the hip will alter the mechanics of the knee joint, indicating the need for hip strengthening in individuals with knee OA.

Due to the pain–inhibition feedback loop, there exists a dependent cycle between the knee extensor strength, knee extension ROM, and knee OA. A dysfunctional cycle begins with injury or pain in the knee, which results in disuse or misaligned weight bearing of the knee, which, over time, causes weakness in the knee extensor (quadriceps) muscles.[13] This quadriceps weakness then transmutes into pain and disability.[22] Furthermore, as knee arthritis progresses, the knee extensor muscles become increasingly weak and knee extension ROM is lost, causing more pain, which feeds right back into the cycle.[8] Thus, in an attempt to break this cycle of pain, knee extension weakness, and loss of ROM, many of the poses in this chapter focus on quadriceps muscle strengthening and improving this muscle group's corresponding ROM.

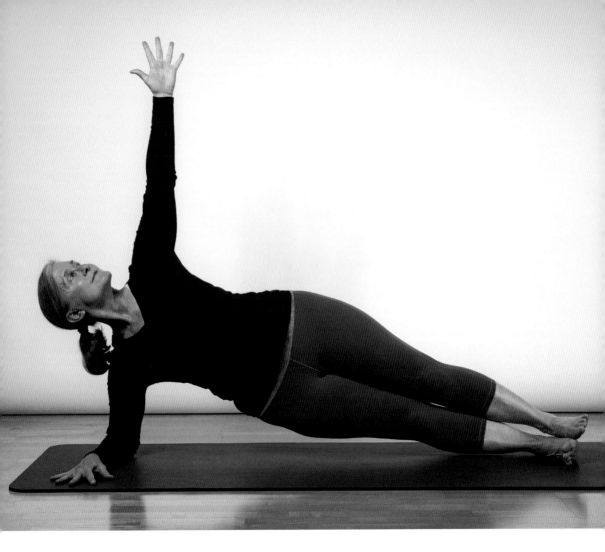

SIDE PLANK ON FOREARM

Vasisthasana

- ✓ Recommended for hip arthritis
- ✓ Recommended for knee arthritis

Hip abductor weakness is common in hip and knee arthritis.[16] The consequence of weak hip abductors is a shifting of the trunk over the affected hip during the swing phase of gait; this causes the pelvis to tilt downward instead of upward on the nonweight-bearing extremity. This position change in the trunk, which is the center of mass (COM), increases compressive forces on the inner aspect of the knee joint, leading to progressive degeneration of the knee[17] and causing a cascade effect of compressive forces from hip to knee. Side Plank is one of the best exercises to strengthen the gluteus medius muscle, which is the primary hip abductor. This is because the hip abductors must resist the body's weight to maintain alignment in body weight, and thus produces greater activation of the hip adductors than any other body weight-bearing exercise.[9] Furthermore, Side Plank is incredibly modifiable, and individuals of all abilities, OA or otherwise, can use it to strengthen the hip abductors.

Benefits

- Strengthens the hip abductors (bottom leg).
- Strengthens the obliques (lower portion).
- Strengthens the knee extensors (both legs).

Precautions

Be careful if you have a history of shoulder injury.

How To

1. From Forearm Plank (pages 100-101), rotate the right forearm so the fingers of the right hand point toward the left hand and your right forearm is at a 45 degree angle to the front edge of the mat.
2. Roll to the outer edge of your right foot, stacking your left foot over the right.
3. Press the hips up and away from the mat, engaging the core and right inner thigh up into the left leg.
4. Lift the left fingertips to the sky and press the right forearm down into the mat as you stack the shoulders.
5. Gaze forward or up to the left hand.
6. Hold for 3 to 5 breath cycles.
7. Repeat on the other side.

Modifications

If this is too hard on your shoulders, lower the bottom knee to the mat for more support.

Variations

Instead of resting on the elbow, you can come up on the hand.

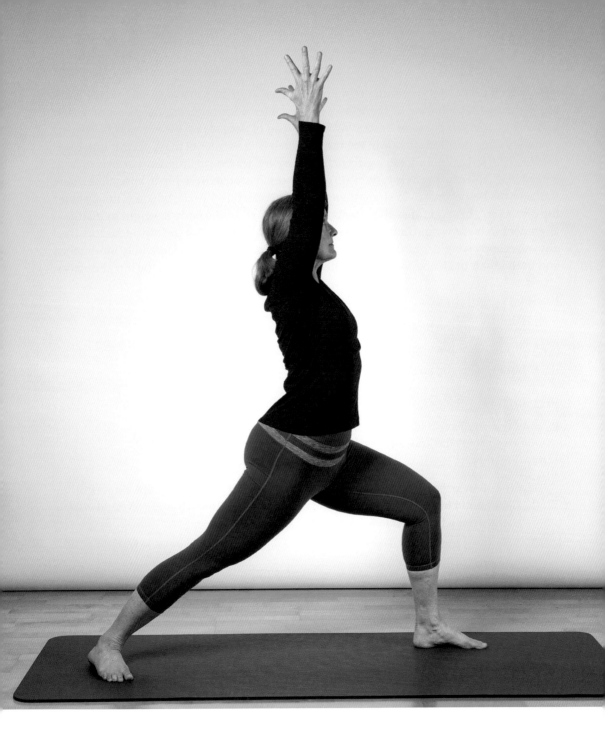

WARRIOR I

Virabhadrasana I

- ✓ Recommended for hip arthritis
- ✓ Recommended for knee arthritis

In hip OA, the strength and muscle mass of the knee extensor are 20 percent and 10 percent lower, respectively, than in the general population.[20] Lunge exercises have been found to be some of the best exercises to activate and strengthen the quadriceps muscle group.[9] In Warrior I, the quadriceps muscles strengthen by maintaining knee stability as the hip, knee, and ankle of the front leg flex. Warrior I also strengthens the hip extensors of the back leg by controlling the degree of hip extension and abduction because of its role in centering the pelvis over the feet.

Warrior I also offers variability because you can control the length of the stance, thus determining the level of challenge (feet further apart for advanced, and closer together for more stability in the beginning stages). Warrior I mimics the terminal stance phase of the gait cycle, with the back knee in extension. However, with knee OA, this same extension is often limited on account of quadriceps weakness.[8] To manage this, the front knee can change its degree of bend, allowing the potential OA-afflicted back knee to better manage its degree of extension.

Benefits

- Strengthens the knee extensors (both legs, primarily the front one).
- Strengthens the hip extensors and abductors (both legs).
- Stretches the hip flexors (back leg).
- Strengthens the knee flexors (both legs).

How To

1. Starting in Downward-Facing Dog (pages 90-91), step the left foot forward between the hands so that it is placed next to the left thumb.
2. Spin the right heel down approximately to a 45 degree angle and spin the outer edge of the right foot down so the entire plantar aspect of the foot grounds down.
3. With your left leg bent and thigh parallel to the floor, inhale your arms up to the sky, hands facing each other, fingers pointing up.
4. The back leg remains straight and strong as you anchor the foot to square the hips forward.
5. Lift the lower abdomen up and in as you lengthen the tailbone down.
6. Draw the shoulders down the back, and gaze forward or slightly up between your hands.
7. Hold for 5 breath cycles.
8. To exit, bring the hands down in a swan dive to frame the foot, and return to Downward-Facing Dog.
9. Repeat on the right side.

Modifications

If this hurts your knee, shorten your stance and back off of the deep knee bend of the front leg.

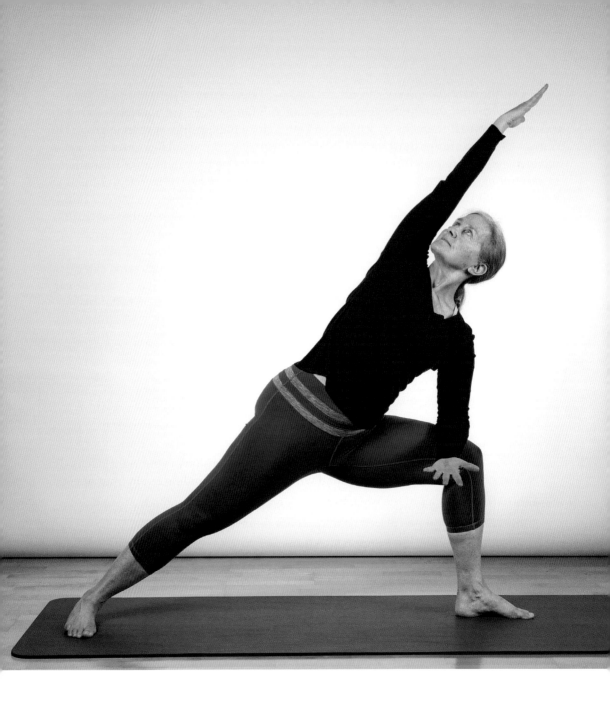

EXTENDED SIDE ANGLE Utthita Parsvakonasana

- ✓ Recommended for hip arthritis
- ✓ Recommended for knee arthritis

In hip OA, the knee flexors have been found to be weaker and lower in muscle bulk.[16] Hamstring strengthening is an important principle in improving muscle strength and decreasing pain in hip OA. Extended Side Angle places the front hip into abduction and external rotation because the torso is extended over the front leg, allowing for increased activation of the hamstrings. This change in the center of gravity, when compared to Warrior I, minimizes the activation of the hip adductor muscles and offers more potential for strength gains in the posterior leg muscles. It is also important to remember to focus on isometrically pulling the front knee toward the trunk in Extended Side Angle to increase hamstring activation.

Benefits

- Strengthens the knee flexors (front leg).
- Strengthens the knee extensors (both legs).
- Strengthens the hip abductors (both legs).
- Strengthens the hip extensors (front leg).

How To

1. Start in Warrior II (pages 104-105), with the left foot forward.
2. Place the left forearm onto the left thigh, or the left hand to the floor or on a block outside your foot.
3. Extend the right arm over the right ear to feel the extension in your right side body. The palm faces down to the ground with the fingers extending out in front of you.
4. Extend both sides of the waist to reach out and over the front thigh.
5. Engage the abdomen to protect the spine and side.
6. Your gaze can extend toward your right hand, to the ground, or straight forward, depending on which is most comfortable for your neck.
7. Hold for 5 breath cycles.
8. To exit the pose, turn the torso to the mat to frame the left foot with your hands, and step back to Downward-Facing Dog (pages 90-91) before switching sides.

Modifications

You can step into Warrior II over the seat of a chair by placing your hand on the chairback for support and resting your front thigh on the seat of the chair for support. Your hands can stay on the chair or extend up to the sky. See the modification for lower extremity amputation on page 153.

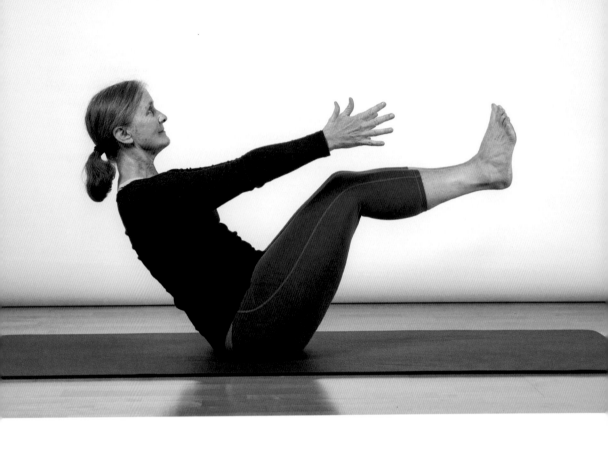

BOAT

Navasana

✓ Recommended for hip arthritis

In hip OA, the muscles of the upper legs are generally weak, particularly the hip flexor muscles.[16] Boat is an excellent exercise to strengthen the hip flexors because it involves flexing the hips and engaging the legs. Additionally, this pose requires a coactivation of the knee extensors and knee flexors. Core strength is paramount in hip OA because it enhances pelvic control and reduces forces on the hip joint. Boat is an ideal core strengthener in its focused activation of the abdominals and spinal extensors.

Benefits

- Strengthens the hip flexors.
- Strengthens the knee extensors.
- Strengthens the knee flexors.
- Stabilizes the core.

How To

1. Start seated with your knees bent and feet flat on the floor.
2. Place your hands behind your knees and start to lean back with the chest lifted, noticing the core activation that is starting to take place.
3. Draw the belly button up and in as you begin to lift the feet off the mat.
4. Engage your abdomen and lift the chest, drawing the shoulders back.
5. Let go of the legs and extend your arms forward alongside your knees with your palms facing each other.
6. Be sure the neck remains comfortable by keeping the chest lifted.
7. Your torso, pelvis, and upper legs will be in a V shape with the hips as the fulcrum.
8. Knees will remain bent and shins parallel to the floor.
9. Feet should be neutral, not flexed.
10. Hold for 3 to 5 breath cycles.

Modifications

- Place the toes on blocks, keeping the heels off the blocks.
- Hold the backs of the knees with the hands.

Variations

To challenge yourself, straighten the legs or bring the arms overhead.

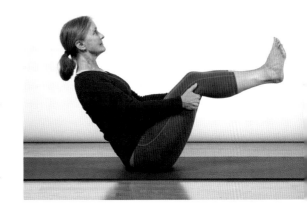

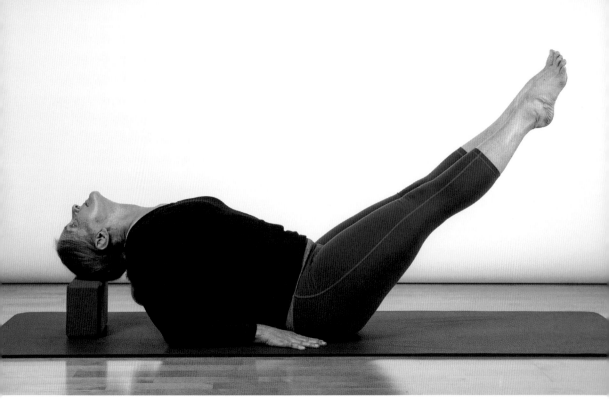

FISH WITH LEGS LIFTED Matsyasana

✓ Recommended for hip arthritis

Forward-flexed posture and exaggerated thoracic kyphosis are common consequences of hip OA and often require activity modification. Some research postulates that these consequences may result from increased sitting because standing and walking may be painful over time as hip OA worsens.[21] This is a prime example of how OA affects the whole body, from posture to lifestyle, and further reinforces the holistic approach of yoga. Yoga is an ideal activity to address these deficits because it focuses on posture and heart opening. This pose incorporates a beautiful thoracic extension that can reverse the action of an exaggerated kyphotic, slumped posture. It also strengthens the hip flexors and knee extensors, similarly to Boat (pages 72-73).

Benefits

- Extends the thoracic spine.
- Strengthens the hip flexors.
- Strengthens the knee extensors.
- Stabilizes the core.

Precautions

This pose may not be appropriate if you have a history of neck injury because of the amount of weight placed on the top of the head as well as the extreme cervical spine extension.

How To

1. Start by lying on your back with the knees bent and feet on the floor.
2. Lift your hips and slide the hands under the buttocks.
3. Scoot the elbows toward each other to lift the torso and head, creating a kickstand with your elbows.
4. Arch the back with the chest puffed out, and walk the elbows farther in toward each other.
5. Release the top of your head to the ground. If it does not reach, place a block under the crown of the head.
6. Lift the legs so that they are at a 45 degree angle from the floor, keeping the quadriceps engaged. You can also keep the knees bent to take the strain out of your hips.
7. Hold for 3 to 5 breath cycles.
8. Release.

Modifications

- Keep the legs on the floor and bend the knees with the feet on the floor; you'll still obtain the benefits of a thoracic backbend.
- Rest the feet on blocks for hip flexor support.
- Place a block under your head if your head is unable to relax on the floor. The head should not be elevated, and the neck should remain relaxed.

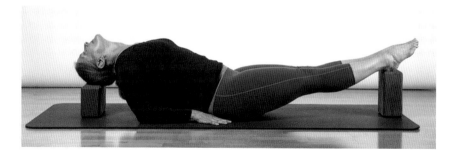

Variations

- *Challenge variation:* Fold the legs into Lotus.
- *Restorative variation:* Place a block lengthwise between your shoulder blades and a block flat behind the back of your head.

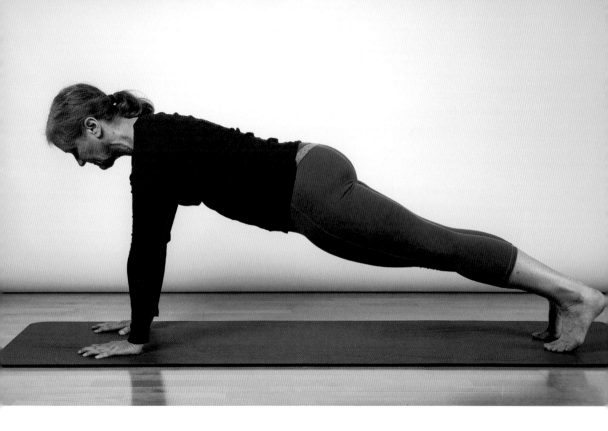

PLANK

Phalakasana

✓ Recommended for hip arthritis
✓ Recommended for knee arthritis

Plank is the quintessential core stabilizer. While pelvic control is beneficial in hip OA, Plank can also be used to strengthen the legs. In Plank, the hip extensors must engage to maintain the hips in neutral extension and the knee extensors activate to straighten the knees. Plank is an excellent example of a weight-bearing, leg-strengthening exercise with upper body support because the hip muscles activate when the joints are bearing body weight.[3] However, weight bearing increases forces on the arthritic joints and may need to be progressed toward; modifications when you first start practicing this pose are encouraged.

Benefits

- Stabilizes and strengthens the core.
- Strengthens the knee extensors and hip extensors.

Precautions

Be careful if you have a wrist injury.

How To

1. Start in Downward-Facing Dog (pages 90-91).
2. Inhale as you extend your chest forward and your heels back, bringing the shoulders over the wrists.
3. Align your body in a straight line from your head to your heels.
4. Engage the abdominal muscles in and up, firming your arms in toward midline.
5. Press into the hands, separating your shoulder blades, drawing your sternum in the direction of your spine, and filling out your thoracic spine.
6. Energize the inner thighs toward each other and up as you press back into your heels and forward with your chest, lengthening the spine and neck.
7. Your gaze should be two feet in front of the hands on the floor for a long neck.
8. Be sure the hips do not sag and are in alignment with the chest and legs.
9. Hold for 5 to 8 breath cycles.
10. Come down to rest in Child's Pose (pages 38-39).

Modifications

- Another way to get into the pose is to start in Table Top (pages 250-251) with the shoulders over the wrists, engage the core, and extend one leg back, and then the other.
- If this hurts the wrists, come down onto forearms for Forearm Plank (pages 100-101), as you will still achieve the core stabilization goals on the forearms.
- *Standing Plank:* Face the wall and extend your arms to place your hands on the wall at chest height. Walk the feet back until the hands are at shoulder height and the abdomen engages. You can walk the feet back farther until you feel the upper arm muscles engage. Be sure you are tucking the tailbone so the hips stay in line with the diagonal of the body.
- *Supported by the knees:* Start with steps 1 to 5 above. In Plank, lower the knees directly to the floor, without moving your hands and chest. Continue engaging the abdominal muscles and hugging the outer arms into midline. Hold for 10 breath cycles and come down to rest in Child's Pose.

Variations

To challenge yourself, lift one foot off the floor, maintaining a neutral position of the hips. Hold for a few breath cycles, release the foot down, and switch to the other foot, holding for the same number of breath cycles.

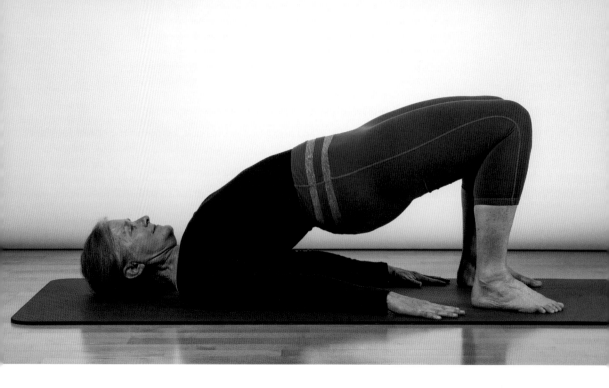

BRIDGE
Setu Bandha Sarvangasana

✓ Recommended for hip arthritis
✓ Recommended for knee arthritis

Reduced strength in the hip extensors is associated with increased pain in hip OA.[18] Bridge is an excellent way to strengthen the hip extensors in a moderate weight-bearing position while the joint is in midrange. Bridge also strengthens the knee flexors and core. An additional benefit of Bridge is that it stretches the hip flexor via the uplifted position of the pelvis.

To understand why hip strength is so important in individuals with knee OA, we must first cover lower extremity biomechanics. With the foot on the ground (closed chain; see chapter 1), hip extension positions the thigh posteriorly (backward), which places the knee joint into extension. The position of knee extension decreases the demand on the knee muscles and therefore reduces the muscle-induced compressive forces on the knee joint.[17] In short, hip extension strength and mobility decrease the workload on the quadriceps and places less force on the knee, which is extremely beneficial for those with knee OA.

Benefits

- Strengthens the hip extensors and the knee flexors.
- Strengthens the core.
- Stretches the hip flexors.
- Increases hip extension mobility.

Precautions

Avoid this pose if you have a current or recent neck injury.

Before You Begin

Have a strap or a block handy for variations.

How To

1. Start by lying on your back with your knees bent, feet flat on the floor, and arms alongside your body with hands facing down.
2. Roll your shoulders underneath you as you begin to lift your hips.
3. Press your feet and shoulders into the mat as you lift your hips.
4. As you rise, walk the feet closer to your buttocks and scoot your shoulders into midline to further elevate the hips and lengthen the tailbone.
5. Keep your knees parallel as you engage the inner thighs.
6. Interlace the fingers on the mat, extend the palms on the floor next to you or hold on to a strap with the hands.
7. Keep your neck neutral by relaxing your chin away from your chest to preserve the natural curve of your cervical spine.
8. Your shoulders, feet, and back of the head support your lift comfortably on the mat because you are using the muscles of your buttocks and back to lengthen your hips.
9. Hold for 5 to 10 breath cycles.
10. To exit the pose, release the hands if interlaced and slowly roll down your spine.

Modifications

- Hold on to a strap with your hands if the fingers cannot reach to interlace.
- Place a block between the knees to keep the thighs parallel and in line with the hips.
- If your neck feels uncomfortable, place a small rolled-up towel behind the neck for support.

Variations

- *Challenge variations:* Bend one knee into the belly, *or* for a further challenge, extend the leg straight up.
- *Restorative variation:* Place a block or bolster directly under your sacrum, allowing the prop to take the weight of your body. Be sure that you continue to lengthen your neck by resting the head's weight on the back of the head and not on the neck. Lift the chest toward your chin, and your chin slightly away from your chest.

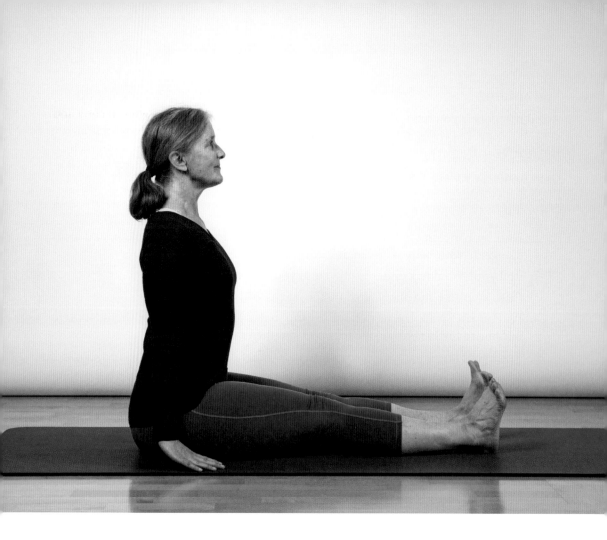

STAFF

Dandasana

✓ Recommended for knee arthritis

Before you can strengthen your knee extensor muscles, you must be able to activate them. Staff provides the opportunity to focus on actively straightening the knee while feeling and actually watching the quadriceps muscles engage. This visual–muscular feedback builds neuromuscular control. Additionally, Staff is performed in an off-loaded position, which provides joint safety and decreases compressive forces on the knee joints. Knee extension mobility is also improved in this pose because it stretches the knee flexors.

Benefits

- Strengthens the knee extensors.
- Stretches the knee flexors.
- Stretches the plantar flexors (calves).

How To

1. Start seated with your legs extended in front of you, hands resting beside your hips with the palms facing down and fingers spread wide.
2. Dorsiflex your feet, extending out through the heels and pointing the toes up and toward your nose.
3. Press the backs of the knees down into the mat as you engage the quadriceps.
4. Roll the shoulders back and engage the belly.
5. Hold for 5 to 10 breath cycles.

Modifications

- Sit facing a wall with your feet flat against the wall to make sure they are dorsiflexed. Press the heels firmly into the wall.
- To emphasize strengthening of the affected side, isolate one leg at a time.

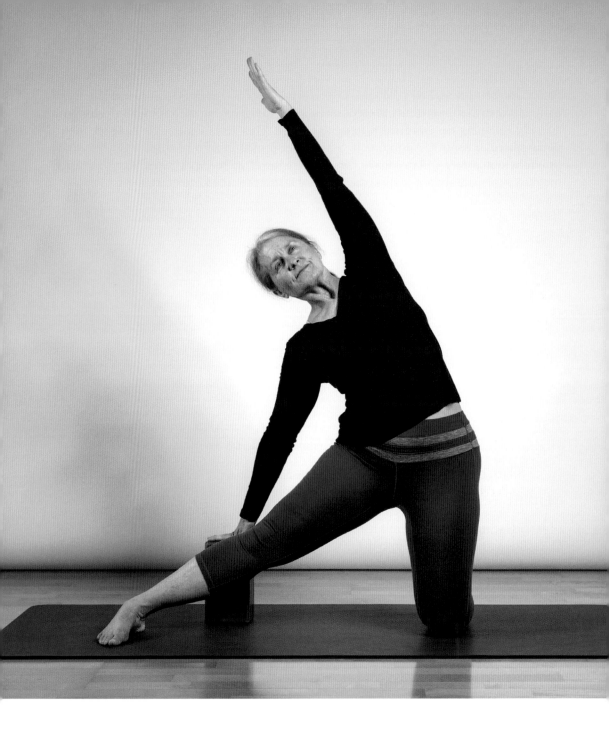

GATE

Parighasana

✓ Recommended for hip arthritis
✓ Recommended for knee arthritis

Studies have shown that hip adductor weakness is common in knee OA. Hip adductor strength is needed to maintain the leg in a neutral position in the lateral plane during dynamic upright activity.[17] Gate creates a strong activation of the hip adductors in the kneeling leg, which keeps the hip in an adducted and internally rotated position. Be sure that the hip adductors engage by isometrically contracting the kneeling leg toward midline. This pose also facilitates strengthening of the hip abductors of the kneeling leg and knee extensors of the extended leg.

With most of the body's weight on the kneeling leg, Gate is an easy progression from Staff because it introduces knee extension of the extended leg, while off-loading the same-side leg muscles. You can still actively engage the knee extensors and, if tolerable, use a hand to apply gentle pressure on the quadriceps of the extended leg to produce more knee extension ROM. This pose enables increased weight to be shifted onto the extended leg based on the amount of side bending in the trunk toward that limb.

Benefits

- Strengthens the hip adductors.
- Strengthens the hip abductors (kneeling leg).
- Strengthens the knee extensors (extended leg).

Precautions

If you have an injury to the patella, avoid kneeling on the side of the injury.

How To

1. Start in a standing kneel (on your knees and shins, but hips lifted). You can place a folded blanket under the knees for cushioning and comfort.
2. Step your right leg out to the side to straighten the knee, with the right toes pointed forward.
3. Make sure your hips are aligned over the knees.
4. Inhale the arms up to the sky and relax your right hand to draw down your right leg toward the ankle, stretching through the left side of the trunk.
5. Continue pressing the hips forward, so as not to let the buttocks bow out.
6. Feel the stretch on the right inner thigh as you ground through the right foot.
7. Bend farther into the side bend, as much as is comfortable but at the same time challenging.
8. Hold for 5 to 10 breath cycles.
9. To exit the pose, reach both arms back up to the sky and step the right knee next to the left.
10. Switch sides.

Modifications

- Place a block behind or in front of the extended shin to support your right hand and your trunk.
- You can also place your extended (left) hand on your waist if the side stretch is too intense.

Increasing joint mobility is one of the key components of rehabilitation in hip OA and has been found to lead to pain reduction and functional improvements.[11] Loss of a joint's flexibility can diminish the amount of loadable surface area. This causes repeated loading in the reduced area, which exacerbates pain and inflammation and accelerates degeneration. Improving flexibility provides rest and reduction of loading stress in specific areas of the joint.[22]

Knee OA often causes reduced ROM in ankle dorsiflexion.[23] This is important because if there is a decreased ROM in the ankle, the tibia (shinbone) will be forced to create increased knee extension to push off the back leg in walking. Since knee OA is characterized by a loss of knee extension ROM, forcing the joint into a position of stiffness can produce pain and inflammation. As demonstrated in this section, both Chair and Downward-Facing Dog focus on increasing ROM for ankle dorsiflexion in order to decrease stress on the knee.

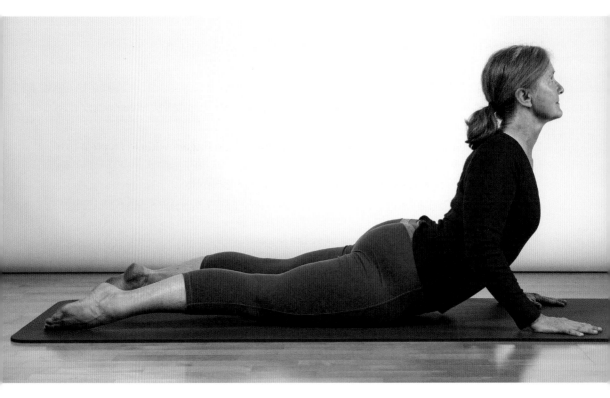

COBRA   Bhujangasana

✓ Recommended for hip arthritis

The most common loss of joint mobility in hip OA is hip extension, likely due to activity modification (increased time sitting). This further causes decreased hip extension during walking, which in turn further worsens OA-related hip pain.[21] Cobra places the hip in a moderate amount of hip extension and stretches the hip flexor muscles, which can improve ROM in hip extension. Keep in mind that moving an arthritic joint into a direction of stiffness may cause pain; thus the lower grade of hip extension in Cobra is an ideal way to initiate increased hip extension safely and comfortably.

Benefits

- Increases hip extension mobility.
- Stretches hip flexors.
- Strengthens hip extensors and knee flexors.

Precautions

Avoid this pose if you are pregnant or if you have a back injury or a wrist injury.

How To

1. Start by lying face down, forehead to the ground, legs extended, and hands directly under the shoulders.
2. Scoop the elbows in toward your body and spread the fingers wide to create a firm foundation with the hands.
3. Press into the hands to lift the chest as you engage the abdominal muscles.
4. Draw the shoulders down your back as you move toward straight arms; it's okay to maintain a bend in your arms for the comfort of your back.
5. Make sure that you continue to engage your abdominal muscles to protect the spine as you lift your heart up and draw the scapulae down your back.
6. Balance the head comfortably in line with the curve of the spine.
7. The pubic bone rests on the mat, but with the action of lifting slightly up toward the chest to lengthen the lumbar spine.
8. Remember, it is about the length and comfort of your spine, not about how high you can lift the chest.
9. Hold for 5 to 8 breath cycles.
10. Release by laying back down on the belly and turn one cheek to the mat.

Variations

- *Challenge variation:* Walk the hands in toward the body to further lift the chest and move toward a more upright spine. Make sure the shoulders continue to draw down the back and away from the ears, and the abdomen remains engaged.
- *Restorative variation:* Place a bolster under the low belly to support the spine.

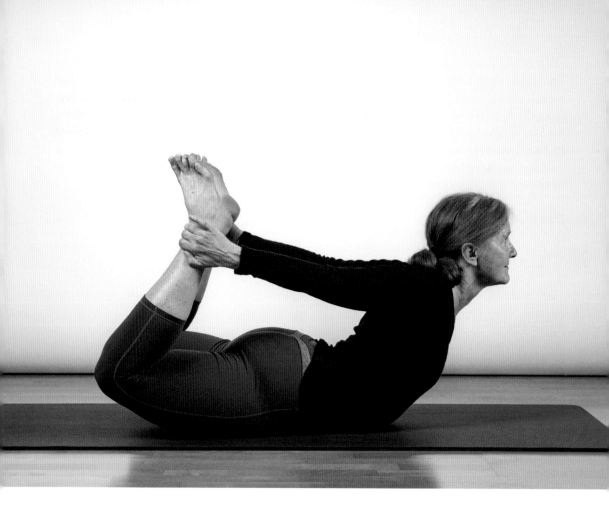

BOW

Dhanurasana

✓ Recommended for hip arthritis

Bow is a progression of hip extension mobility. This pose allows movement into end range hip extension in a nonweight-bearing position, eliminating compressive forces on the hip joint. Progress the amount of hip extension gradually so as to reduce potential pressure on the hip. An added bonus is that this pose is an excellent strengthener of the hip extensors and knee flexors.

Benefits

- Increases hip extension mobility.
- Stretches the hip flexors.
- Strengthens the spinal extensor muscles.
- Strengthens the hip extensors.
- Strengthens the knee flexors.

Precautions

Be careful if you have high blood pressure or are prone to headaches.

How To

1. Start by lying face down, arms alongside your body with the palms facing up.
2. Bend the knees and lift your chest and head to reach back for your ankles.
3. Wrap your hands around your ankles and kick the ankles back to lift your chest.
4. Keep the knees no wider than hip width apart as you continue to kick the feet back and lift the knees to open your chest.
5. Engage the belly button up toward the spine to support the low back.
6. Draw your shoulder blades down your back to enhance the opening of your chest.
7. Hold for 5 breath cycles.
8. Exhale to release and turn one cheek to the mat.

Modifications

Wrap straps around the ankles and hold the straps in your hands if you cannot reach your feet.

Variations

As a restorative option, place a bolster under the low belly to support the spine.

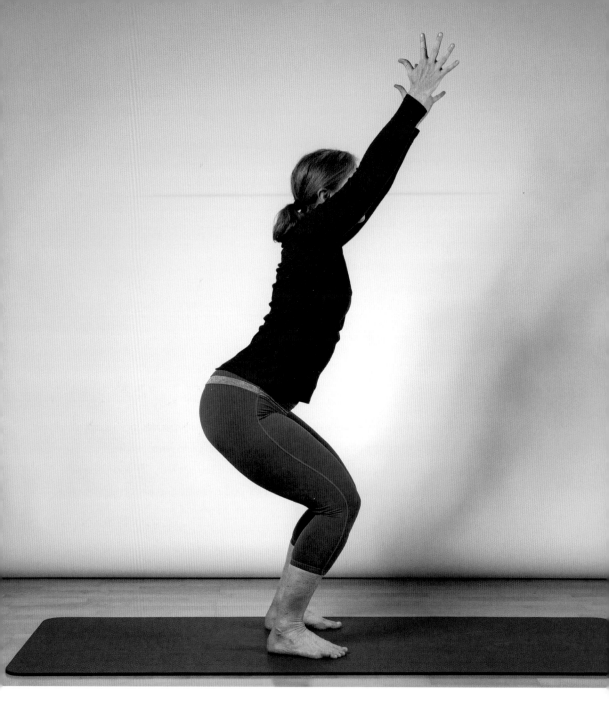

CHAIR

Utkatasana

✓ Recommended for knee arthritis

Because of poor ROM in ankle dorsiflexion, most people cannot perform a full squat without lifting the heels off the ground. Chair deliberately positions the ankle into dorsiflexion and transitions the COM forward of the ankle joint, which improves mobility for ankle dorsiflexion. In doing so, the improved ankle dorsiflexion will off-load and decrease stress on the knees when walking. You should go only as low as you can while keeping your heels in full contact with the ground.

Benefits

- Increases ankle dorsiflexion mobility.
- Strengthens the knee extensors.
- Strengthens the core stabilizers.
- Strengthens hip extensors.

How To

1. Start in Mountain (pages 150-151).
2. Bend your knees to sit the hips back, trying to bring your thighs parallel to the floor.
3. Reach your arms overhead alongside your ears and engage your abdomen.
4. Ground through all four corners of the feet.
5. Notice that you are bent at the ankles, knees, and hips.
6. Hold for 5 to 10 breath cycles.
7. To exit the pose, press down into your feet to straighten your legs and stand upright. Relax your arms alongside your body as you return to Mountain.

Modifications

Practice with different arm positions, such as prayer at the chest or hands on the hips.

Variations

To challenge yourself, place a block between your knees to engage the inner thighs. Be sure that you still place even weight between both feet so that you do not collapse into the arches of the feet.

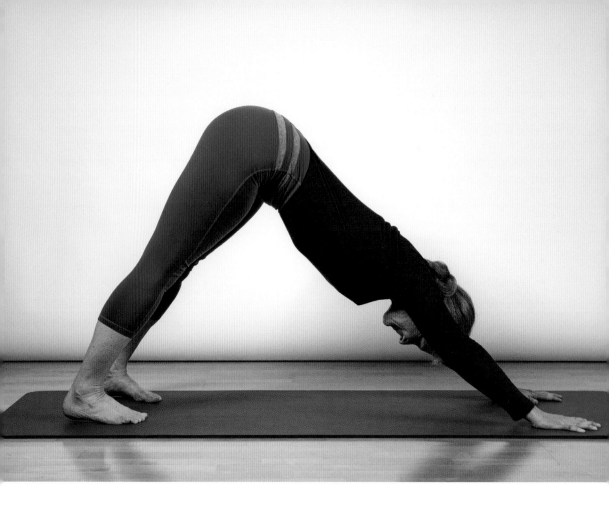

DOWNWARD-FACING DOG   Adho Mukha Svanasana

✓ Recommended for knee arthritis

In order to increase the mobility of a joint, it should be placed into its end range while maintaining a weight-bearing position. Downward-Facing Dog does just that for ankle dorsiflexion, thereby decreasing stress on osteoarthritic knees. Because the ankle is placed in this position by your body weight shifting back into the heels, it also facilitates pliant stretching of the ankle plantar flexor muscles. Focus on ankle dorsiflexion while in this position both with your knees straight and knees bent, because each of these positions targets different plantar flexor muscles in the ankle.

Benefits

- Stretches the ankle plantar flexors.
- Strengthens the knee extensors.

Precautions

Avoid this pose if you have an active or recent wrist injury.

How To

1. Start in Table Top (pages 250-251), with your hips aligned above your knees and shoulders above your wrists.
2. Walk the hands forward about half a hand's length with the wrists aligned parallel to the front of the mat.
3. Tuck the toes under and lift your hips up and back to create an upside-down V shape with your body.
4. Spiral the upper arms toward the ears to open the shoulders and midback.
5. It's okay to keep the knees bent initially to take strain off of your hamstrings and calves. The goal is to lengthen your spine.
6. Spread the collarbone wide and slide the shoulder blades down away from your neck.
7. Move toward straighter legs, but it's okay to keep the knees bent to maintain a lengthened spine.
8. Hold for 5 to 10 breath cycles.
9. To exit the pose, bend the knees down to the floor. You can relax in Child's Pose (pages 38-39) or sit back on your heels.

Modifications

Practice against a wall by facing the wall, then placing the hands at shoulder height and walking the feet back. This allows both the spine to lengthen and the hamstrings to stretch, but without bringing the head below the heart.

Variations

- *Challenge variation:* Lift one leg at a time.
- *Restorative variation:* Place a bolster under the crown of the head for further support.

Balance training is recommended for individuals with hip OA because it increases joint proprioception, which is integral for joint stability. Additionally, balance training increases muscle strength. Single leg exercises can significantly increase core and hip muscle activation.[4] Balance, as a general rule, is founded upon strength and stability, and the poses we recommend to improve balance in hip OA should be practiced with attention to improving strength and stability.

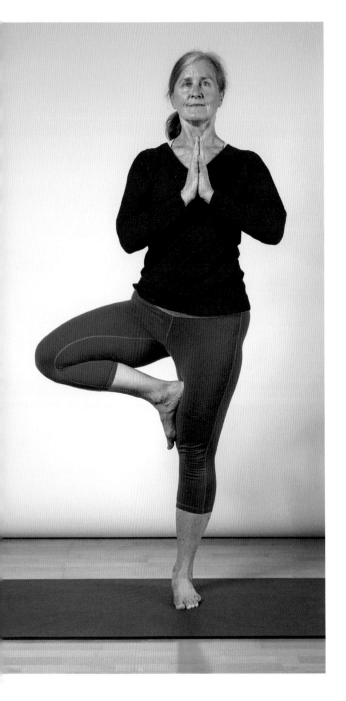

TREE Vrksasana

✓ Recommended for hip arthritis
✓ Recommended for knee arthritis

In order to improve function, you must exercise and strengthen the knee in functional positions. Tree helps achieve many of the goals of knee OA rehabilitation: knee extension mobility, knee extensor strengthening, hip abductor strengthening, and increased core stability. Tree requires significant muscle activation of the knee extensors and knee flexors to keep the knee in neutral extension in this single leg stance. It also produces a strong activation of the hip abductors to keep the pelvis level. The lifted leg strengthens the hip flexors and hip external rotators of the bent leg to maintain the same-side hip in line with the pelvis. With the knee flexors bending the knee, it also provides excellent hip opening because it stretches the internal rotators. As we have discussed, hip muscle weakness is quite common in hip OA, making the traditional Tree very challenging; modifications will likely need to be made initially.

We ask that you be mindful in Tree. It can place compressive loads on the standing knee because the full body weight is on the stance leg and the knee extensors in the straightened knee are strongly contracted. This is a pose that should be worked toward and modified initially.

Benefits

- Improves hip joint proprioception (standing leg).
- Strengthens the hip abductors and knee extensors (standing leg).
- Strengthens the knee flexors (lifted leg).
- Strengthens the hip external rotators and hip flexors (lifted leg).
- Stretches the hip internal rotators (lifted leg).
- Increases core stability.

Precautions

Be careful if you have knee instability.

How To

1. Start in Mountain (pages 150-151), with a firm footing on the ground and your gaze focused on an object in front of you.
2. Shift all of your weight to your left leg and bend your right knee up into your chest, catching hold of the knee with your hands.
3. Hold your right ankle with your right hand and fold the foot into your inner thigh.
4. Press the left thigh back into your right foot so the foot does not overpower the standing leg or cause it to bow out.
5. Reach your arms overhead or keep the hands to prayer at heart center.
6. Lengthen through your tailbone and engage the abdomen as you draw the shoulder blades down the back and open the heart space.
7. Hold for 5 to 10 breath cycles.
8. To exit the pose, step your right foot down and shake it out.
9. Repeat on the opposite side.

Modifications

- Stand next to a wall, at the side of your standing leg. Place your hand on the wall for extra support.
- Keep the toes on the ground, with the heel on the ankle.
- Place the lifted foot on the calf muscle rather than on the inner thigh.

Variations

To add a balance challenge, reach the arms overhead.

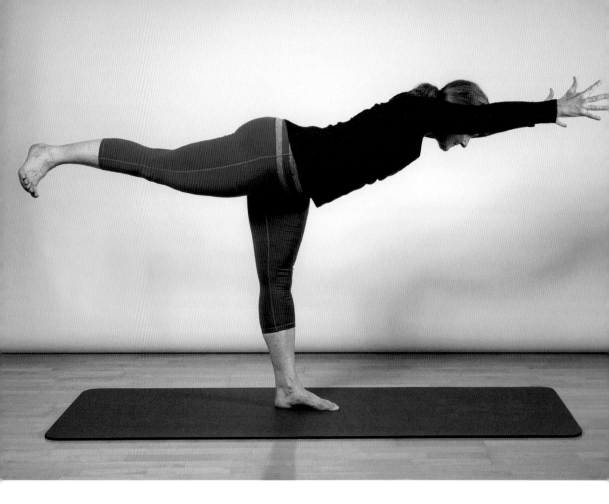

WARRIOR III

Virabhadrasana III

✓ Recommended for hip arthritis
✓ Recommended for knee arthritis

Warrior III is a progression of the single leg stance balance and strength from Tree because it positions the trunk (your COM) in front of the foot (your base of support). This stance requires significant activation of the standing leg's hip extensors to control the amount of hip flexion. The knee extensors must engage to maintain a neutral knee extension. Hip abductors also work to keep the pelvis level (many of us must open our hips in this pose because our hip abductors are not strong enough).

Benefits

- Increases proprioception of the hip joint (stance leg).
- Strengthens the hip extensors (both legs).
- Strengthens the knee flexors (both legs).
- Strengthens the knee extensors (stance leg).
- Strengthens the hip abductors (stance leg).

Precautions

Be careful if you have an ankle injury to the standing leg.

How To

1. Start in Warrior I (pages 68-69) or Crescent Lunge (pages 42-43), with the left foot forward and arms overhead.
2. Put all your weight into your left foot and start to lean the torso and arms forward.
3. Push off of the right foot, lifting it straight back behind you.
4. Bring the torso and right leg parallel to the ground, creating a T shape with the body.
5. You can bring your arms alongside the body, overhead, or in prayer.
6. Straighten your standing leg by engaging the left quadriceps muscles.
7. Dorsiflex the right foot to point the toes down to the ground, and internally rotate the right hip joint so the foot and knee point down toward the ground.
8. Continue pressing the foot into the ground so as not to collapse into the right hip socket and engage the core muscles.
9. Hold for 3 to 5 breath cycles.
10. Exit the pose the same way you entered it, by stepping the foot back into Crescent Lunge or Warrior I or by stepping the feet together into Mountain (pages 150-151).
11. Repeat on the right side by first coming into Warrior I or simply switch your feet.

Modifications

- Stand next to a wall, at the side of your standing leg. Place your hand on the wall for extra support.
- Place the hands on the hips, or the arms alongside the torso, instead of overhead.
- If balance or strength is not quite there yet, use the back of a chair to rest your hands while you extend the back leg. You will still get all the benefits of strengthening the leg muscles.

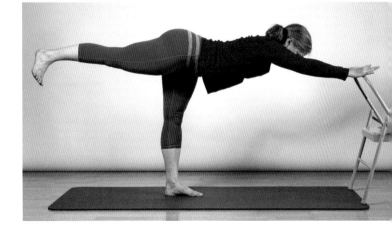

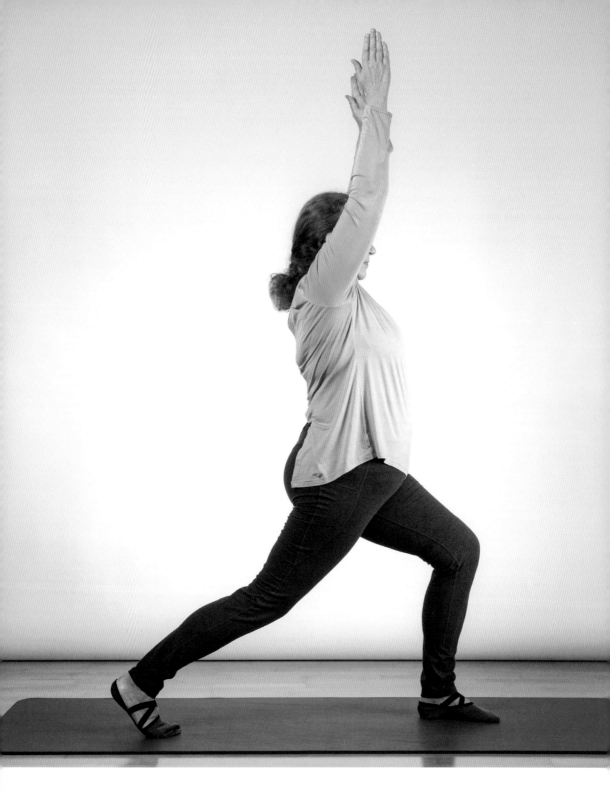

CHAPTER 5

Rheumatoid Arthritis

Rheumatoid arthritis (RA) is a systemic, inflammatory, peripheral polyarthritis. It is an autoimmune disease with an unknown cause. It typically leads to deformity through the stretching of tendons and ligaments and the destruction of joints through the erosion of cartilage and bone.[7] If it is untreated or is unresponsive to therapy, inflammation and joint destruction lead to loss of physical function and difficulty carrying out daily tasks of living.[24]

The most distinctive signs of RA are joint erosions, rheumatoid nodules, symptoms for more than six weeks, and swollen and tender joints in three or more joints, particularly the hands and knuckles.[10] Additionally, RA is often accompanied by other inflammatory diseases such as inflammatory bowel disease and fibromyalgia.[18]

Often, patients with RA are on medications such as disease-modifying antirheumatic drugs (DMARDs), steroids, and ibuprofen.[4] Despite advances in medical therapies, many patients continue to experience ongoing disease activity with the risk of developing resultant disability. Many of these risks can be substantially reduced by a comprehensive management program for RA, including appropriate use of rest, exercise, medication, and counseling.[5]

Pain and stiffness often lead students with RA to avoid using the affected joints. This lack of use can result in loss of joint motion, contractures, and muscle atrophy, thereby decreasing joint stability and further increasing fatigue and weaker muscles. Therefore, it is important for patients to exercise and move regularly to prevent and potentially mitigate these disabling problems.[21]

Regular exercise for patients with RA improves muscle function, joint stability, aerobic capacity, and physical performance. This can result in improved overall pain control and quality of life, without an increase in disease activity.[20] Physical activity has also been shown to decrease the level of fatigue in patients with RA.[17]

Exercise programs should be tailored for each individual's disease, body build, and previous activity level. High-intensity weight-bearing exercises and repetitive, high-impact activities may not be appropriate for patients with preexisting structural damage of lower limb joints.[15] Less intense or nonweight-bearing exercises, such as yoga, are excellent alternatives for such patients.[2]

Regular yoga practice has many benefits for patients with RA, including increasing muscle strength and endurance, proprioception, and balance, and emphasizing movement through a full range of motion (ROM) to increase flexibility and mobility. Additional benefits of yoga include improved breathing, relaxation, body awareness, and meditation, which can reduce stress and anxiety and promote a sense of calmness, general well-being, and improved quality of life. Research suggests that yoga may even help decrease inflammatory markers that signal the severity and activity of disease.[3]

In early stages of RA, relaxation, imagery, and biofeedback, as adjuncts to conventional therapy, can improve pain and mood as well as physical functioning and coping.[1] Mindfulness has been shown to decrease stress, as well as improve mood in RA.[16] Other aspects of yoga may be particularly important for individuals with musculoskeletal concerns, including the emphasis on acknowledging and accepting day-to-day variability in well-being and energy, enhancing body awareness, respecting limits, and modifying exercise (mode, duration, frequency) in response to transient changes in disease activity.

The physical exercise associated with yoga also may build strength in the lower extremities. In this chapter, we include three common poses (Crescent Lunge, Warrior II, and Tree) that simultaneously target five functionally important muscle groups: hip flexors, hip extensors (glutes), knee flexors (hamstrings), knee extensors (quadriceps), and ankle plantar flexors (calves). Notably, strengthening of these muscle groups can prevent collapse of the center of mass (COM) during standing and walking.[22]

The goals of yoga in RA are pain relief, reduction of inflammation, and preservation of joint integrity and function. The yoga therapy plan should involve specific modalities targeted to the following problem areas.

- Passive and active poses to improve and maintain joint mobility.[6]
- Dynamic exercise to improve aerobic capacity and strength.[8]
- ROM exercises to preserve flexibility and general mobility.[9]
- Rest as needed to reduce pain and improve function.[12]
- Relaxation techniques.[23]

Since RA produces fatigue, the performance of many normal tasks may be difficult. We highly recommend resting an inflamed joint when it feels fatigued, as well as the entire body; you can alternate these rest periods with exercise.[14]

We also emphasize ROM exercises because this helps to preserve and restore joint motion.[19] Exercises to increase muscle strength, performed even once or twice a week, have the potential to improve function, without worsening RA disease activity.[13]

Whether you have RA, or are a teacher of a student with RA, we hope you can incorporate these guided poses into your practice. The approach taken in yoga, with an emphasis on mindfulness and stress reduction, improves psychological well-being, reduces pain, enhances function and participation, and can be an invaluable part of a comprehensive approach to RA.

GENERAL GUIDELINES

- Any weight on the head is largely contraindicated in RA. While those with little to no musculoskeletal manifestations may be able to tolerate weight, patients with RA have an increased risk of axial (high cervical spine) instability. Therefore, avoid extreme neck extension and head standing, or bearing weight on the top of the head. This is absolutely contraindicated in patients with advanced RA.
- Note that weight bearing on the hands may be difficult because RA commonly affects the wrists and finger joints. Therefore, prolonged Plank or Sun Salutes may be difficult, but you can modify with knees down or forearms down. Place cushioning such as a folded blanket or a wedge under the wrists if needed.
- The joint mobility of a person with RA is typically most limited in the morning, so morning classes can help that person move and stretch.
- Joint protection is very important, so avoid end range positions (especially while weight bearing) such as a deep lunge on the knee joint (e.g., Warrior I with a long stance).
- Flowing movements are ideal, with an emphasis on stability via slow and controlled movements.
- The recommended joints to move during stretches vary from person to person (based on which joints are affected); the commonly affected joints are knees, ankles, elbows, and hands, especially the knuckles.

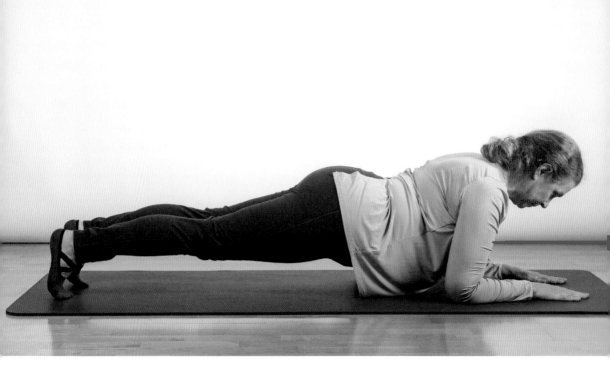

FOREARM PLANK

Phalakasana

Individuals with RA tend to have a lower level of physical activity, and less active individuals tend to possess less core strength. The core muscles create a foundation for the strength of the body. Modifying Plank to the forearms protects the hands and wrists while strengthening many of the core muscles: spinal extensors, abdominals, and obliques. This pose greatly strengthens the legs because it activates the hip extensors, knee extensors, and plantar flexors. Weight bearing through the arms also activates the shoulder muscles.

Benefits

- Strengthens the core.
- Strengthens the hip extensors.
- Strengthens the knee extensors.
- Strengthens the knee flexors.
- Strengthens the plantar flexors.
- Strengthens the shoulder flexors.
- Strengthens the rotator cuff muscles.
- Strengthens the scapular muscles.

Precautions

Avoid this pose if you have an injured elbow, shoulder, or rotator cuff.

How To

1. Start in Downward-Facing Dog (pages 90-91).
2. Walk the elbows down to rest on your forearms, keeping them parallel to each other.
3. Inhale as you extend your chest forward and your heels back and bring the shoulders over the wrists.
4. Align your body in a straight line from your head to your heels.
5. Engage the abdominal muscles in and up, firming your arms in toward midline.
6. Press into the hands, separating your shoulder blades, drawing your sternum in the direction of your spine, and expanding your thoracic spine.
7. Energize the inner thighs toward each other and up as you press back into your heels and forward with your chest, lengthening the spine and neck.
8. Your gaze should be two feet in front of the hands on the floor for a long neck.
9. Be sure the hips do not sag and are in alignment with the chest and legs.
10. Hold for 5 to 8 breath cycles.
11. Come down to rest in Child's Pose (pages 116-117).

Modifications

- Another way to get into the pose is to start in Table Top (pages 250-251) with the shoulders over the wrists, engage the core, extend one leg back and then the other, and then walk down onto your forearms.
- *Standing:* Face the wall and extend your arms to place your hands on the wall at chest height. Walk the feet back until the hands are at shoulder height and the abdomen engages. You can walk the feet back further until you feel the upper arm muscles engage. Be sure you tuck the tailbone so the hips stay in line with the diagonal of the body. You can keep the hands on the wall, or walk down onto your forearms if preferred.
- *Supported by the knees:* Start with steps 1 to 5 above. In Forearm Plank, lower the knees directly to the floor, without moving your arms and chest. Continue engaging the abdominal muscles and hugging the outer arms into midline. Hold for 5 to 10 breath cycles and come down to rest in Child's Pose.
- Place a block under the hips across the width of the hips to support the core, and lift the hips up an inch from the block when you are ready for more strengthening.
- You can perform Plank on your hands instead of your forearms if you feel that you have the strength. However, remember that RA often affects the finger and wrist joints, so be mindful that if you experience pain practicing Plank on your hands, you should walk back down onto your forearms.

Variations

To challenge yourself, lift one foot off the floor, maintaining a neutral position of the hips. Hold for a few breath cycles, then release the foot down and switch to the other foot, holding for the same number of breath cycles.

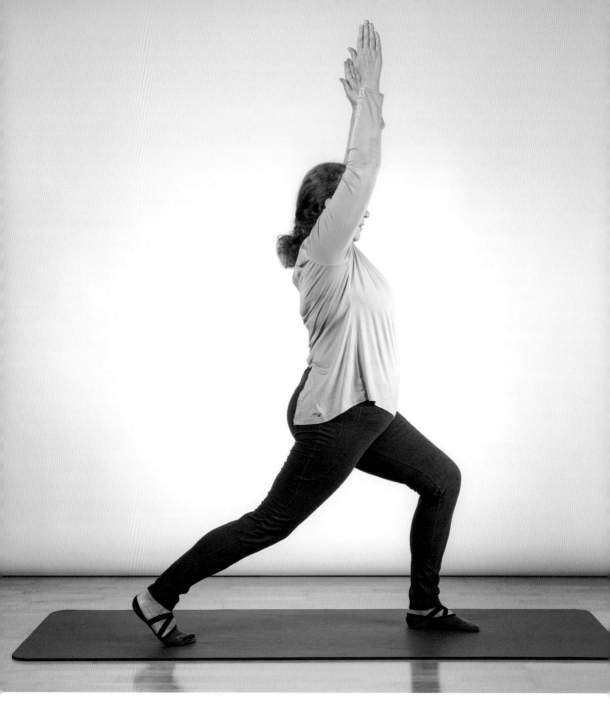

CRESCENT LUNGE   Anjaneyasana

A lunge is one of the best ways to strengthen the knee extensors. The knee extensors are considered one of the most functionally important muscle groups because they aid in standing from a seated position, going up and down stairs, walking, and protecting the knee joint. With the arms above the head, Crescent Lunge opens the chest to increase breath volume and strengthens the shoulder flexors.

Benefits

- Strengthens the knee extensors (both legs).
- Strengthens the hip adductors (front leg).
- Strengthens the knee flexors (both legs).
- Strengthens the plantar flexors (back leg).
- Strengthens the hip extensors (back leg).
- Stretches the hip flexors (back leg).
- Increases breath volume.
- Strengthens the shoulder flexors.

Precautions

Avoid bending the knee past 90 degrees.

How To

1. Starting in Downward-Facing Dog (pages 90-91), step the left foot forward between the hands so that it's next to the left thumb.
2. Keep the back heel up and firm up the strength in your back leg by engaging your right quadriceps muscles.
3. With your left leg bent and thigh parallel to the floor, inhale your arms up to the sky, hands facing each other, fingers pointing up.
4. Keep your back leg straight and strong; your right heel will remain up, but use the action of extending it straight back to the ground as though you are in Downward-Facing Dog.
5. Lift the lower abdomen up and in as you lengthen the tailbone down.
6. Draw the shoulders down the back, and gaze forward or slightly up between your hands.
7. Hold for 5 breath cycles.
8. To exit, bring your hands down in a swan dive to frame the foot and return to Downward-Facing Dog.
9. Repeat on the right side.

Modifications

- If this hurts your front knee, shorten your stance and back off of the deep bend of the front knee.
- Drop the back knee down onto the floor with a blanket or bolster underneath it; you will still get the benefits of quadriceps strengthening (front leg) and hip stretch (back leg).
- If your arms feel strained, place your hands on your waist or into Prayer Hands (pages 118-119).

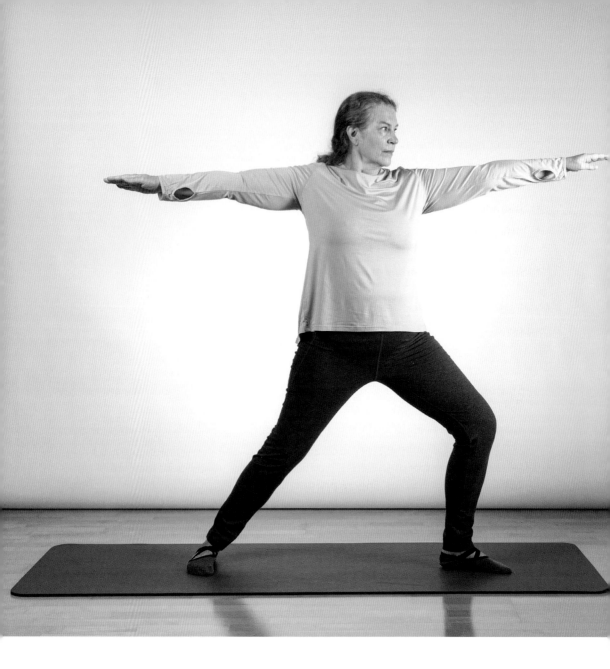

WARRIOR II

Virabhadrasana II

Warrior II strengthens several muscle groups that are beneficial to those with RA. This pose strengthens the hip extensors, knee flexors, knee extensors, and plantar flexors, all of which are needed to maintain a normal gait pattern. This pose also strengthens the shoulder flexors and scapular muscles, which can help keep the shoulder functioning properly and pain free.

Benefits

- Strengthens the hip and knee extensors.
- Strengthens the hip flexors (front leg).
- Strengthens the knee flexors.
- Strengthens the plantar flexors.
- Strengthens the shoulder flexors.
- Strengthens the scapular retractors.

Precautions

If you have knee issues, be careful not to bend farther than the ankle.

How To

1. Start with your feet wide (3.5 to 4 feet depending on your height) on the mat, left toes in front and pointing forward, and right foot with toes pointing toward the long edge of the mat.
2. Ground all four corners of the feet down, creating a strong base for your legs.
3. As you inhale, extend your arms straight out to the sides, parallel to the floor.
4. Relax the shoulders down and extend the neck long as you gaze over the left fingertips.
5. Bend the left knee forward with the goal of extending it in line over the left ankle. You can shift the position of your feet to make space.
6. Roll the inner thigh toward the outer hip so you can see the left big toe (it should be obscured in vision by your left knee). This will maintain alignment of the knee with the ankle.
7. Ground the outer edge of your right foot into the floor.
8. Extend the fingertips out with strength and purpose, while relaxing the shoulders down your back.
9. Hold for 5 to 8 breath cycles.
10. To exit the pose, place the hands on the hips, straighten the legs, and shift the feet to turn to the other side of the mat so your right foot is forward.
11. Repeat on the right side.

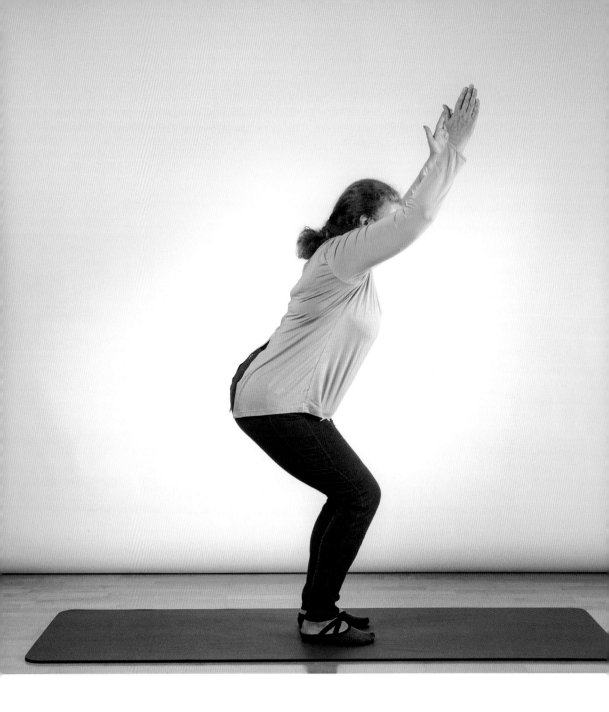

CHAIR

Utkatasana

The squat position of Chair is a staple of lower body strengthening programs. Squatting strengthens the knee extensors, hip extensors, hip adductors, knee flexors, and plantar flexors. Chair is particularly favorable for those with RA because it can be performed despite a decreased ROM in the lower extremities.

Benefits

- Strengthens the hip extensors.
- Strengthens the hip adductors.
- Strengthens the knee extensors.
- Strengthens the knee flexors.
- Strengthens the plantar flexors.

How To

1. Start in Mountain (pages 150-151).
2. Bend your knees to sit the hips back, trying to bring your thighs parallel to the floor.
3. Reach your arms overhead alongside your ears and engage your abdomen.
4. Ground through all four corners of the feet.
5. Notice that you are bent at the ankles, knees, and hips.
6. Hold for 5 to 10 breath cycles.
7. To exit, press down into your feet to straighten your legs and stand upright. Relax your arms alongside your body as you come back into Mountain.

Modifications

- Practice with different arm positions, such as Prayer Hands (pages 118-119) or hands on the hips.
- Stand next to a wall if needed for balance.

Variations

To challenge yourself, place a block between your knees to engage your inner thighs. Be sure that you still place even weight between both feet so that you do not collapse into the arches of the feet.

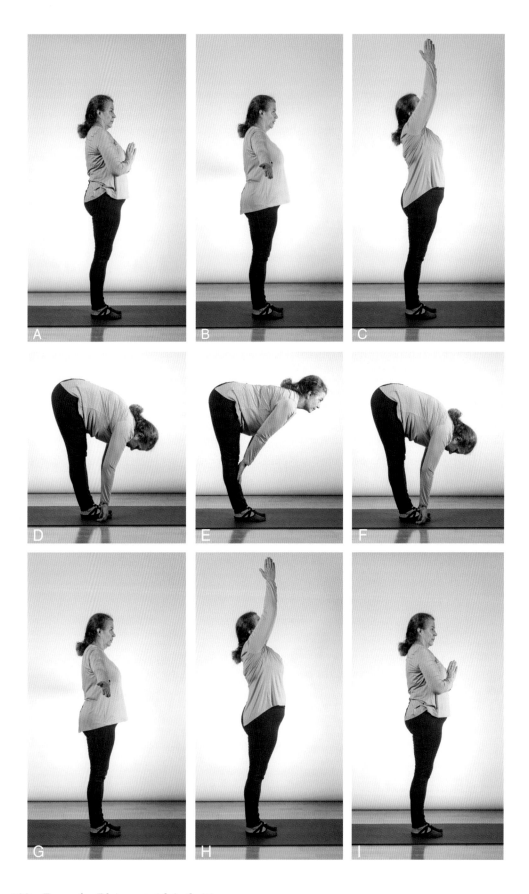

HALF SUN SALUTATION Ardha Surya Namaskar

The flowing motion of Half Sun Salutation provides many benefits for people with RA. One of the benefits is that the constant movement of the body improves aerobic capacity. Additionally, connecting with the breath teaches an important principle of exercise, which is that attention to breath during exercise reduces fatigue. The focus on taking long, deep breaths during the entire movement into each pose also exercises our diaphragm, and thus, strengthens our pulmonary system. Further benefits include minimizing pressure on the joints through flowing movement. Finally, the forward bend and half-lift movement offer a stretch in the knee flexors and improve spinal mobility.

Benefits

- Improves aerobic capacity.
- Teaches the pairing of breathing with movement.
- Strengthens the upper body.
- Stretches the knee flexors.
- Increases mobility of the spine.

Precautions

Be mindful and modify if you have back pain; in general, if you have low back pain symptoms, avoid deep forward bending.

How To

1. Start in Mountain (pages 150-151).
2. Inhale and bring the arms overhead.
3. Exhale and bend forward over the legs, with the knees slightly bent to protect your back.
4. Inhale and extend your chest forward.
5. Exhale and bend forward again.
6. Inhale and sweep the arms up and out, standing up with the arms overhead.
7. Exhale and bring the hands to the heart.
8. Repeat for a total of 5 to 8 breath cycles.

Modifications

- Place blocks under the hands to support the back when folding forward.
- If you have back pain or shooting pain down the legs, minimize the forward bend.

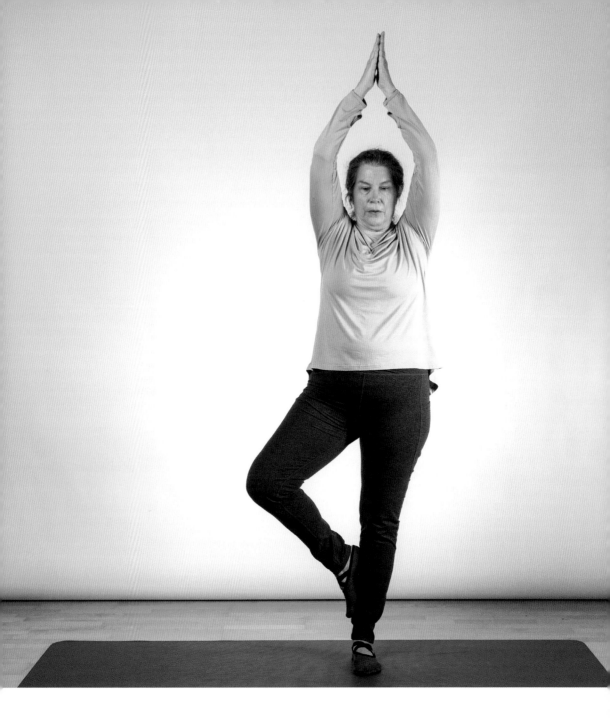

TREE

Vrksasana

Balance is often compromised in those with RA. Tree and its variations allow you to improve single leg balance while strengthening the knee extensors and hip abductors. Single leg balance requires a constant activation of the muscles of the stance leg to microadjust the COM (the trunk) over the base of support (the foot). This occurs not only at the hip but also at the ankle and in the foot, effectively strengthening our foundation of balance.

Benefits

- Improves balance.
- Strengthens the hip flexors (lifted leg).
- Strengthens the knee flexors (lifted leg).
- Strengthens the hip extensors (standing leg).
- Strengthens the knee extensors (stance leg).
- Strengthens the hip abductors (stance leg).
- Strengthens the ankle muscles.
- Strengthens the intrinsic foot muscles.

Precautions

Avoid this pose if you have knee instability or poor balance.

How To

1. Start in Mountain (pages 150-151), with a firm footing on the ground and your gaze focused on an object in front of you.
2. Shift all of your weight to your left leg and bend your right knee up into your chest, catching hold of the knee with your hands.
3. Hold your right ankle with your right hand and fold the foot into your inner calf muscle.
4. Press the left calf back into your right foot so the foot does not overpower the standing leg or cause it to bow out.
5. Reach your arms overhead or keep the hands to prayer at heart center.
6. Lengthen through your tailbone and engage the abdomen as you draw the shoulder blades down the back and open the heart space.
7. Hold for 5 to 10 breath cycles.
8. To exit the pose, step your right foot down and shake it out.
9. Repeat on the opposite side.

Modifications

- Stand next to a wall, at the side of your standing leg. Place your hand on the wall for extra support.
- Keep the toes on the ground with the heel propped against the ankle rather than the inner calf if balance is difficult with the foot on the calf.
- Try practicing next to a wall if you have poor balance.

Variations

- To challenge yourself, place the foot on the inner thigh.
- To challenge yourself, reach the arms overhead to increase your balance difficulty.

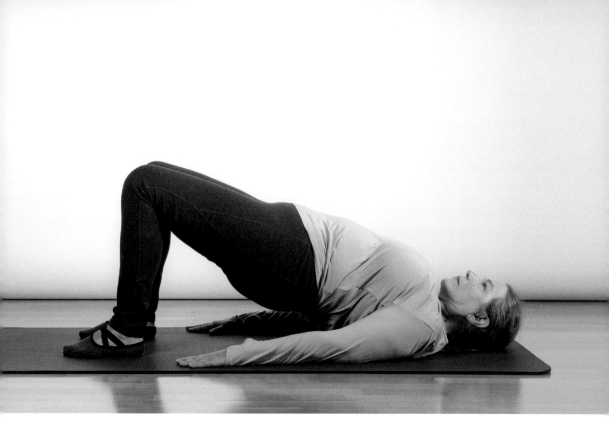

BRIDGE Setu Bandha Sarvangasana

Bridge is another example of an excellent pose that is ideal for building strength in the legs. This pose strengthens the knee extensors, knee flexors, hip adductors, and hip extensors while keeping the ankles and knees (two joints commonly affected by RA) in a safe, mid-range position.

Benefits

- Strengthens the hip extensors.
- Strengthens the hip adductors.
- Strengthens the knee flexors.
- Strengthens the knee extensors.
- Stretches the hip flexors.
- Improves mobility of the spine.

Precautions

Avoid this pose if you have a neck injury.

Before You Begin

Have a strap or a block handy for variations.

How To

1. Start by lying on your back with your knees bent, feet flat on the floor, and arms alongside your body with the palms facing down.
2. Press your feet and shoulders into the mat as you lift your hips.
3. As you rise, walk the feet closer to your buttocks and scoot your shoulders into midline, creating a slight shelf to further elevate the hips and lengthen the tailbone.
4. Keep your knees parallel as you engage the inner thighs.
5. Interlace the fingers, extend the palms on the mat, or hold on to a strap with your hands.
6. Relax your chin away from your chest to preserve the natural curve of your cervical spine.
7. Your shoulders, feet, and back of the head support the lift of your pelvis comfortably on the mat as you use the muscles of your buttocks and back to lengthen your hips.
8. Hold for 5 to 10 breath cycles.
9. To exit the pose, release the interlacing of the hands and slowly roll down your spine.

Modifications

Wrap a strap around the upper thighs to relax the quadriceps and keep the knees in line with the hips to focus on spinal extension.

Variations

- *Challenge variations:* Bend one knee into the belly, *or* for a further challenge, extend one leg straight up.
- *Restorative variation:* Place a block or bolster directly under your sacrum and allow the prop to take the weight of your body. Be sure that you continue to lengthen your neck by resting the head's weight on the back of the head and not on the neck. Lift the chest toward your chin, and your chin slightly away from your chest.

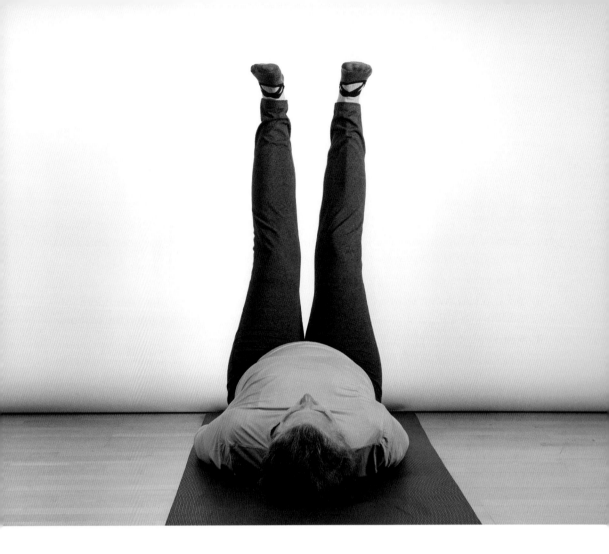

LEGS-UP-THE-WALL
Viparita Karani

This pose helps to reduce swelling in your feet and to stimulate the lymphatic system, which cleanses the body of toxins. You also obtain a change of perspective with your feet elevated above your heart and can flush blood into new areas of your body where it may have felt stagnant before. This is also an inverted pose, thus reversing the pull of gravity on your body and decompressing the spine and the ankle and knee joints.

Benefits

- Decompresses the joints of the lower body and the spine.
- Calms the mind.
- Stimulates deep breathing.
- Relieves swelling in the lower limbs.
- Offers new perspective by inverting the body.

Precautions

- Avoid this pose if you are in advanced stages of RA because it requires that you get on the floor, roll onto your back and shoulders, and swing your legs up the wall.
- Avoid this pose if holding your weight on your elbows is a challenge.

Before You Begin

Have a strap handy for the modifications, and clear a space on the floor next to an empty part of the wall.

How To

1. Sit next to the wall with your left or right side against the wall, with your knees bent and feet on the floor.
2. Rest on your elbow and turn onto your back, while simultaneously stepping your feet up onto the wall, keeping the knees bent.
3. If you would like to adjust closer to the wall, you can scoot your buttocks farther in.
4. The back and head rest on the floor while your legs extend up the wall to rest the heels against the wall; your body will form an L shape.
5. The head and neck remain in a neutral position and the legs should be relaxed.
6. Hold for 10 to 20 breath cycles.
7. To exit the pose, bend your knees, place the feet on the wall, and tuck your knees into your chest. Roll onto one side and use your elbow to sit back up.

Modifications

- If your legs do not feel completely relaxed or your hips feel strained, wrap a strap around your thighs to keep your legs no more than hip width apart.
- You can also place a blanket under the head and shoulders for cushioning.

Variations

- *Challenge variation:* To further stretch your inner thighs, bend the knees into your chest and roll the knees out to each side so that the bottoms of the feet touch.
- *Restorative variation:* You can place a bolster lengthwise against the wall before you start, and sit on it so that the hips are lifted up. Note that this may make it more challenging to roll your back onto the floor.

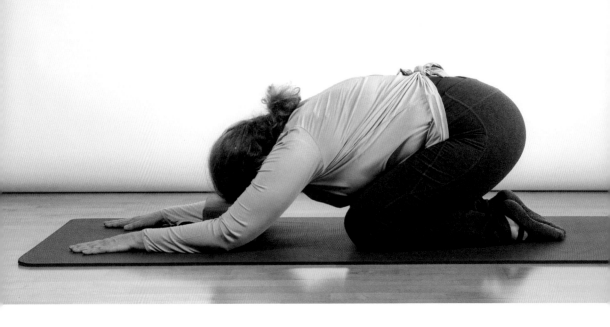

CHILD'S POSE Balasana

As mentioned earlier, fatigue is often a limiting factor for participating in exercise for those with RA. Child's Pose is a restful pose that can be utilized regularly in a yoga practice. This pose allows you to rest and catch your breath while stretching many areas vital to RA: wrist and hands into extension, the hamstrings, and buttocks; it also provides a gentle traction or decompression effect to the spine.

Benefits

- Provides spinal traction or decompression.
- Stretches the spinal extensors.
- Stretches and relaxes the hip extensors.
- Stretches the hip external rotators.
- Stretches the wrist and finger extensors.

Precautions

Be careful in this pose if you have a knee injury or ankle injury.

How To

1. Start in Table Top (pages 250-251).
2. Lower your torso to the thighs and rest your forehead on the floor or a block.
3. Rest your elbows, forearms, and palms on the floor in front of you. You can also stack the hands under the forehead or place a block under the forehead to make sure your neck is comfortable.
4. Direct your breath to your lower back and side ribs, expanding the back of your body when you inhale and releasing into the mat on your exhale.
5. Hold for 10 breath cycles.

Modifications

- If this causes knee or chest discomfort, perform Child's Pose on your back. To do so, lie on your back and draw your knees into your chest.
- If your forehead does not reach the floor, place a block or folded blanket under the forehead to relax the neck.
- If keeping your knees together causes pain in your back because of spinal flexion, you can draw the knees wide apart and lay the belly between the thighs to obtain a more neutral position.
- Rest the arms alongside your body instead of forward if that feels more relaxed for you.

Variations

- *Challenge variation:* Child's Pose is meant to be a restful pose; we do not recommend creating a challenge.
- *Restorative variation:* From a wide-knee Child's Pose, place a bolster far up into the thighs and under the belly to completely support your weight.

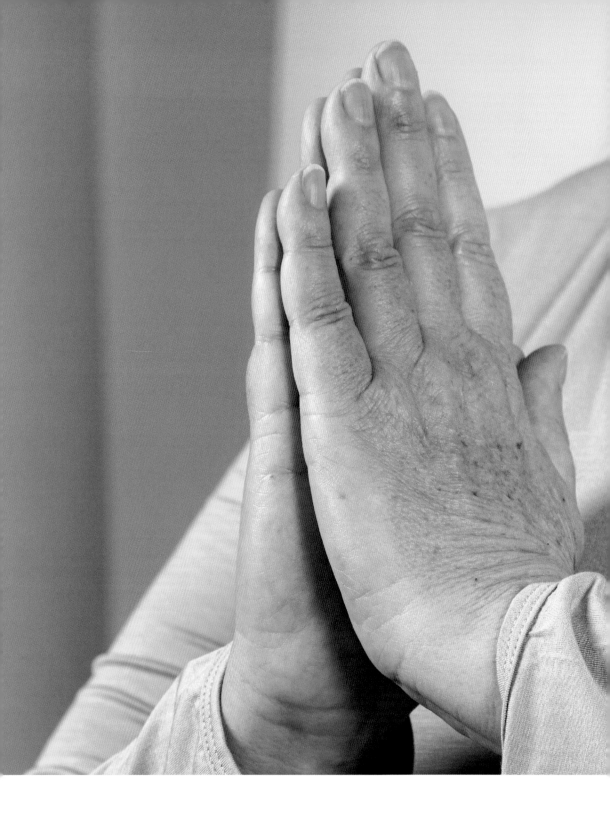

PRAYER HANDS

Anjali Mudra

It is quite common for individuals with RA to lose ROM in their wrist and fingers. The most common ROM loss in RA is in wrist extension, limiting the ability to open the hands fully. Prayer Hands is an effective form of self-stretching that can be applied to several poses. Because it is not weight-bearing, there is no risk of joint damage.

Benefits

- Stretches the wrist into extension.
- Stretches the fingers into extension.

How To

1. Place the palms of the hands together in front of your heart space.
2. Seal the palms together.
3. Hold for 5 to 10 breath cycles.

Variations

To challenge yourself, lift the arms overhead with elbows bent or straight.

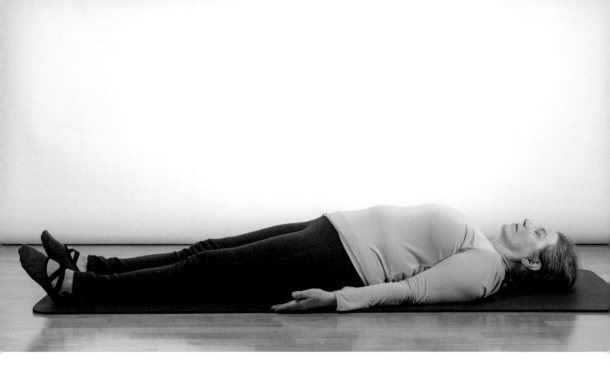

BODY SCAN

Yoga Nidra

Yoga Nidra combines intentional relaxation, a self-inquiry, and a meditation to achieve a relaxed state. This state of relaxation activates the parasympathetic nervous system (the rest and digest part of your autonomic nervous system), and thus reduces stress in the moment and inflammation in the long term. This practice relieves pain by suppressing stress hormones and inflammation.[14] Those who practice Yoga Nidra experience feelings of well-being, lightness in the body, and improvement in mental tension, muscular tension, and emotional tension.[14] Make sure you have a quiet space to practice before you begin, and feel free to use audio accompaniment; many guided Yoga Nidra practices are available online for free.

Benefits

- Promotes deep relaxation and rest.
- Decreases muscular and emotional tension.
- Decreases pain sensitivity.

How To

1. Lie on your back in a bed, on a couch, or on your yoga mat.
2. Stretch your arms alongside your body.
3. Place pillows and bolsters under your neck, head, or knees for comfort.
4. Close your eyes and start to take long, deep, intentional breaths.
5. Starting with the right side, bring your awareness to all the parts of your body, limb by limb, noticing small details like the fingernails as well as large areas like the thighs.
6. Follow this progression: each finger, palm of the hand, back of the hand, hand as a whole, forearm, elbow, upper arm, shoulder joint, shoulder, neck, each section of the face (forehead, eyes, nose, and so on), ear, scalp, throat, chest, side of the rib cage, shoulder blade, waist, stomach, lower abdomen, genitals, buttocks, whole spine, thigh, top and back of knee, shin, calf, ankle, top of foot, heel, sole, toes.
7. Allow yourself to sleep and rest as long as it feels good. If you fall asleep, so be it. Just rest.

Variations

To challenge yourself, depending on how long you want to practice, you can become more specific by scanning each part of the body in more detail (e.g., the fingernail, the top of the finger, the bottom of the finger, the webbing of the hands).

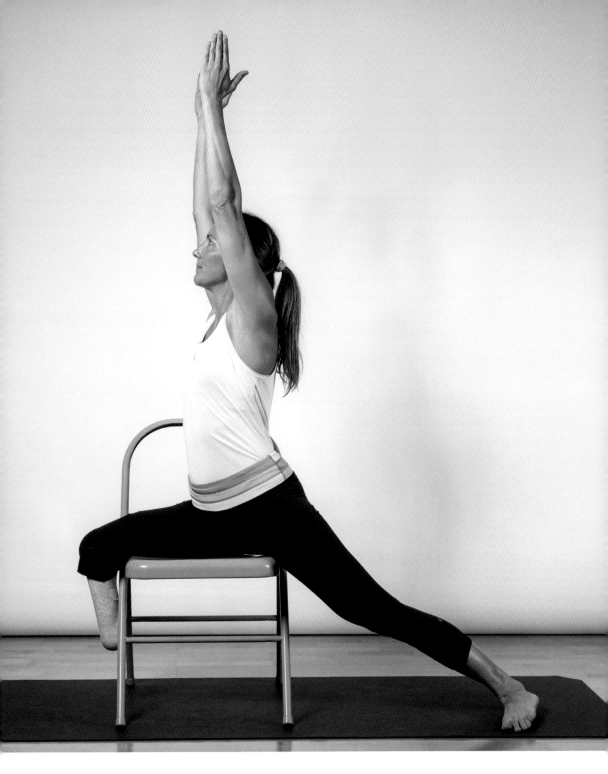

CHAPTER 6

Lower Limb Amputation

Lower limb amputation (LLA), the removal of part or all of a lower extremity, is one of the oldest known surgical procedures. Today, 130,000 LLAs are performed in the United States every year.[2] In 2005, more than a million Americans were living with LLAs and this number is expected to almost triple by 2050.[9] LLAs due to vascular disease comprise the majority of amputations, at 93.4 percent, owing to conditions such as diabetes, peripheral vascular disease (PVD), and infections.[2] Trauma accounts for 5.8 percent and cancer for 0.8 percent of LLAs.[2]

The following are the most common locations for LLA.[2]

- 33 percent—toe
- 28 percent—transtibial (through the lower leg bone), commonly referred to as below knee amputation (BKA)
- 26 percent—transfemoral (through the thigh bone), commonly referred to as above knee amputation (AKA)

This chapter focuses on BKAs and AKAs because they are more common and have a greater functional impact than amputations involving the foot or toes.

In recent years, yoga for individuals with LLA has been growing in popularity. Books have been written on adapting yoga for those living with LLA, websites offer videos and trainings on the subject, and even popular social media accounts feature yogis with LLA. Not only is yoga incredibly accessible for individuals with LLA, but the principles of yoga seem uniquely to fit the improvement of function for amputees. The cornerstone of a physical yoga practice (strength, flexibility, and balance) are essential across the lifespan for anyone with an LLA. Muscle strengthening and balance exercises have demonstrated improvements in walking mechanics and speed in people with LLA.[14]

From the day the decision is made to undergo amputation, the goal is to return to walking functionality with the use of a prosthetic leg. Within weeks of amputation, focus on strength and flexibility of both the intact and residual limb are integral. From surgical techniques, wheelchair components, and preparing and fitting the prosthetic leg, the majority of activities performed in therapy are directed toward the goal of walking with a prosthetic device. As you will see in this chapter, yoga is an extremely valuable therapeutic modality that can facilitate improvements in strength and flexibility in preparation for and during gait training.

Because it is hard to find access to safe exercise in the community or in a local gym, many individuals with LLA report difficulty performing regular exercise after inpatient rehabilitation and prosthetic training.[3] Yoga is a safe and effective way for people with LLA to engage in regular physical activity in order to maintain the strength, flexibility, and balance to retain maximal function and walking in the community.

Even after completing a rehab program, individuals with LLA experience decreased balance, fear of falling,[11] and decreased strength and coordination both in their residual and in their intact limb.[3] Consequently, walking ability and participation in the community are significantly affected after LLA, regardless of whether the amputation was a result of PVD or trauma, and whether it is above or below the knee.[6]

Aerobic capacity, strength, balance, and flexibility are needed to walk successfully with a prosthetic device in the community.[10,12] Research suggests that training to promote walking with a more normal gait pattern while using the prosthesis can prevent falls and improve community engagement.[6,10] Walking with an abnormal gait pattern decreases efficiency and increases the risk of pain and injury. The poses in this chapter were chosen to target muscles that are commonly found to be weak or tight in those with LLA and that lead to gait abnormalities.

GENERAL GUIDELINES

- Prioritize poses that promote strength and flexibility of the residual limb.
- Gradually increase weight bearing through the residual limb.
- Hip strength and flexibility are beneficial to individuals with BKAs and AKAs.
- Utilize walls, chairs, or any props to provide the upper body with support when performing standing poses.
- Focus on your breath when practicing yoga. Connecting breath with movement is key to getting the most out of your yoga practice.

Whether owing to illness before amputation, to side effects from surgery, to decreased activity after amputation, or to a combination of the above, bilateral lower extremity muscle weakness and tightness are very common in people with LLA. Weakness or tightness in a single muscle group results in altered gait mechanics while walking with a prosthetic device. Gait abnormalities can result in increased energy expenditure, decreased gait speed, pain, and decreased community involvement. The following poses primarily focus on targeting the muscle groups that are weak or tight in the residual limb, leading to common gait abnormalities while using a prosthetic device.

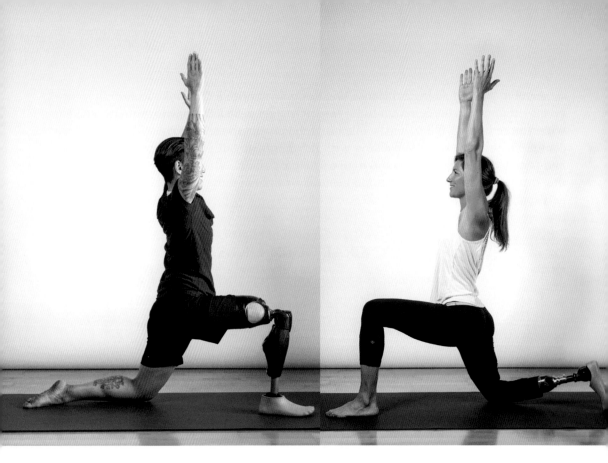

CRESCENT LUNGE WITH KNEE DOWN

Anjaneyasana

- ✓ Recommended for BKA
- ✓ Recommended for AKA

Maintaining knee flexion (bending) of a prosthetic device while bearing weight through the residual limb can be challenging (especially for those with AKA). Lowering the back leg in Crescent Lunge provides the stability needed to strengthen the muscles of the front leg, which makes this pose accessible while still improving flexibility of the back leg. For people with BKA, decreased knee extension strength (quadriceps) can lead to excessive knee flexion in the prosthetic limb while stepping forward with the intact limb.[8] With the prosthesis forward, Crescent Lunge strengthens the knee extensors required to maintain stability in gait. For those with AKA, stepping the prosthesis forward produces a strong contraction of the hip extensors (glutes). Weakness in the hip extensors can result in external rotation (knee and foot pointing outward) of the prosthetic limb.[8] This rotation can cause compensatory muscle use at the hip and over time can lead to pain while walking. Crescent Lunge helps those with both BKA and AKA build the strength needed in quadriceps and gluteal muscles respectively to enable a steady and stable gait.

Benefits

- Strengthens the knee extensors (front leg).
- Strengthens the hip extensors (back leg).
- Stretches the hip flexors (back leg).

How To

1. From Downward-Facing Dog (pages 90-91), raise your prosthetic leg up and back to extend the leg.
2. Step the prosthetic foot forward between your hands. If it doesn't make it far enough with your step, catch the ankle with your hand and assist it forward so it aligns with your hands.
3. Lower the back knee to rest on the ground; you can place a blanket or towel under the knee for cushioning.
4. Bring your upper body upright and bend the prosthetic knee.
5. Make sure your knee is above the ankle, not forward of the ankle.
6. Extend your arms up with the palms facing each other.
7. Expand your chest to the sky as you draw your arms further behind your ears and lift the chest up to deepen the stretch at the front of the hip.
8. Gaze directly in front of you or slightly up to where the wall meets the ceiling, with the goal of extending the back of your neck.
9. Hold for 5 breath cycles.
10. To exit the pose, release your hands down to the mat to frame the foot and step the front leg back to Downward-Facing Dog.
11. Repeat on the other side.

Modifications

Your hands can be on blocks, on your hips, or in Prayer Hands (pages 118-119), depending on the support you need.

Variations

- *Challenge variation:* Practice with the back knee off the mat for leg strengthening. Note that this tilts the pelvis forward; you can add a slight bend in the back knee to neutralize the pelvis. This will significantly increase the balance challenge with the prosthetic limb forward.
- *Restorative variation:* Place a bolster in front of the back knee and rest the quadriceps on the bolster.

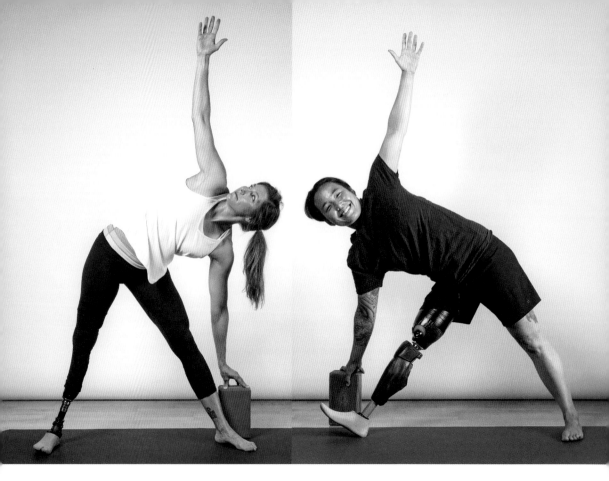

TRIANGLE

Trikonasana

✓ Recommended for BKA
✓ Recommended for AKA

Tightness in the hip abductors (muscles on the outside of the hip and buttocks) is common in individuals with an AKA and can lead to several gait abnormalities.[13] The bilateral knee extension intrinsic to Triangle provides stability while strengthening the knee extensors and stretching the knee flexors (hamstrings) in the front and back of the legs. Positioning the weight of the torso over the front leg provides a stretch to the hip abductors of the back leg. Furthermore, the ability to place a hand on your leg or on a block reduces the challenges of standing asymmetrically with a prosthesis. Because this pose benefits both the intact and prosthetic sides, it should be practiced on both sides.

Benefits

- Strengthens the hip abductors (back leg).
- Strengthens the knee extensors (both legs).
- Strengthens the hip extensors (front leg).
- Strengthens the knee flexors (back leg).
- Strengthens the core.

- Stretches the hip abductors (back leg).
- Stretches the knee flexors (both legs).

Precautions

Avoid looking up if you have a neck injury.

How To

1. Start in Warrior II (pages 104-105), with the right foot forward (right foot pointing forward, left foot parallel to the short edge of the mat).
2. Keep the arms extended.
3. Straighten the right leg and extend the right fingertips forward, lengthening both sides of your waist.
4. Continue to extend your torso forward in line with your right leg, grounding through the left foot and leg to anchor your movement.
5. Rotate the torso, hinging at the right hip and extending both sides of the waist.
6. Your left hip will roll slightly down, which is okay. Make sure that both sides of the torso extend equally long and that you are not rounding the left side waist.
7. Rest your hand on a block or on your shin and engage your abdominal muscles to support your spine.
8. Point the left arm to the sky, in line with your shoulder and with your palm facing forward.
9. Maintain extension of your neck in line with your spine and look up (or forward or down if looking up strains your neck).
10. Hold for 5 breath cycles.
11. To exit the pose, bend the right knee slightly and press firmly into the feet to lift your torso upright again.
12. Switch sides by pivoting your heels or resetting in Downward-Facing Dog (pages 90-91).

Modifications

- Practice with a wall behind you for additional support and a chair in front of you to rest your hand.
- Avoid looking up if you have a neck injury; you can perform this pose with your gaze down toward the floor.
- Make sure that you are still maintaining equal weight on both sides, no matter which leg has the prosthetic device.

Variations

To challenge yourself, hover the bottom hand in front of the shin, rather than on the shin, to engage the abdominal muscles and increase core strength.

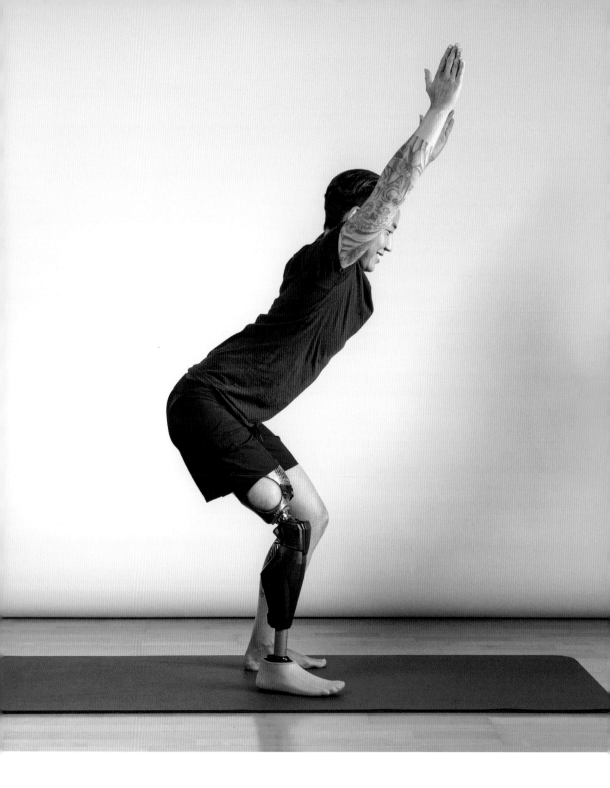

CHAIR Utkatasana

✓ Recommended for BKA
✓ Recommended for AKA

Strong hip and knee extensors are integral to walking efficiently with a prosthesis. For those with AKA, the hip extensors are used to stabilize the prosthetic knee when the heel touches the ground. Weakness in these hip extensors can lead to knee instability and can cause the device to buckle.[8] For individuals with BKA, the knee extensors control the degree of knee extension on the prosthetic leg when the opposite leg is stepping forward. Weakness in the knee extensors can lead to hyperextension of the knee joint.[8] Chair strengthens both the knee and the hip extensors, making this an ideal pose for improving walking efficiency in those with LLA.

Benefits

- Strengthens the hip and knee extensors.
- Strengthens the knee flexors.
- Improves balance.

How To

1. Start in Mountain (pages 150-151), with a chair behind you for safety if needed.
2. Bend your knees to sit the hips back, trying to bring your thighs parallel to the floor.
3. Reach your arms overhead alongside your ears and engage your abdomen.
4. Ground through all four corners of the intact foot and try to maintain equal distribution of weight through both lower limbs.
5. Notice that you are bent at the ankles, knees, and hips.
6. Hold for 5 to 10 breath cycles.
7. To exit the pose, press down into your feet to straighten your legs and stand upright. Relax your arms alongside your body as you come back into Mountain.

Modifications

- Practice with different arm positions, such as Prayer Hands (pages 118-119) at the chest or hands on the hips.
- Keep a chair behind you so you have the security of the chair to back into if you lose your balance.
- Perform through a small range of motion, barely bending at the knees and hips.

Variations

To challenge yourself, place a block between your thighs or knees and gently squeeze the block to engage your inner thighs. Make sure you are still placing even weight between both feet.

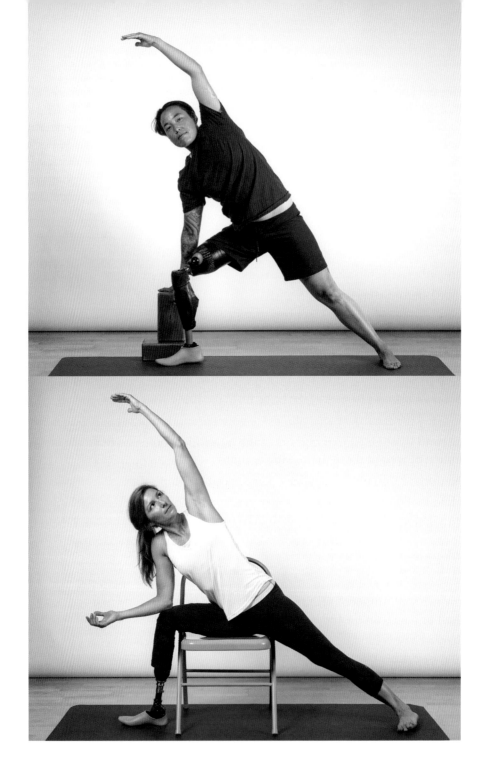

EXTENDED SIDE ANGLE   Utthita Parsvakonasana

✓ Recommended for BKA
✓ Recommended for AKA

Extended Side Angle is another example of a challenging yet attainable pose that improves bilateral leg strength and flexibility. One notable muscle group that this pose strengthens is the hip abductors. Weakness in the hip abductors can cause the trunk to lean toward the prosthetic device (BKA or AKA) during the single leg phase of walking.[8] Hip abductors provide stability during the single leg stance portion of walking on the prosthetic device. Additionally, Extended Side Angle stretches the hip adductors (groin muscles) of the back leg. This is important because hip adductor tightness can lead to standing with the prosthetic foot too wide,[13] causing instability in gait.

Benefits

- Strengthens the hip abductors (both legs).
- Strengthens the hip extensors (front leg).
- Strengthens the knee extensors (both legs).
- Strengthens the knee flexors (both legs).
- Strengthens the core.
- Stretches the hip adductors (back leg).

How To

1. Start in Warrior II (pages 104-105), with the right foot forward.
2. Bend the right elbow and place the forearm on the right thigh or bring the right hand to the floor or onto a block outside your right foot.
3. Extend the left arm over the ear to feel the extension in your left side body. The palm faces down to the ground with the fingers extending out in front of you.
4. Extend both sides of the waist to keep the trunk parallel to the floor.
5. Engage the abdomen to protect the spine and side stretch.
6. Your gaze can be directed to your left hand, to the ground, or straight forward, depending on how your neck is comfortable.
7. Hold for 5 breath cycles.
8. To exit the pose, turn the torso to the mat to frame the right foot with your hands, and step back to Downward-Facing Dog (pages 90-91) before switching sides.

Modifications

If it helps, have the seat of a chair under the front thigh, as pictured.

The following poses can be performed on the mat by people with BKAs or AKAs with or without the use of the prosthesis. Remember that performing the poses like the photos is not the goal of yoga; focus on what you are trying to do for your body and find a way to do it, with or without the prosthesis. The challenges will vary from person to person. An important part of yoga's role is to help you mindfully identify your challenges and allow you to meet them or let it go. As long as you're breathing and moving mindfully, you are doing it right.

SIDE PLANK Vasisthasana

✓ Recommended for BKA
✓ Recommended for AKA

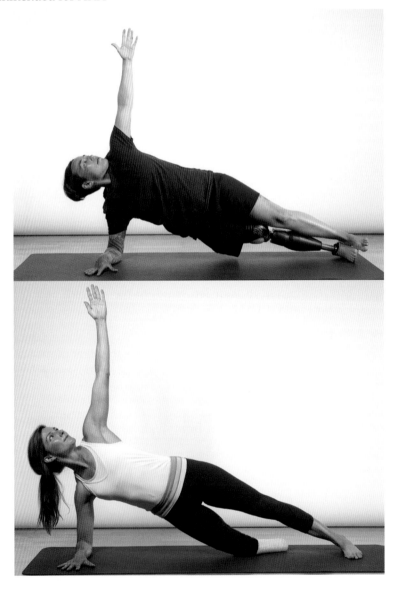

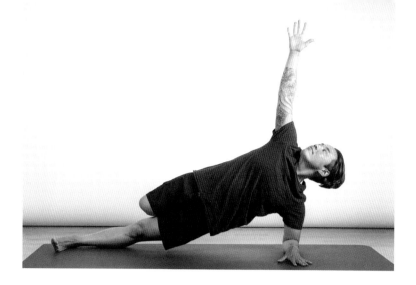

As discussed in chapter 4, Side Plank activates the high hip abductor muscles. To achieve the goal of strengthening the hip abductors, Side Plank should be performed with the residual limb on the bottom. Maintaining strong hip abductors on the side of the residual limb is important because weakness in this muscle group can make it harder to stand on the prosthesis for any length of time.[8]

Benefits

- Strengthens the hip abductors.
- Strengthens the core.

Precautions

Avoid this pose if you have a shoulder or wrist injury.

How To

1. From Forearm Plank (pages 100-101), roll onto the side of your residual limb, propping yourself up onto that forearm.
2. Press up onto that forearm, lifting the hips and engaging the abdomen.
3. Your intact limb's inner foot will press into the mat and lift you up into a Side Plank.
4. Lift your residual limb up into the intact side's leg to press the inner thighs toward each other. This will engage the hip adductors and groin; you want these muscles to push the residual limb into the mat to engage the hip abductors.
5. Lift the top arm to the sky and press the bottom arm into the mat as you stack the shoulders.
6. Gaze forward or up toward the lifted arm.
7. Hold for 3 to 5 breath cycles.
8. You can also practice this pose on the other (intact) side for balance and strength.

Variations

To challenge yourself, come up onto your hand instead of resting on your elbow.

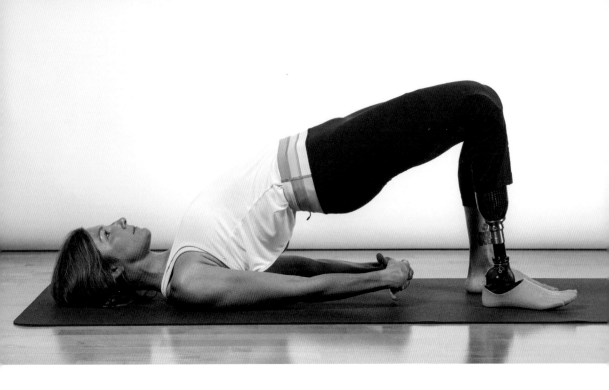

BRIDGE Setu Bandha Sarvangasana

✓ Recommended for BKA
✓ Recommended for AKA

When performed with or without a prosthesis, Bridge is a great exercise to strengthen the posterior muscles of the intact limb. This pose can also be performed with the use of the prosthetic device to strengthen the hip extensors and knee flexors. Weakness in the knee flexors is associated with knee hyperextension when walking with a below knee prosthesis.[4] Additionally, hip flexor tightness is a very common problem following LLA, and performing Bridge with a prosthesis increases flexibility of the hip flexors. For those with BKA, tight hip flexors may decrease the amount of time they can stand on the prosthesis, and for those with AKA, tight hip flexors may decrease the step length with the prosthesis.[8] Bridge strengthens and stretches several key muscle groups that have been shown to improve function in individuals with LLA.

Benefits

- Strengthens the hip extensors.
- Strengthens the knee flexors.
- Stretches the hip flexors.
- Improves mobility of the spine by spinal extension.
- Strengthens the spinal extensors.
- Opens the chest when fingers are interlaced.

Precautions

Avoid this pose if you have a neck injury.

Before You Begin

Have a strap or a block handy for the modifications and variations.

How To

1. Start by lying on your back with your knees bent, feet flat on the floor, and arms alongside your body with the palms facing down; your knees will be directly over your feet. If you are practicing without your prosthetic device, place your residual limb on a bolster, block, or folded blankets.
2. Press your feet and shoulders into the mat as you lift your hips.
3. As you rise, walk the feet closer to your buttocks and scoot your shoulders into midline, creating a slight shelf to further elevate the hips and lengthen the tailbone.
4. Keep your knees parallel as you engage the inner thighs.
5. Interlace the fingers underneath you or hold onto a strap with your hands.
6. Relax your chin away from your chest to preserve the natural curve of your cervical spine.
7. Your shoulders, feet, and back of the head support the lift of your pelvis comfortably on the mat as you use the muscles of your buttocks and back to lengthen your hips.
8. Hold for 5 to 10 breath cycles.
9. To exit the pose, release the interlacing of the hands and slowly roll down your spine.

Modifications

Wrap a strap around the upper thighs to relax the quadriceps and allow the lower body to focus on spinal extension.

Variations

- *Challenge variations:* Bend one knee into the belly, *or* for a further challenge, extend the residual leg straight up.
- *Restorative variation:* Place a block or bolster directly under your sacrum and allow the prop to take the weight of your body. Be sure that you continue to lengthen your neck by resting the head's weight on the back of the head and not on the neck. Lift the chest toward your chin, and your chin slightly away from your chest.

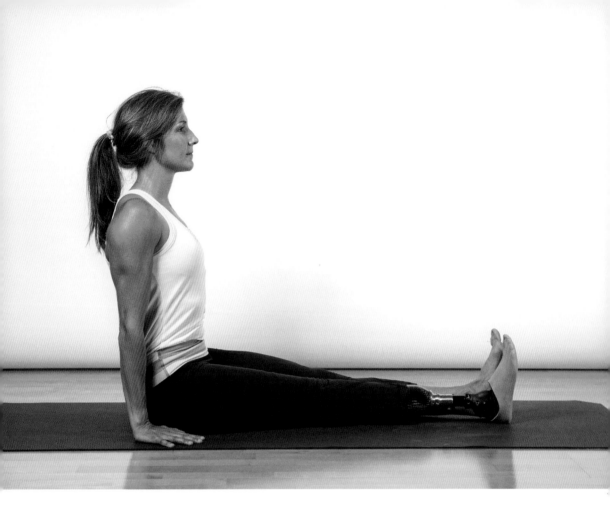

STAFF Dandasana

- ✓ Recommended for BKA
- ✓ Recommended for AKA

Hip flexor strength is needed to lift the residual limb and prosthesis in order to step forward. Weakness in the hip flexors can lead to compensation by leg circumduction (swinging the leg to the side to advance the foot) during walking.[8] With the hips positioned at a 90 degree angle, this pose places the legs into an ideal position for strengthening the hip flexors. At this joint angle, the hip flexors will activate when you engage the leg muscles. Strengthening the hip flexors is needed to ensure the prosthetic device clears the ground while walking.

Benefits

- Strengthens the hip flexors.
- Strengthens the knee extensors.
- Stretches the knee flexors.

How To

1. Start seated with your legs extended in front of you, hands resting beside your hips with the palms facing down and fingers spread wide.
2. Dorsiflex the intact limb's foot, extending the back of your knee into the floor.
3. Engage your quadriceps and press the hands down into the earth next to your hips.
4. Lift the belly button up and in to engage the core and strengthen the hip flexors.
5. Roll the shoulders back and engage the belly.
6. Hold for 5 to 10 breath cycles.

Modifications

- Sit facing a wall with the foot of your intact limb flat against the wall to make sure you are dorsiflexing that foot. Press the heel firmly into the wall.
- To emphasize strengthening of the affected side, isolate one leg at a time.

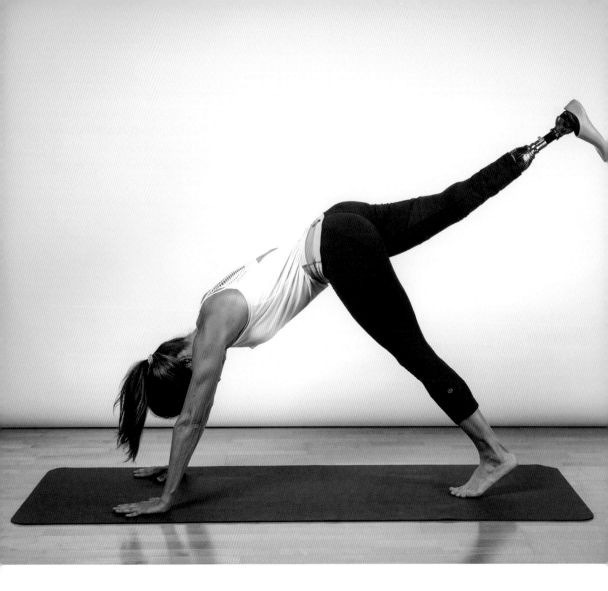

ONE-LEGGED DOWNWARD-FACING DOG

Eka Pada Adho Mukha Svanasana

✓ Recommended for BKA
✓ Recommended for AKA

One-Legged Downward-Facing Dog is a great exercise to strengthen the hip extensors of the lifted leg (especially if you use the prosthesis for resistance). The standing leg provides strengthening of the knee extensors while stretching the knee flexors. Additionally, because the knee of the residual limb has a tendency to remain bent while the person is sitting, knee flexor tightness is common in those with BKA. Loss of knee flexor flexibility prohibits full knee extension, leading to a shortened stride length and decreased walking speed.[13] This pose also offers stretching of the residual limb's hip flexors.

Benefits

- Strengthens the knee extensors (standing leg).
- Strengthens the hip extensors (lifted leg).
- Strengthens the knee flexors (lifted leg).
- Stretches the knee flexors (standing leg).
- Stretches the knee extensors (standing leg).
- Stretches the hip flexors.

How To

1. Start in Downward-Facing Dog (pages 90-91).
2. Lift the residual limb (with or without prosthesis) to the sky, keeping your hip in line with your knee or prosthetic foot.
3. Hold for 5 breath cycles.
4. To exit the pose, come down onto the hands and knees.

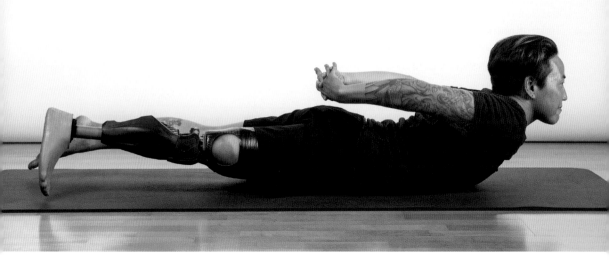

LOCUST Salabhasana

✓ Recommended for BKA
✓ Recommended for AKA

Locust improves the function of several targeted muscle groups for those with LLA. It strengthens the knee and hip extensors and facilitates stretching of the hip flexors and knee extensors. It also strengthens the spinal extensors, contributing to pelvic control. Strengthening these muscle groups helps to facilitate a normalized gait pattern, which improves quality of life and increases interaction with the community.

Benefits

- Strengthens the knee extensors.
- Strengthens the hip extensors.
- Strengthens the core.
- Stretches the hip flexors.
- Stretches the knee extensors.
- Strengthens the spinal extensors.

Precautions

Avoid this pose if you are pregnant or if you have severe stenosis of the lumbar spine.

How To

1. Start by lying face down with your forehead on the mat, hands alongside your hips, palms facing upward.
2. Inhale, and with the action of dragging your shoulder blades down your back, extend your head, chest, and arms up and back off the mat.
3. Lifting the belly button up and in, start to lift your legs off the mat and extend the thighs long behind you and slightly toward each other.
4. Firm and strengthen the legs and buttocks as you extend your arms farther back toward your feet, and your legs higher.
5. Interlace the fingers behind your back as you squeeze the shoulder blades closer toward each other.
6. Allow the gaze to extend on the ground or to the space in front of you.
7. You should be balancing on your belly and pelvis.
8. Hold for 5 to 8 breath cycles.
9. Rest by releasing the body down and turning one cheek to the mat.
10. Take a few restful breaths and repeat three more times.

Modifications

- To avoid neck strain, rest your forehead on the mat.
- Place the hands on the ground alongside the body and just lift the legs or keep the legs on the mat and extend the arms only.
- Unlock the hands and extend the arms at your side.

Variations

- *Challenge variations*: Reach the arms forward like Superman flying, lifting the hands and feet up and away from the mat.
- *Restorative variation:* Place a bolster under the chest and rest the chest on the bolster. This still allows you to experience spinal extension.

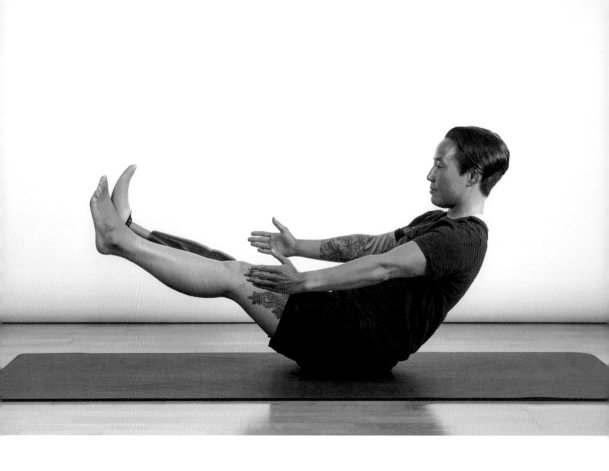

BOAT Navasana

✓ Recommended for BKA
✓ Recommended for AKA

Boat assists in strengthening the knee extensors and the hip flexors, but the main benefit for those with LLA is that it activates and strengthens the core. Core strength is crucial for those walking with a prosthetic device. With decreased core stability, individuals with LLA may compensate by shifting the location of the trunk or default into an exaggerated lumbar lordosis while walking. Additionally, a weak core may cause an overshifting of weight at the trunk toward the prosthesis while standing still.[13] Such gait abnormalities require increased energy expenditure and lead to fatigue and decreased endurance. The benefits of strengthening the core muscles makes Boat a key pose for individuals with LLA.

Benefits

- Strengthens the core.
- Strengthens the hip flexors.
- Strengthens the knee extensors.

How To

1. Start seated with your knees bent and feet flat on the floor (with the prosthesis on or off).
2. Place your hands behind your thighs and start to lean back with the chest lifted, noticing the core activation that is starting to take place.
3. Draw the belly button up and in as you begin to lift the feet off the mat.
4. Engage your abdomen and lift the chest, drawing the shoulders back.
5. If you can, let go of the legs and extend your arms forward alongside your knees with your palms facing up. If letting go of the legs causes you to lose your balance, keep your hands behind the thighs.
6. Be sure your neck remains comfortable by keeping your chest lifted.
7. Your torso, pelvis, and upper legs will be in a V shape, with the hips as the fulcrum.
8. Knees will remain bent and shins parallel to the floor, or you can extend the legs (as pictured).
9. The feet should be neutral, not flexed.
10. Hold for 3 to 5 breath cycles.

Modifications

Place the feet on blocks for hip flexor support while still achieving core activation.

Variations

To challenge yourself, straighten the legs or bring the arms overhead.

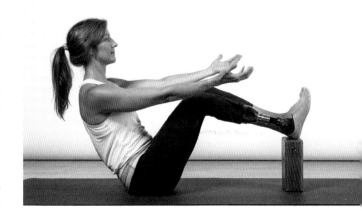

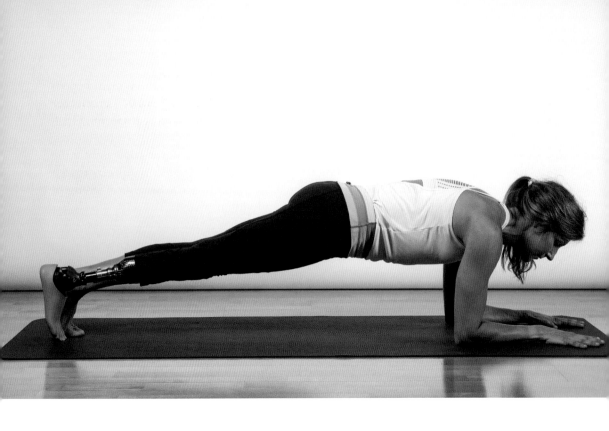

FOREARM PLANK Phalakasana

- ✓ Recommended for BKA
- ✓ Recommended for AKA

Forearm Plank is another great all-purpose pose for those with LLA. Performing this pose strengthens the hip and knee extensors, stretches the knee flexors, and is an excellent core stabilizer. Furthermore, Forearm Plank is very modifiable because it can be performed with or without a prosthesis and can even be shifted to the hands or knees.

Benefits

- Strengthens the core.
- Strengthens the hip extensors.
- Strengthens the knee extensors.
- Stretches the knee flexors.

How To

1. Start in Table Top (pages 250-251) or in Sphinx (pages 162-163), with the hips over the knees and the shoulders over the wrists.
2. Walk your elbows down so you are supported by your forearms.
3. Walk the feet back so your body is in a straight line from your head to your heels. (If you don't have your prosthesis on, place your residual limb on a bolster.)
4. Engage the abdominal muscles in and up, firming your arms in toward midline.
5. Press into the forearms, separating your shoulder blades, drawing your sternum in the direction of your spine, and expanding your thoracic spine.
6. Energize the inner thighs toward each other and up as you press back into your heels and forward with your chest, lengthening the spine and neck.
7. Your gaze should be a few feet in front of the hands on the floor for a long neck.
8. Be sure the hips and shoulder blades do not sag and are in alignment with the chest and legs.
9. Hold for 5 to 8 breath cycles.
10. Come down to rest in Child's Pose (pages 38-39).

Modifications

- You can do this standing, by facing the wall and extending your arms to place your forearms on the wall at chest height. Walk the feet back until the abdomen engages. You can walk the feet back further until you feel the upper arm muscles engage. Be sure you are tucking the tailbone, so the hips stay in line with the diagonal of the body.
- You can also support yourself on your knees. Start with steps 1 to 5. In Forearm Plank, lower the knees directly to the floor, without moving your hands and chest. Continue engaging the abdominal muscles and hugging the outer arms into midline. Hold for 10 breath cycles, then come down to rest in Child's Pose.

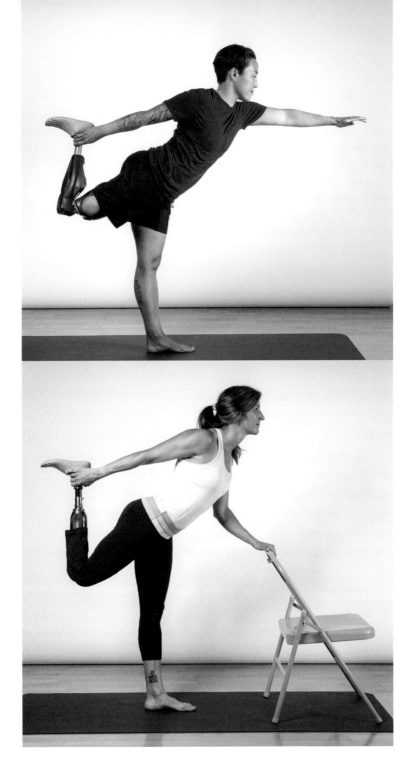

DANCER Natarajasana

✓ Recommended for BKA
✓ Recommended for AKA

Because single leg standing on a prosthesis is incredibly difficult, Dancer should only be performed unilaterally by individuals with LLA, with the intact leg as support on the ground and the prosthetic leg lifted. Dancer lets you isolate the hip extensors of the residual limb. Whether you have a BKA or an AKA, you need hip extensor strength on the residual limb to avoid compensating with excessive lumbar lordosis while standing.[13] Weakness in the hip abductors of the intact limb can cause the trunk to lean away from the prosthesis when you step it forward.[4] Single leg standing on the intact limb strengthens the hip abductors, which provide medial–lateral support of the pelvis. Dancer is an ideal exercise to strengthen the hip muscles to improve balance and control when standing or walking with a prosthesis.

Benefits

- Strengthens the hip abductors (standing leg).
- Strengthens the hip extensors (lifted leg).
- Strengthens the knee flexors (lifted leg).
- Stretches the hip flexors (lifted leg).

How To

1. Start standing at the front of your mat in Mountain (pages 150-151), with the hand on the side of your intact limb resting on the wall, a chair, or a table in front of you.
2. Focus the weight of your body on your intact limb as you bend the knee of your residual limb to bring the prosthetic foot toward the same-side buttock.
3. Catch the inner ankle of the prosthetic leg with your same-side hand to bend the knee more deeply so you feel a stretch in your quadriceps.
4. Make sure you feel balanced on your intact leg as you begin to kick the prosthetic foot back, maintaining a steady grip of the ankle in your hand.
5. Extend the prosthetic leg back, aiming to get the upper thigh close to parallel to the floor.
6. Extend your chest forward and slightly down to arch your back as you kick the foot back farther away from your body; you will enjoy a stretch in your pectorales (chest muscles).
7. Hold for 5 breath cycles.
8. To exit the pose, lift your chest and bring the prosthetic foot back toward your buttocks to regain the center of gravity over your pelvis, and release the foot back to the ground.

Modifications

If your prosthetic device is too heavy, perform the pose without using it.

Balance training is one of the foundations of rehabilitation after LLA. In early phases of rehab this occurs with just the use of the intact limb. However, walking with a prosthesis requires learning new motor coordination and balance strategies,[1] which is why balance training while using the prosthetic limb is essential. LLA results in lost sensory input from the ankle or knee and a modified center of gravity. Balance training is needed not only to learn new coordination and balance strategies but also to gain trust in the prosthetic device. In those with LLA, low balance confidence has been found to correlate with the use of an assistive device (e.g., walker, crutches, cane) while walking.[6] On the other hand, people with LLA who score higher on balance tests tend to participate more in the community.[5] With this in mind, we felt it important to present balancing poses with the prosthesis on specifically to help you gain skills and balance with the prosthetic device.

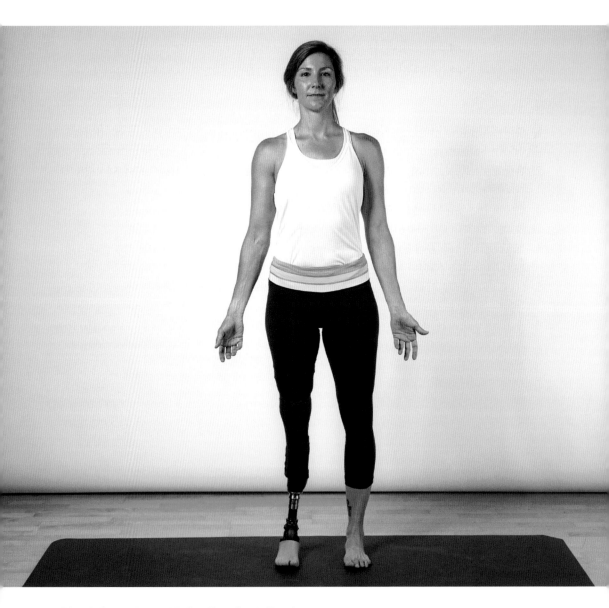

MOUNTAIN *Tadasana*

✓ Recommended for BKA
✓ Recommended for AKA

In Mountain, equal weight is placed between both feet, which is often a challenge for those with LLA because body weight is instinctively shifted to the intact limb. To avoid loss of balance, the residual limb must compensate by activating the hip muscles. Mountain provides an opportunity to begin shifting your weight onto the prosthetic device and to facilitate trust and reliance on it.

Benefits

- Improves balance.
- Improves posture.
- Tones the hips and abdomen and helps to gain control over core strength and gait.

How To

1. Standing with feet hip width apart, ground all four corners of your intact foot into the mat.
2. Roll the shoulders down your back, palms facing slightly forward and rotating the inner elbows slightly out.
3. Firm the thighs and lengthen the tailbone to engage the abdomen.
4. Open the heart and broaden the collarbones.
5. Try to maintain even weight between the legs, even and especially with the prosthesis on.
6. Hold for 5 to 10 breath cycles, or use this as the beginning point for your vinyasa flow practice.

Modifications

Practice with a wall behind your back for safety.

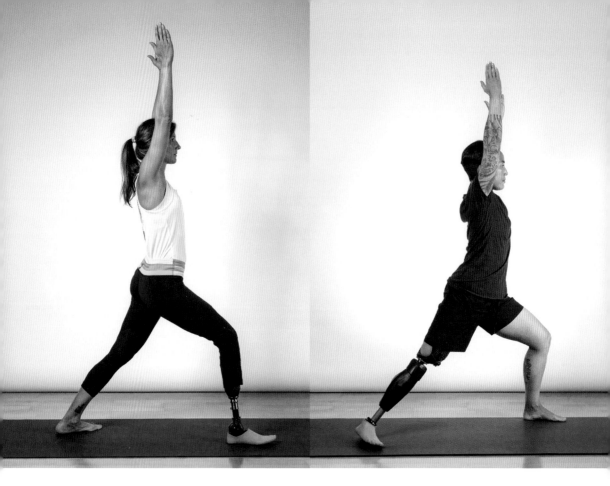

WARRIOR I

Virabhadrasana I

✓ Recommended for BKA
✓ Recommended for AKA

Warrior I with the prosthetic limb forward places a significant amount of weight bearing through the prosthetic limb. To achieve the pose, you may need upper body support, but once you are in position, this pose not only activates muscles of the hip and thigh but requires microadjustments to movements of the prosthetic device. This can help build the trust in the prosthesis needed to develop and maintain a fluid walking pattern. This pose can also be performed with the residual limb as the back leg (as pictured), or with the residual limb (without prosthesis) on the seat of a chair (pictured on page 153). This will help to stretch the hip flexors and further strengthen the residual limb.

Benefits

- Improves balance.
- Strengthens the knee and hip extensors.
- Strengthens the knee flexors.
- Stretches the hip flexors.

How To

1. Start in a wide-legged stance facing the long edge of a mat with hands on the hips and feet parallel.
2. Turn your residual limb's foot to point forward and bend that knee.
3. Turn the intact limb's foot to a 45 degree angle (so the toes point toward the front corner of the mat). The entire plantar aspect of that foot should ground down.
4. Bend the knee of the residual limb so that the thigh comes as close to parallel to the floor as possible.
5. Inhale your arms up to the sky, hands facing each other, fingers pointing up.
6. Keep the back, intact limb straight and strong as you anchor the foot to square the hips forward.
7. Lift the lower abdomen up and in as you lengthen the tailbone down.
8. Draw the shoulders down the back, and gaze forward or slightly up between your hands.
9. Hold for 5 breath cycles.

Modifications

If you prefer to practice this without your prosthesis, start by standing next to a chair with your residual limb side next to the chair. Place your hand on the back of the chair for support and your residual limb on the seat of the chair, as pictured. You can keep your hands on the back of the chair or extend them up to the sky.

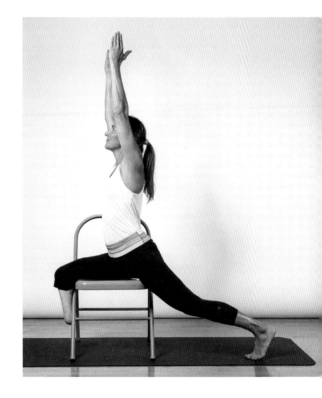

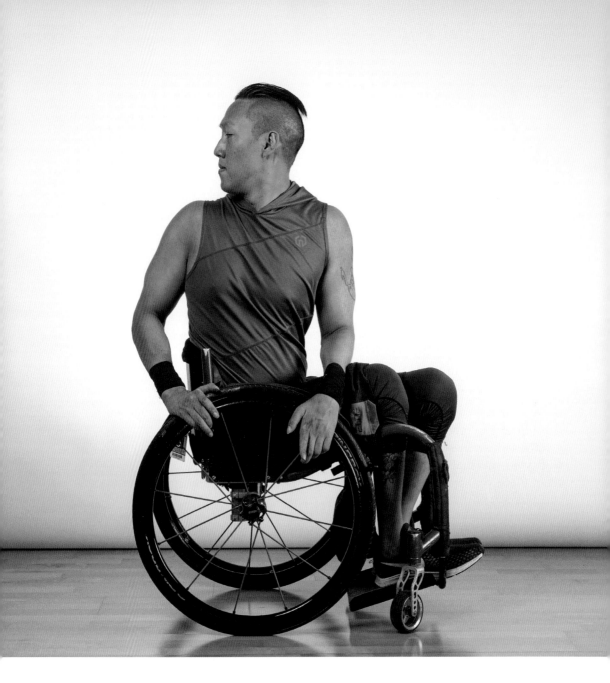

Spinal Cord Injury

The spinal cord is a long bundle of nerves that extends from the brainstem to the low back via the spinal column. The spinal cord is a direct extension from the brain, and its function is to transmit nerve signals between the brain and the body. Descending signals from the brain to the body connect the motor cortex of the brain to the muscles in order to control movement. Ascending signals from the body to the brain connect sensory nerves to the sensory cortex of the brain to enable us to feel sensations such as touch, temperature, and vibration. An event that causes damage to this structure is considered a spinal cord injury (SCI).

SCI causes partial or complete paralysis and impaired sensation, and affects several of the body's organ systems, including the respiratory and cardiovascular systems. The National Spinal Cord Injury Statistical Center[9] estimated that there are 17,700 newly acquired SCIs every year in the United States and that there are currently approximately 288,000 people living with SCI.[9] The average age of injury is 43 and about 78 percent of cases are male. Vehicle crashes (38.3 percent) are the leading cause of injury, closely followed by falls (31.6 percent). Acts of violence (13.8 percent), primarily gunshot wounds, and sports and recreational activities (8.2 percent) are also common causes.[9]

An individual's function and presentation are largely predicated on the location and severity of the injury. Location is determined by where the spinal cord was damaged. The nerves (and therefore strength and sensation) below the location of the injury will be affected, and thus unable to transmit the signals required for sensation (sensory function) or for activating a muscle (motor function). For example, if there is an injury to the spinal cord at the low back, there will be significant or complete weakness and loss of sensation in the legs. If the injury occurs higher up at the midback (i.e., between the shoulder blades), strength and sensation of the core and legs may be lost. If injury occurs at the neck, strength and sensation of the arms, core, and legs can be lost.

The severity of the injury also affects how one functions after SCI. An injury to the spinal cord is considered *complete* when there is total loss of strength and sensation below the location of the injury to the spine. The injury is considered *incomplete* if there is still partial muscle activation and sensation below the location of the injury. This can range from near-full muscle strength with little weakness to just barely having the ability to activate the corresponding muscles.

There are several additional physical effects associated with SCI besides the loss of strength. One of the most common is the presence of joint contractures, which are permanent movement limitations of the joints due to prolonged sitting, lack of movement, or muscle spasticity (involuntary muscle contractions that cause stiffness or tightness of the muscles). Muscles that have been denervated (the connection severed or lost between the nerves and the muscles) will demonstrate atrophy, and osteoporosis of the leg bones may also develop due to the lack of weight being placed on the body. Furthermore, compromised respiratory function may increase the risk of respiratory infections, congestion, and shortness of breath. Neuropathic pain is common, even years after the initial trauma or illness. Sensory deprivation (an inability to accurately determine the nature of stimuli at or below the level of injury) is also common.

The main focus of rehabilitation after a spinal cord injury is to improve function. The goal of early rehabilitation is to teach skills to improve the ability to participate in specific life situations (transfer in and out of a car, get in and out of bed, transfer from a wheelchair to a bed, etc.). These functional activities require adequate strength, joint range of motion (ROM), and muscle flexibility.[11] Reductions in passive joint movement are not always acknowledged and addressed in traditional exercise programs. You can use yoga to maintain and increase joint mobility and to increase the strength of muscles weakened from SCI.

Functional improvement can occur via the learning of compensatory strategies, restoring strength, or a combination of the two. The strategies used are determined by the individual's ability to activate the muscles below the level of injury to the corresponding portion of the spinal cord. When muscle activation is absent below the injury, functional independence is optimized through compensatory measures. New motor skills (compensatory movement strategies) are learned and utilized to perform tasks using the remaining working muscle groups. For example, using the arms to move the legs into and out of bed when the legs are paralyzed is a quintessential compensatory movement strategy. In contrast, individuals with muscle activation that is restored after injury, whether completely or incompletely, have the potential to return to normal movement. For these individuals, the goal is to restore normal motor patterns and minimize compensatory movements.[11] It is important to know that recovery occurs most rapidly within the first six months and then typically plateaus, at the latest, after two years.[4] Understanding this timeline aids in choosing the exercises that are recommended for individuals with SCI as compensatory or restorative.

Yoga's basic principles of meditation, breath control, mindful relaxation, and poses are uniquely tailored toward the goals of rehabilitation for SCI. While many types of exercise can benefit individuals with SCI, they are often predicated on limiting movement to only a few joints within one plane of motion, such as in cycling (hips and knees) and swimming (shoulders and hips). In yoga, the goal is to maintain mobility in all the joints of the body (even the toe joints!).

The goal of yoga for SCI is to promote physical and mental well-being through stretching and activating all of the available muscle groups to gain strength, flexibility, and physical balance to improve and maintain functional mobility. Adopting some of the therapeutic tenets of yoga can promote natural relaxation and give individuals with SCI the tools to look inside themselves and concentrate on their breathing. Thus they become aware of a deep and positive mind–body experience.

For individuals with SCI, we recommend using passive or assisted yoga poses first, especially for those with tone abnormalities (stiffness or rigidity of the muscles). This slow introduction will invoke a relaxation or release phenomenon throughout the trunk and extremities.[9] For some individuals, there may be resistance to movement in some joints. This resistance can be alleviated with prop support and repositioning, so be sure to adjust as needed. Your pose does not need to look exactly as it does in the photo. Eventually, gently stretching and elongating the muscles will prompt release and your body will accept relaxation. If you experience pain, be sure to modify or choose a different position.

The poses recommended in this chapter have been selected to improve the strength and flexibility of muscle groups that can improve function in SCI. These poses are intended to improve or maintain your ability to perform the specific activities and obtain the positions needed to maximize independence and wellness after SCI. We note that poses can and should be modified as needed to meet individual needs, because no two spinal cord injuries are the same. Props such as blocks, sandbags, blankets, and chairs are strongly encouraged.

The recommendations in this section are tailored to individuals whose SCI requires them to use a wheelchair for mobility, making these poses appropriate for those with complete paraplegia. We also note that the instructions and modifications include options for those who do have some lower extremity strength and wish to utilize yoga as a way to strengthen their legs as well. Finally, for those who may have incomplete tetraplegia (have most of their arm function, but with core weakness), you can also practice these postures, with modifications noted in the instructions.

GENERAL GUIDELINES

- Individuals with SCI often utilize leg loops (a Velcro-looped positioning aid that is placed around the thigh and lower leg) to assist them in moving their legs; these would be great to use during yoga. They serve a similar function to a yoga strap, or a yoga strap can be used in its place.
- Shoulder blade positioning is integral for shoulder injury prevention in SCI, so correct positioning, movement, and control of the scapulae should be emphasized when practicing yoga.
- The backrest of a wheelchair is used to support the trunk; to challenge core strength and sitting balance you can scoot forward so your trunk is not supported by the backrest.
- If you have a history of spinal fusion, ease into poses requiring spinal rotation or flexion.
- Improving the mobility of knee extension (hamstring flexibility) is essential as prolonged use of a wheelchair for mobility often leads to hamstring tightness.
- Integrate strengthening of core muscles that remain functional in all poses when possible because core stability is almost always weakened after SCI.
- If practicing in a wheelchair, perform with the brakes locked while wearing a seat belt for safety.

Strengthening exercises are an essential component of living with SCI. After SCI, greater upper extremity strength is associated with increased levels of independence.[3] Due to postural changes from prolonged use of a wheelchair and substituting the arms for mobility rather than the legs, there is a high incidence of shoulder pain and dysfunction after SCI, and strengthening the upper extremities has been shown to reduce shoulder pain in SCI.[2,10] Muscles of the trunk and lower extremities with some preserved function should also be strengthened to enhance function.

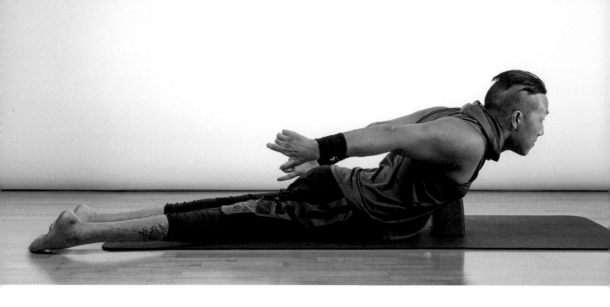

LOCUST

Salabhasana

In Locust, the scapulae are moved into a depressed and retracted position, promoting strength of the shoulder and upper back muscles, and allowing control of and focus on the position of the scapulae. This scapular motor control is vital in wheelchair users because it ensures that the appropriate muscles are used to move the shoulder, thus preventing shoulder injury. Additionally, strength in the scapular depressors (lower trapezius muscles) is required to perform transfers and push downward through the arms to help lift the body for the transfer. Scapular retraction (middle trapezius and rhomboids) strength also reduces the risk of shoulder injury. This pose also facilitates strength of the functioning spinal extensors (paraspinals).

Benefits

- Strengthens the elbow extensors.
- Strengthens the scapular retractors.
- Strengthens the scapular depressors.
- Strengthens the shoulder adductors.
- Strengthens the spinal extensors.

Before You Begin

Have a strap close by.

How To

1. Start by lying face down with your forehead on the mat, with hands alongside your hips, palms facing upward.

2. Inhale, and with the action of dragging your shoulder blades down your back, extend your head, chest, and arms up and back off the mat. Place a block under your chest if you do not have the paraspinal strength to lift the chest, and work toward lifting the chest off the block.

3. Use a strap between your hands to draw the shoulder blades closer to each other, or if you don't have a strap, interlace the fingers as you squeeze the shoulder blades closer toward each other.

4. Allow your gaze to relax forward or upward, or you can look down if this is uncomfortable for your neck.

5. The goal is to lift the chest and engage the back and abdominal muscles.

6. Hold for 5 to 8 breath cycles.

7. Rest by releasing the body down and turning one cheek to the mat for a few breaths.

8. Repeat three more times.

Modifications

To perform the pose while sitting in a wheelchair, extend the trunk, retract (depress) the shoulder blades, and straighten the elbows while lifting the chest up and rolling the shoulders back.

Variations

- If you have the flexibility in your shoulders, reach the hands forward to strengthen the shoulder flexors, but don't let this compromise your neck. It is better to maintain comfort in your neck and keep the arms back rather than try to reach them forward if that causes strain. This version strengthens the elbow extensors, shoulder flexors, and spinal extensors.

- *Challenge variation:* If you have the strength in your legs, lift your feet (and maybe even your knees) off the mat with the action of reaching the feet behind you and slightly toward each other. Firm and strengthen the legs and buttocks as you extend your arms further back toward your feet and lift your legs higher.

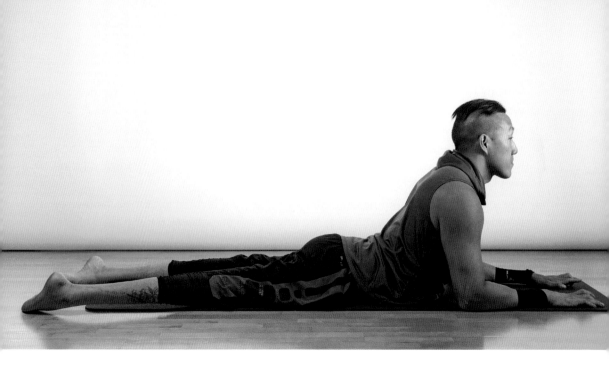

SPHINX Salamba Bhujangasana

Weight bearing through the upper extremities is a common strategy to improve scapular stabilization. This position activates several muscles that attach to the scapulae; one in particular is the serratus anterior. This muscle assists in the upward rotation of the scapulae (required for raising the hand above the head); strengthening this muscle is emphasized in Sphinx and can assist with the prevention of shoulder injury.

Benefits

- Stabilizes the core.
- Strengthens the scapular stabilizers.
- Stretches the hip flexors.
- Stretches the knee flexors.

How To

1. Start by lying face down with the forehead on the mat.
2. Walk the elbows underneath your chest to rest on your forearms, keeping them parallel to each other if possible. Your shoulders should be directly above the elbows.
3. Roll your shoulders down your back, away from your ears.
4. Start to firm up your abdominal muscles, engaging the belly button up toward the spine.
5. No matter the degree to which your body is lifted from the floor, be sure you are engaging the abdominal muscles in and up, firming your arms in toward midline.
6. Press into the forearms, opening the collarbones out to the sides, lifting your sternum up and open.
7. Gaze forward one or two feet on the ground for a long neck.
8. Hold for 5 to 8 breath cycles.
9. Come down to rest in Child's Pose (pages 38-39).

Modifications

To perform the pose when sitting in a wheelchair, face a wall and extend your arms to place your forearms on the wall at chest height. Be sure you are opening through your chest and using your abdominal muscles so the hips stay in line with the diagonal of the body.

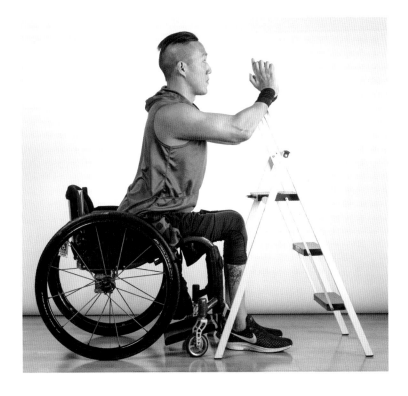

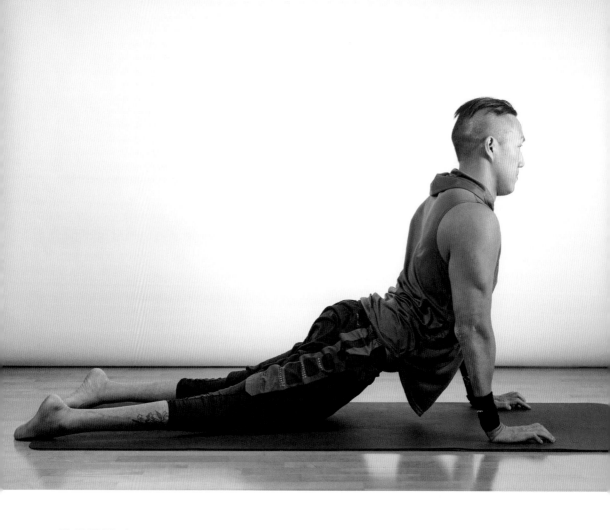

COBRA   Bhujangasana

The muscle group that enables elbow extension is key to performing transfers. To transfer to and from the wheelchair or another surface (bed, car, shower chair, etc.), one hand is placed on the wheelchair and the other hand is situated on the second surface. Then, to enable the transfer, you must push down, utilizing the elbow extensors (triceps) and shoulder depressors to perform a "squat-pivot" onto the target surface. Cobra strengthens both the elbow extensors and the shoulder depressors, which assists in training for the squat-pivot technique. Cobra also helps to improve flexibility. Flexibility of the hip and knee flexors is lost due to the prolonged sitting that accompanies wheelchair use. These muscle groups, however, are needed to move easily while in bed and lying on the mat. Cobra places the body in the opposite position of sitting in a wheelchair; it stretches the hip flexors and promotes lumbar extension. In facilitating this lumbar extension, Cobra can also address and improve low back pain. Additionally, Cobra stretches the knee flexors for those specifically with complete paraplegia. Contracted knee flexion caused by prolonged wheelchair sitting can be countered by the knee straightening action of Cobra. Thus, Cobra provides the stretch needed simply by placing the knees in gravity-assisted extension.

Benefits

- Strengthens the shoulder flexors and adductors.
- Strengthens the elbow and spinal extensors.
- Increases lumbar extension.
- Strengthens the scapular depressors.
- Stretches the hip flexors.
- Stretches the knee flexors for those with no motor function in the legs (contracts the knee flexors for those with leg strength).

Precautions

Be careful if you have a shoulder injury or a wrist injury.

How To

1. Start by lying face down with the forehead to the ground, legs extended behind you, and hands directly under the shoulders, elbows bent.
2. Scoop the elbows in toward the midline behind your back and spread the fingers wide to create a firm foundation with the hands.
3. Press into the hands to lift the chest and engage the abdominal muscles as best you can.
4. Move toward straight arms (it's okay to maintain a bend in your arms for the comfort of your back).
5. Make sure you continue to engage your core muscles to protect the spine as you lift your heart up and draw the shoulder blades down your back.
6. The head balances comfortably in line with the curve of the spine.
7. The pubic bone lifts off the mat and slightly up toward the chest to lengthen the lumbar spine.
8. Hold for 5 to 8 breath cycles.

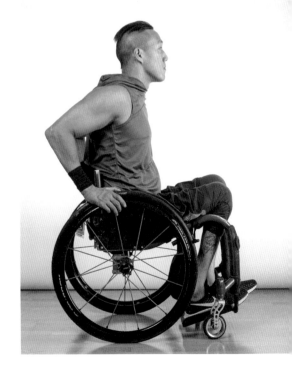

Modifications

To perform this pose when sitting in a wheelchair, roll the shoulders back, drawing the shoulder blades down the back, and lift your chest on an inhale. Hold for 5 breath cycles. This pose strengthens the scapular depressors.

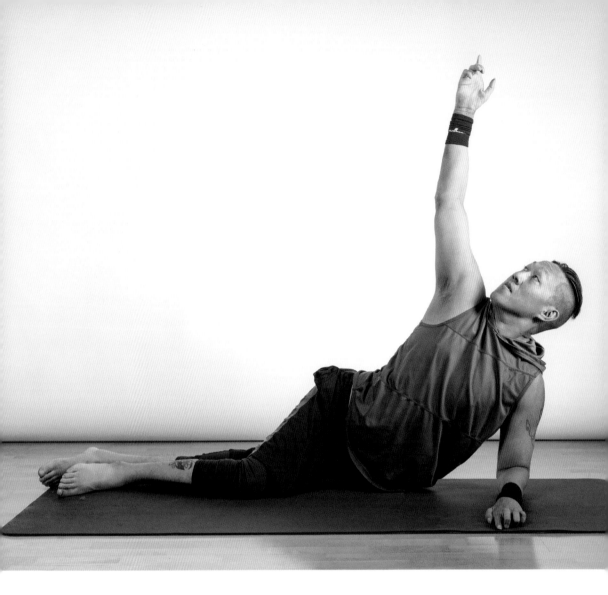

SIDE PLANK Vasisthasana

Side Plank is another pose that promotes strength of the entire shoulder complex. Again, strengthening the shoulders assists in general mobility and helps reduce the risk of shoulder injury. As the core muscles are significantly weakened below the level of the injury, it is also important to strengthen the core muscles that remain functional. Side Plank activates the oblique muscles that assist in rotational movements of the spine used to position the torso for several functional movements, such as transfers, dressing, and bathing.

Benefits

- Strengthens the scapular stabilizers.
- Strengthens the shoulder flexors and adductors.
- Stabilizes the core.

Precautions

Be careful if you have a shoulder injury.

How To

1. Start on your left side, propping yourself up on your left elbow and using your right hand in front of you for stability.
2. If possible, stack the right leg over the left (you can use a wall behind your back to keep from rolling all the way over).
3. Press into the left elbow to lift the trunk off the mat as high as possible.
4. Engage the core.
5. Your right hand can rest on the waist or extend up to the sky.
6. Continue to press the left forearm into the mat as you stack the shoulders.
7. Gaze forward or up to the right hand.
8. Hold for 3 to 5 breath cycles.
9. Repeat on the other side.

Modifications

- Use the top hand to steady yourself by placing it on the floor.
- To perform this pose when sitting in a wheelchair, remove the armrest, place another chair directly to the left of the wheelchair, and place the left forearm on the seat of the chair next to you.

Variations

To challenge yourself, come up on the hand instead of resting on the elbow.

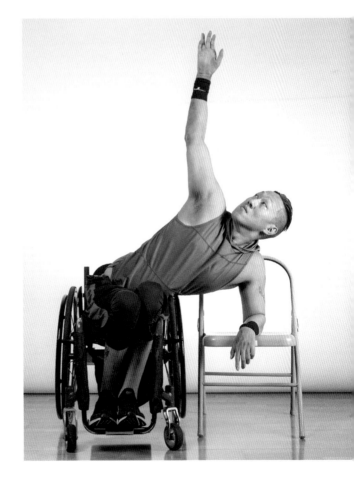

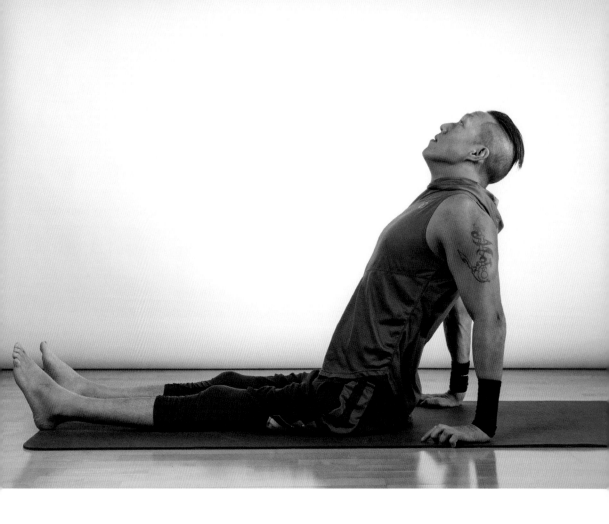

REVERSE PLANK

Purvottanasana

Reverse Plank facilitates strengthening of the elbow extensors (triceps). These muscles are utilized in many functional movements including transfers and transitioning from lying on the back to sitting. Lying to sitting is achieved by pushing down with the hands and rocking the trunk from side to side as the elbows straighten. The higher the location of the injury in the spine, the less core strength is available and the greater the need for triceps strength. Those whose injury occurred higher in their cervical spine do not have use of the elbow extensor muscles, which makes it challenging to straighten or lean on the elbows to assist with sitting balance. Sitting balance can be achieved via compensation by placing the hands on a mat or bed with the fingers pointing backward and engaging the shoulder muscles to lock the elbows. By recreating this position, Reverse Plank can assist in training the muscles to improve this sitting balance maneuver.

Benefits

- Strengthens the scapular depressors.
- Strengthens the scapular retractors.
- Strengthens the elbow extensors.

Precautions

Be careful if you have a shoulder injury.

How To

1. Start seated on the mat with your legs extended in front of you in Staff (pages 176-177).
2. Walk your hands behind your hips with the fingers pointing toward the toes.
3. Inhale, press your hands down into the ground to straighten the arms, and lift your hips up as high as you can. Keep the chin toward the chest to start out.
4. Lift the chest up and breathe into straighter arms.
5. Keep the gaze upward.
6. Hold for 3 to 5 breath cycles.
7. Exhale to bend the elbows and lower your hips back down into Staff.

Modifications

For those with complete paraplegia, you may not be able to lift your hips at all. That's okay. Focus on engaging the core, opening the chest, and straightening the elbows.

Variations

If you have incomplete paraplegia and some activity in your legs, engage the leg and buttock muscles, and point the toes.

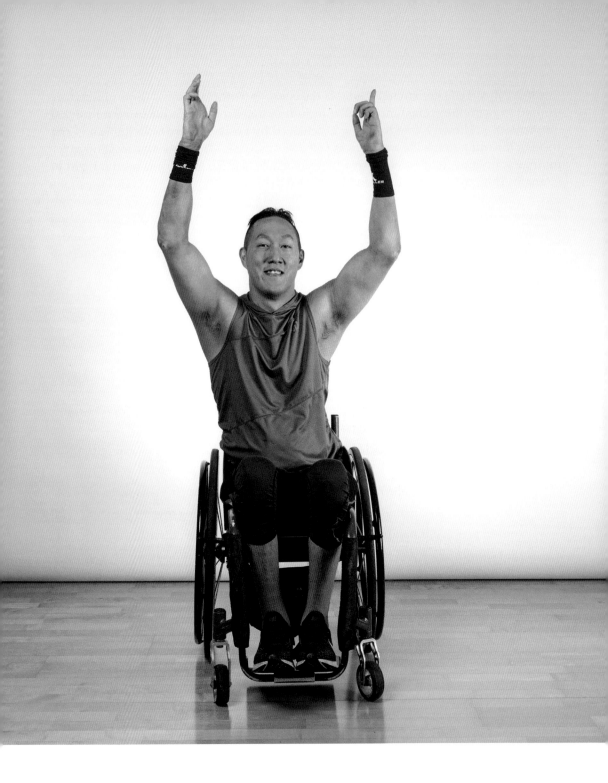

UPWARD SALUTE

Urdhva Hastasana

Elevating the hands above the head activates and strengthens a key muscle of shoulder flexion, the deltoid. Significant shoulder flexion strength is needed after SCI because you must flex your shoulders to lift your legs with your arms (e.g., when getting into and out of bed or dressing). Additionally, if you use a wheelchair for mobility, your body's center of mass (COM) is significantly lower. Upward Salute increases shoulder flexion ROM to increase the ease of overhead reaching activities.

Benefits

- Strengthens the scapular upward rotators.
- Strengthens the shoulder flexors.
- Increases thoracic extension.
- Strengthens the core and spinal extensors.

How To

1. Start by sitting in your wheelchair or any comfortable seat.
2. Raise your arms overhead, alongside your ears.
3. Spread the fingers wide and lift the fingertips high, engaging the arm muscles, and relaxing the shoulders down and away from your neck.
4. Lift your abdominal muscles up and in, while simultaneously softening the ribs back in.
5. Hold for 5 to 10 breath cycles.

Variations

To challenge yourself, use a block between the hands overhead and press the hands into the block for increased trapezius and upper back muscle strengthening.

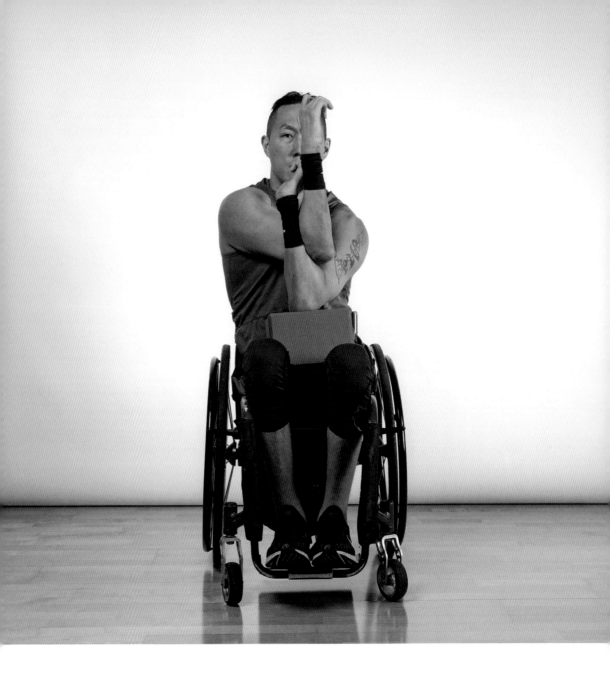

SEATED EAGLE

Garudasana

Seated Eagle promotes flexibility and strength of the shoulder complex. In particular, this pose is one of the few yoga poses that promotes strength of the elbow flexors (biceps). It also increases strength in the shoulder horizontal adductors (pectoralis major). The biceps and the pectoralis major are essential muscles used for propelling a wheelchair. The position of the arms, pulled tightly together in front of the chest, also stretches the muscles behind the shoulder.

Benefits

- Strengthens the elbow flexors.
- Strengthens the scapular upward rotators.
- Strengthens the shoulder horizontal adductors.
- Stretches the shoulder extensors.

How To

1. Start by sitting in your wheelchair or any comfortable seat.
2. Extend your arms straight in front of your body with the hands facing each other.
3. Hook the elbow of the left arm under your right arm, with elbows bent.
4. If you can reach, wrap your arms and hands, and press your palms together (or as close as you can get them).
5. If unable to reach, bring the backs of the hands or forearms to touch, or use a strap.
6. Lift the forearms so that the elbows are as close as possible to the height of your collarbones.
7. Keep your shoulder blades pressing down the back, toward your waist.
8. Allow the gaze to fall onto your fingertips.
9. Hold for 5 to 10 breath cycles and then switch sides.

Variations

Lift the elbows up to throat height and wrap the wrists around each other to touch the palms together to deepen the pose, and open and stretch your upper back.

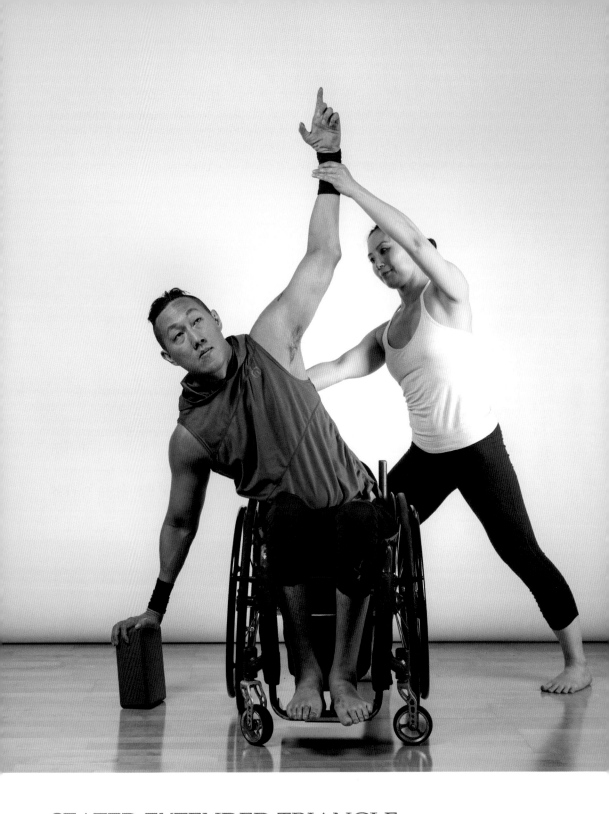

SEATED EXTENDED TRIANGLE   Utthita Trikonasana

Reaching the arm overhead strengthens the muscles of the scapular upward rotators and the shoulder flexors. In this manner, Seated Extended Triangle works to improve functional mobility and assists in avoiding shoulder injury. Additionally, this pose promotes strength of the oblique muscles. It's vital to strengthen the remaining functional core muscles to promote better sitting balance and to execute many other functional tasks.

Benefits

- Strengthens the shoulder flexors.
- Strengthens the scapular upward rotators.
- Strengthens the core.

Precautions

If you have had a past cervical spine injury, be careful not to let the head hang down, and maintain the neck in a neutral position.

How To

1. Start by sitting in your wheelchair or any comfortable seat.
2. Stretch your arms out to the sides in line with your shoulder sockets.
3. Side bend at the torso down to your right to bring the right hand down and the left hand up.
4. Make sure that both sides of the torso extend equally long and you don't collapse into the right side of your waist.
5. Rest your hand on a block or a chair beside you, or grasp the wheel of your chair.
6. Engage your abdominal muscles to support your spine.
7. Point the left arm to the sky, in line with your shoulder with your palm facing forward.
8. Maintain extension of your neck in line with your spine and look up, forward, or down if looking up strains your neck.
9. Hold for 5 breath cycles.
10. Switch sides by rotating to the other side of the chair.

Modifications

Keep your arms at the waist if it is too much to try to extend arms out while side bending at the torso.

Variations

- To challenge your core strength, scoot forward in your wheelchair so the backrest of the chair is not supporting your trunk.
- To challenge yourself, remove the arms of the wheelchair for further side bending if your spine has the flexibility and you want to go deep into the lateral stretch.

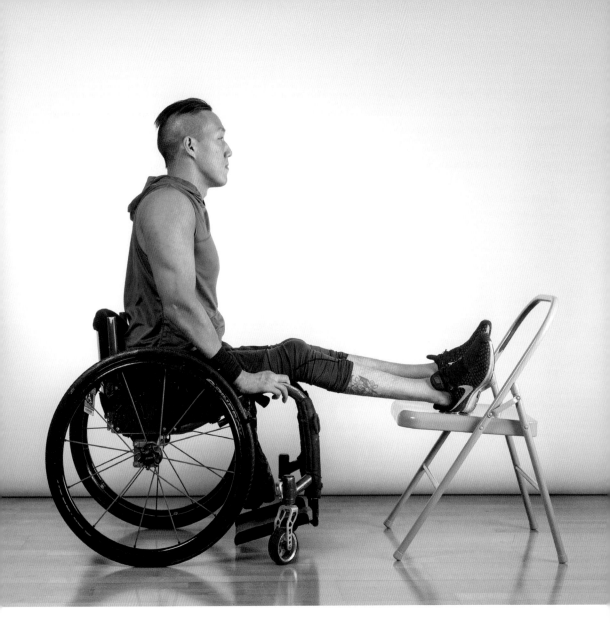

STAFF

Dandasana

Protracted and elevated scapulae (rounded shoulders) can increase the risk of shoulder pain or injury in those with SCI.[8] Staff is an exemplary pose that assists in strengthening the elbow extensors and shoulder depressors. This pose can be utilized to reinforce the desired resting position of the scapulae, which should be slightly retracted and depressed. The knee flexor muscles, also known as the hamstrings, are attached to the sit bones (ischial tuberosities), cross behind the hip joint, and pass behind the knee joint before attaching to the back of the tibia. Therefore, straightening the knees in a seated position stretches the knee flexors at the hip and knee joints, making Staff an excellent pose to stretch this muscle group.

Benefits

- Strengthens the scapular retractors and depressors.
- Strengthens the elbow extensors.
- Stretches the knee flexors.

How To

1. Start seated in your wheelchair with a chair at the same height in front of you.
2. Place and extend the legs onto the chair in front of you.
3. Rest your hands beside your hips in the seat of the wheelchair with the palms facing down and fingers spread wide.
4. Roll the shoulders back and engage the belly.
5. Push your hands into the seat, drawing your shoulder blades down and straightening the elbows, depressing the shoulders down away from your ears.
6. Lift the belly button up and in to engage the core and strengthen the hip flexors.
7. Hold for 5 to 10 breath cycles.

Modifications

Sit on the mat with legs extended out in front of you and push your hands down into the mat next to you.

Variations

Sit with the bottoms of your feet against the wall to assist with dorsiflexion and stretch the anterior tibialis muscles.

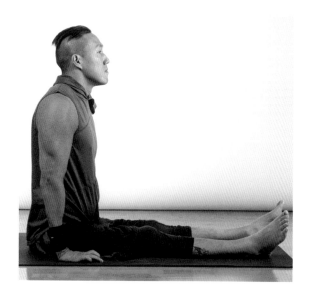

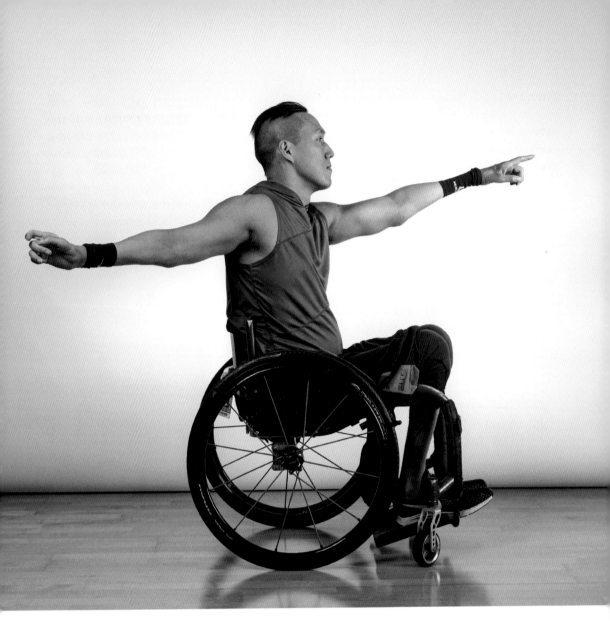

SEATED WARRIOR II

Virabhadrasana II

Seated Warrior II places the arms into a position to activate and strengthen the muscles of shoulder flexion and elbow extension. A point of emphasis for this pose is to make sure the arms are lifted with awareness and control of the movements of the scapulae. Developing and maintaining scapular control decreases risk of pain from shoulder overuse or developing poor shoulder mechanics over time.

Benefits

- Strengthens the scapular upward rotators.
- Strengthens the shoulder flexors.
- Strengthens the elbow extensors.

How To

1. Start by sitting comfortably in your wheelchair.
2. Extend arms out to the sides, in line with the shoulder sockets, reaching strongly out through the fingertips.
3. Rotate the torso in the direction of your front fingertips, while maintaining extension through your back hand.
4. Hold for 3 to 5 breath cycles.
5. Switch sides by rotating toward the other side of your chair and repeating the arm extension with the opposite arm in front.

Variations

Sit with the bottoms of your feet against the wall to assist with dorsiflexion and stretch the anterior tibialis muscles.

Maintaining or improving appropriate ROM is critical in SCI. Development of joint stiffness can slow the rehabilitation process or, if severe enough, seriously limit function.[6] Indeed, ROM exercises are initiated as soon as possible after SCI and are recommended throughout the life span.[6] Generally, normal joint ROM and muscle flexibility will enhance function. However, after SCI, ROM and flexibility in specific muscle groups and joints have a greater functional significance. These specific muscle groups and joints, and how to improve their function and ROM, will be discussed in detail in this section.

Spinal surgery is common after SCI. We recommend that you obtain permission from your physician prior to engaging in any exercise intended to improve spinal mobility.

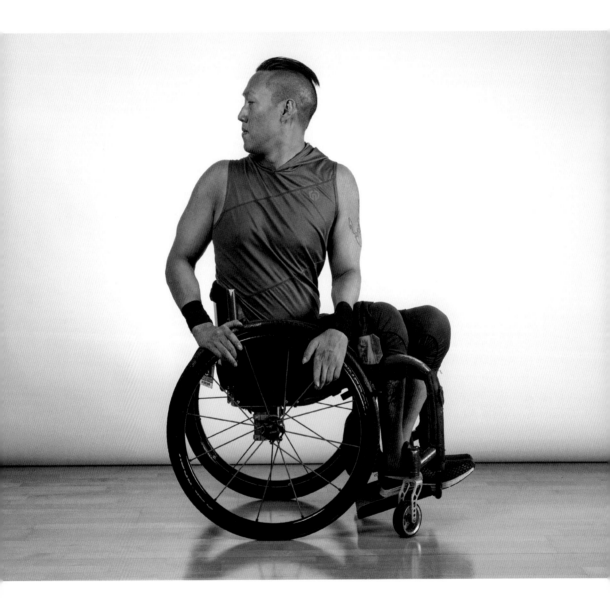

SEATED REVOLVED SIDE ANGLE

Parivrtta Parsvakonasana

Rotational movements of the spine are needed for rolling in bed and to allow the torso to twist while using the arms to roll from lying on your back up to a sitting position. Seated Revolved Side Angle improves spinal rotation mobility of the mid and low back. We recommend you obtain clearance from your physician prior to performing poses that incorporate spinal rotation.

Benefits

Improves spinal rotation.

Precautions

Avoid this pose if you have a current or recently herniated disc.

How To

1. Start by sitting in your wheelchair with the seat belt on.
2. Twist to the right at the trunk to hold onto the armrests or wheel of the right side of your chair with both hands.
3. Inhale as you lift your belly in and elongate the spine. Exhale to twist toward the back of the chair.
4. Optionally, turn your gaze over your right shoulder to gaze behind you.
5. Hold for 5 to 8 breath cycles.
6. Switch sides by turning in the chair.

Variations

- To challenge your core strength, scoot forward in your wheelchair so the backrest of the chair is not supporting your trunk.
- For a lateral stretch, lift the left arm and reach it overhead for a stretch of the left side of your body.

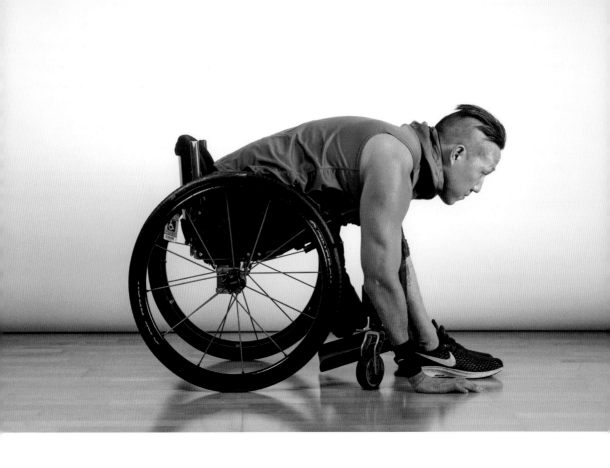

FORWARD BEND, SEATED

Uttanasana

Hip extensor and ease of low back flexion are required for several functional positions and movements. Both are required when reaching forward to perform lower body dressing, especially putting on shoes and socks. Significant forward bending is required when performing transfers; Forward Bend places the trunk, which is your COM, over the feet, which are used as a pivot point when transferring. We recommend you obtain clearance from your physician prior to performing poses that incorporate spinal flexion, particularly if you have a history of spinal surgery.

Benefits

- Stretches the hip extensors.
- Increases lumbar flexion.

Precautions

Avoid this pose if you have a current or recently herniated disc.

How To

1. Sit on the edge of your wheelchair with feet firmly planted on the ground, hip width apart.
2. Exhale to bend forward over your legs.
3. Rest your hands on blocks, your shins, your ankles, the wheelchair frame, or the floor.
4. Let the head hang heavy.
5. Hold for 5 to 10 breath cycles.
6. Come up slowly to avoid light-headedness.

Modifications

- If your feet are not comfortable resting on the floor, you can use blocks under the feet.
- If your back feels strained or your hands do not rest comfortably on your shins or on the floor, place blocks under the hands.

Variations

- *Challenge variation:* If you want to go deeper into the pose, you can bring the feet and knees further apart, and bend the torso between the thighs.
- *Restorative variation:* Place a bolster or blanket on the thighs to decrease the forward bend and take tension out of your back.

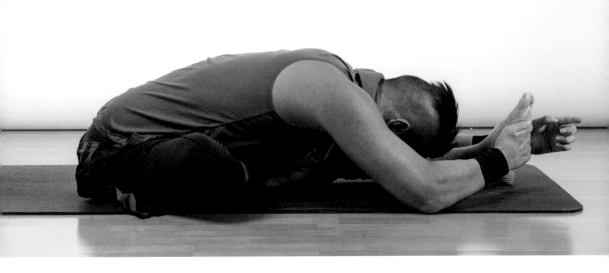

HEAD-TO-KNEE Janu Sirsasana

Head-to-Knee assists in stretching multiple muscle groups that improve function and mobility in SCI. *Long sitting* means sitting with both legs straight in front while the torso is vertical; it is a very functional position for those with SCI. This position is used to get into and out of bed, for lower body dressing, and for transitioning between a wheelchair and the floor. Long sitting requires flexibility of the knee flexors (hamstrings), which is improved with Head-to-Knee. Additionally, because individuals with SCI do not stand, plantar flexor tightness is common, which can affect the ability to perform transfers. In Head-to-Knee, the plantar flexors are stretched, one leg at a time, allowing focus on the individual muscle group. Furthermore, stretching the knee flexors is also useful in reducing muscle spasms and allows for an anteriorly tilted pelvis, which promotes an upright sitting posture and assists with breathing. Head-to-Knee also assists in stretching the knee flexors when the pose is performed with attention to dorsiflexing the foot of the extended leg.

Benefits

- Stretches the knee and plantar flexors.
- Stretches the hip internal rotators.
- Stretches the hip extensors.

Precautions

Avoid this pose if you have a current or recently herniated disc.

Before You Begin

Have a strap or a block handy for modifications.

How To

1. Start in Staff (pages 176-177).
2. Sitting on the mat, bend your right knee and place the foot to the inside of the left thigh.
3. Rotating from the hip, bring the right knee down to the mat or onto a block.
4. Extend the spine and, if able, press the back of the right thigh into the mat.
5. Inhale to lengthen the spine and rotate your torso toward the left foot. (You can use your hands on the mat to assist the mild spinal rotation.)
6. Exhale to walk your hands toward the left ankle or foot to bend forward at the hips.
7. Dorsiflex the left foot (left toes point straight up to the sky) with a strap or clasping with your hands.
8. Make sure that you are not rounding the spine but are maintaining an extended spine.
9. Continue to walk the hands forward as much as is comfortable for your forward bend; your hands can rest on the floor, on a strap (see the following modification), or on your shin, ankle, or foot.
10. You can rest your forehead on your shin, a block, or a folded blanket, or you can keep your gaze forward on the ground with an extended neck.
11. Hold for 5 to 10 breath cycles.
12. Inhale to sit upright, and switch sides.

Modifications

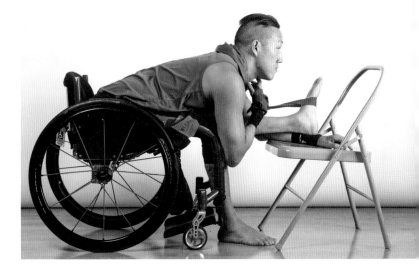

- If you can't reach the floor or your shin (or ankle or foot) comfortably, wrap a yoga strap around the ball of your foot and hold onto the strap with both hands.
- You can perform the pose in your wheelchair by placing your extended leg onto a chair in front of your wheelchair and placing the other foot onto your extended knee or keeping it on the floor for support, as pictured.

Variations

Place a bolster or blanket on or inside the extended leg and allow your torso to rest on it.

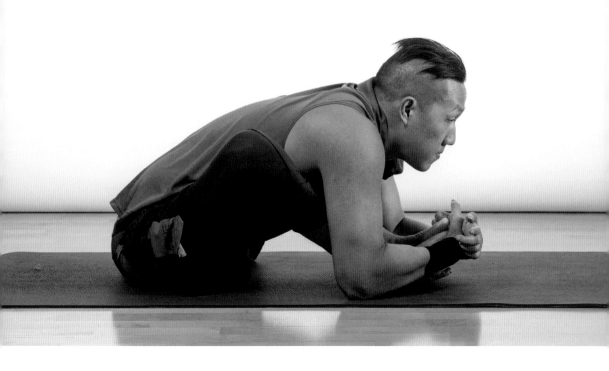

BOUND ANGLE Baddha Konasana

Bound Angle is an excellent way to stretch the hip internal rotators. Flexibility in these muscles is required to obtain a *ring sitting* position (sitting with the hips externally rotated and the knees bent). This pose increases the base of support and improves balance to enable the hands to be free to manage the lower extremities while getting into and out of bed, or while dressing and undressing. Additionally, this position is commonly used for females to perform self-catheterization.

Benefits

- Stretches the hip internal rotators.
- Strengthens the core.
- Promotes upright posture.

How To

1. Start seated on the mat in whatever leg position is comfortable for you.
2. Use the hands to bend the knees into your chest and the feet flat on the ground.
3. Roll the knees out to the sides, supporting the outer knees with the hands and keeping the bottoms of the feet together.
4. Ground the sitting bones and inhale to lengthen the spine.
5. Hold the feet or ankles with the hands.
6. If your body allows, hinge from your hips to bend forward, maintaining an elongated spine.
7. Hold for 5 to 10 breath cycles.
8. Come up slowly; you can use your hands on your thighs or next to you on the ground to help you push up to a straight spine again.

Modifications

- Place blocks under your knees to relieve tension in the hips.
- Bring the feet farther away from the pelvis to decrease the flexion in your knees.
- You can do this pose in a wheelchair by placing your feet on a chair positioned in front of you.

Variations

For a more intense inner thigh stretch, bring the feet closer to the pelvis.

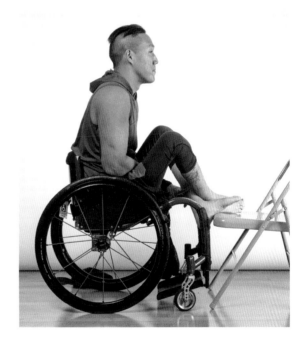

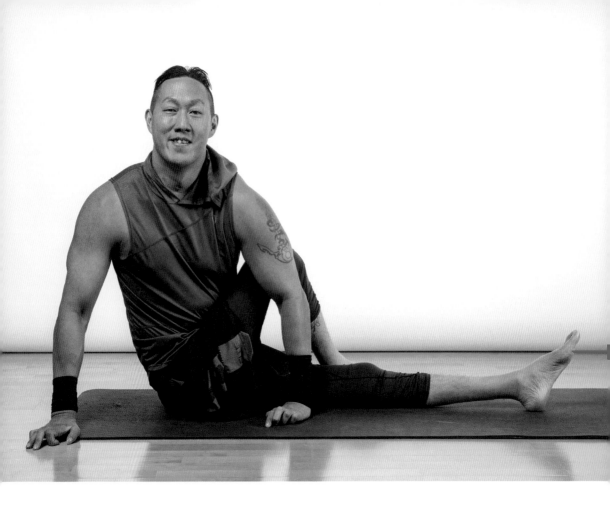

MODIFIED HALF LORD OF THE FISHES

Ardha Matsyendrasana

Spinal rotation is important for functional mobility. Modified Half Lord of the Fishes incorporates lumbar spine rotation and allows for an emphasis on rotation of the cervical spine. Good mobility of the cervical spine is needed for environmental awareness, upper body dressing, and to obtain a proper sitting posture. This pose also provides the opportunity to stretch the wrist flexors. Maintaining flexibility in this muscle group is needed to perform transfers.

Benefits

- Promotes full spinal rotation.
- Stretches the wrist flexors.

Before You Begin

We recommend you obtain clearance from your physician prior to performing poses that incorporate spinal rotation.

Precautions

Avoid this pose if you have a current or recent herniated disc.

How To

1. Start in Staff (pages 176-177).
2. Use your hands to lift the right leg and bend the knee to place the right foot outside of your left knee.
3. Hug the right knee into your body with your left arm and inhale to elongate the spine.
4. Place the right hand, palm down, behind your back to offer stability and leverage for your twist.
5. Make sure both sitting bones remain grounded to the earth; don't let one hip hike up.
6. Exhale, and rotate the torso to the right as you hug the knee in.
7. Optionally, gaze over your right (back) shoulder to rotate through the cervical spine.
8. Continue to inhale and exhale in your twist, elongating your spine with every inhale, and twisting deeper with every exhale.
9. Hold for 5 to 8 breath cycles.
10. To exit the pose, untwist the spine, extend the legs, and switch sides.

Modifications

If one hip wants to lift, sit on blankets or a bolster to lift the hips and even out the pelvis.

Variations

To challenge yourself, bend the bottom leg before you twist.

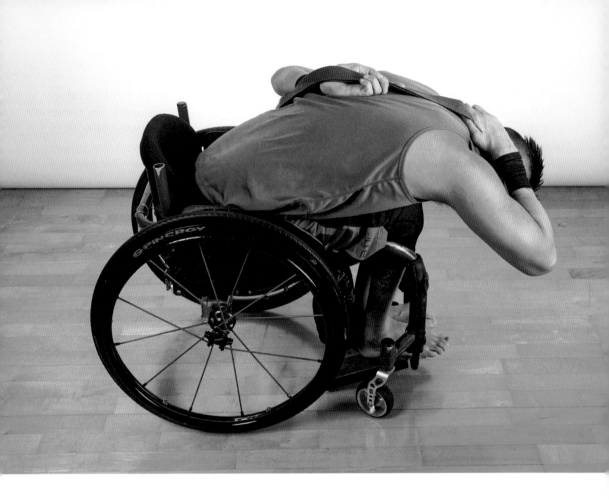

UPPER BODY COW FACE   Gomukhasana

To decrease risk of shoulder injury, upper extremity flexibility is also important in SCI. Upper Body Cow Face stretches the elbow extensors (triceps); these muscles must be flexible in order to fully bend the elbow. Full elbow flexion is required for certain wheelchair skills and to transfer between the wheelchair and the floor. This pose also stretches the shoulder flexors, which are used to reach the hand up and back when transferring onto a higher surface. This pose also helps to facilitate increased thoracic and cervical extension, which can enhance your breathing.

Benefits

- Stretches the elbow extensors.
- Stretches the shoulder protractors and flexors.
- Improves extension of the thoracic spine.

Precautions

Avoid this pose if you have a current or recent rotator cuff injury or a history of shoulder dislocations.

Before You Begin

Have a strap handy for modification.

How To

1. Start seated in a chair with an elongated spine.
2. Extend your arms out to the sides with the thumbs pointing up.
3. Rotating from your left shoulder, turn the left thumb down so that the palm faces back.
4. Bend the left elbow and rotate the hand behind your back.
5. Turn the right palm up and rotate the right thumb back behind you.
6. Stretch the right arm up to the sky and bend the elbow.
7. Reach your fingertips behind your back toward each other (the fingers do not have to touch; please see the following modification using a strap).
8. Relax the shoulders down your back and gaze forward.
9. Hold for 5 to 8 breath cycles.
10. To release the hands, slowly unbind and extend the arms back out to the sides and into your lap.
11. Switch sides.

Modifications

- Use a strap between the hands (most people need this).
- You can also perform this pose bent forward over your legs if that is more accessible to you.

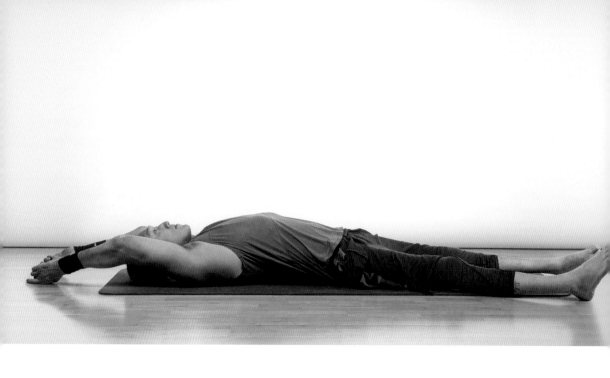

MODIFIED RECLINING HERO Supta Virasana

Wheelchair propulsion is typically achieved with the use of the pectoralis and elbow flexor muscles. Frequent use of these muscles can lead to tightness and consequent shoulder and rotator cuff pathology. Modified Reclining Hero promotes stretching of the pectoralis and elbow flexors. Full flexibility of the elbow flexors is essential for performing transfers, for moving in bed, and to execute certain wheelchair skills. Additionally, thoracic kyphosis, which can contribute to shoulder stiffness and make breathing more difficult, is common in wheelchair users. This pose counteracts the exaggerated kyphosis by opening the chest and reaching the arms overhead in a supine position.

Benefits

- Stretches the shoulder adductors.
- Improves extension of the thoracic spine.
- Stretches the elbow flexors.

Precautions

- Avoid this pose if you have a current or recent rotator cuff injury.
- Please do not perform this as the traditional yogic pose with the knees bent and ankles next to the hips. Because of the lack of sensation in the lower extremities, you will be prone to ligament tears in the knees if they are placed into extreme flexion. Practice this pose with the arms portion only.

How To

1. Lying supine on the mat, extend your arms overhead as much as is comfortable.
2. You can keep the arms parallel or bend the arms to hold onto the opposite elbows above your head.
3. Hold for 8 to 10 breath cycles or as long as is comfortable for you.

Modifications

- Place a bolster or blocks behind you (above your head) to rest the arms on if you are unable to reach the arms all the way to the mat.
- You may also reach for the opposite elbows to gain more traction in the side body stretch.

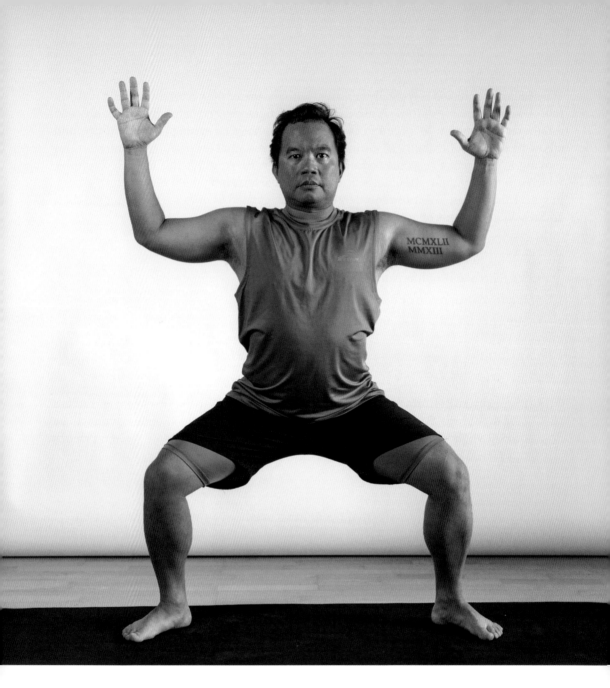

Parkinson's Disease

First described by James Parkinson in his classic 1817 monograph, "An Essay on the Shaking Palsy,"[20] Parkinson's disease (PD) is a progressive neurodegenerative disease that affects between 100 and 200 per 100,000 people over 40, and over 1 million people in North America alone.[30] It is the second most common neurodegenerative disease after Alzheimer's disease.

Regular exercise is especially valuable because of the chronic nature of PD and its associated progressive motor limitations. Exercise may not slow the progression of akinesia, rigidity, or gait disturbance, but it can alleviate some secondary orthopedic effects. Specifically, exercise can assist in improving rigidity and flexed posture, and improve joint pain, motor task function,[8] and even some nonmotor symptoms.[3]

Many patients engaged in regular physical activity gain lasting confidence and a sense of control over the physical aspect of the disease, even if they have never engaged in physical activity in the past. Working with a physical therapist, practicing yoga, or joining exercise groups may be a good way to get started in such activities.

Yoga and meditation cultivate mindfulness in patients with PD and have, in recent years, become a subject of in-depth study among neuroscientists.[5,14,29] In fact, yoga programs including mindfulness can even lead to similar improvements in motor function and disability compared with stretching and resistance training exercise, with superior results on measures of depression, anxiety, well-being, and quality of life.[14]

Yoga is one of the most beneficial complementary therapies for PD, helping to increase flexibility, improve posture and balance, loosen tight muscles, and build confidence. This helps patients with PD to improve general function and thus enhances quality of life.[18,27]

Mobility and balance are important components of yoga and can help to decrease fall risk. It is cited that as many as 60 percent of Parkinson's patients will fall.[2] Mobility and balance have important implications for falls in PD, and yoga participation has been shown to improve functional mobility and how a person with PD walks.[7] Standing yoga poses target the hip extensors, knee extensors, and ankle plantar flexors, which improves control of one's center of mass (COM) during walking and may improve overall stability. Research has also shown yoga-related improvements in balance (both in tandem and one-legged stances) and an associated reduction in fear of falling; this can also help people with PD remain active in their community.[18] Additionally, greater hip mobility gained from yoga may translate into improvements in the shuffling gait experienced by many living with PD.

Strength is also an integral component of postural stability in individuals with PD.[4] Yoga requires isometric contractions in which joint angle and muscle length do not change. These isometric contractions stabilize the body and may mimic isokinetic contractions, in which variable resistance to movement is performed at constant speed. Transitioning from one pose to the next achieves stabilization through the isometric and isokinetic contractions. These mechanisms may be the reason why yoga improves muscular strength.

Yoga also assists in improving flexibility and range of motion (ROM), which are integral to improving function in patients with PD because rigidity is one of the hallmarks of the disease. Research shows improvements in flexibility and ROM of the shoulder, hip, and spine in patients with PD who practice yoga.[23] Additionally, patients with PD often exhibit an exaggerated kyphosis in the spine (stooped posture), which can be related to short spinal flexors and weak spinal extensors. Yoga supports an upright posture by improving shoulder and spinal flexibility.

Although the psychosocial benefits associated with yoga may be obvious, they deserve some attention in this chapter. Depression occurs in approximately 40 percent of patients with PD, and medications often do not adequately treat the depression and social withdrawal commonly associated with the disease.[9] Because exercise promotes a feeling of physical and mental well-being, yoga can provide a sense of purpose, hope, community support, and confidence to those with PD.[6] The calming effect of yoga (by enhancing parasympathetic output) has also been demonstrated to lessen stress, enhance relaxation, and improve sleep in PD.[24]

GENERAL GUIDELINES

- Utilize poses that require large amplitude movements (taking up as much space as possible).
- Integrate spinal rotation and extension.
- Incorporate lifting the hands above the head as able.
- Use props liberally to assist in achieving the poses safely.
- Repeatedly move into and out of poses. For example, you can perform several cycles of Mountain to Five Pointed Star.
- If in a group class, visual demonstration of poses by the instructor is helpful.
- Use voice and chanting when possible to improve voice control.

Rigidity is one of the primary motor symptoms of PD. Rigidity is caused by stiff or inflexible muscles due to the muscles' inability to relax, and can contribute to pain and reduced ROM. This can affect the muscles of the extremities, neck, and trunk. The poses that follow were selected to improve flexibility of the shoulders, hips, and spine muscles that are commonly stiff in individuals with PD.

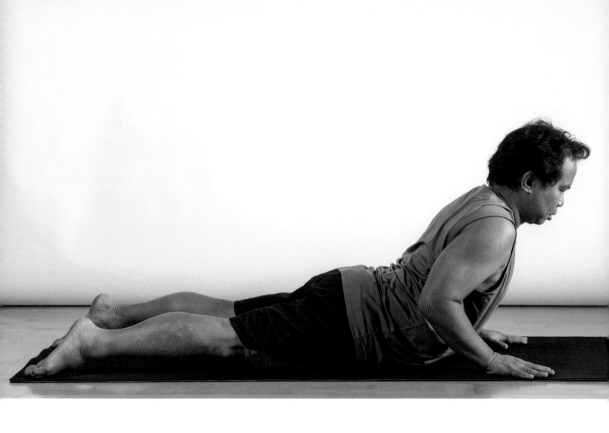

COBRA

Bhujangasana

One symptom of PD is that the spine is bent forward during standing and walking, but this resolves when lying down. Clinically, this phenomenon is known as *camptocormia*, and presents as forward flexion of the thoracic and lumbar spine only when upright.[1] Cobra can be used to improve flexibility of the spine in extension and stretch the abdominal muscles. Rigidity combined with a general decrease in activity levels commonly leads to tightness in the hip flexors, which can also be improved with this pose.

Benefits

- Improves lumbar and thoracic spinal extension.
- Stretches the hip flexors.
- Stretches the chest and abdominal muscles.

Precautions

Avoid this pose if you are pregnant or be careful if you have a current or recent wrist injury.

How To

1. Start prone with the forehead to the ground, legs extended, and hands directly under the shoulders.
2. Scoop the elbows in toward your body and spread the fingers wide to create a firm foundation with the hands.
3. Press into the hands to lift the chest as you engage the abdominal muscles.
4. Draw the shoulders down your back as you move toward straight arms (it's okay to maintain a bend in your arms for the comfort of your back).
5. Make sure that you continue to engage your abdominal muscles to protect the spine as you lift your heart up and draw the shoulder blades down your back.
6. The head balances comfortably in line with the curve of the spine.
7. The pubic bone rests on the mat, in conjunction with the action of lifting slightly up toward the chest to lengthen the lumbar spine.
8. Hold for 5 to 8 breath cycles.

Modifications

Place a bolster under the belly to take the weight off the arms and shoulders.

Variations

- *Challenge variation:* Walk the hands farther in toward the body to lift the chest higher and move toward a more upright spine. Make sure the shoulders continue to draw down the back and away from the ears, and the abdomen remains engaged.
- *Restorative variation:* Place a bolster under the low belly to support the spine as in the modification.

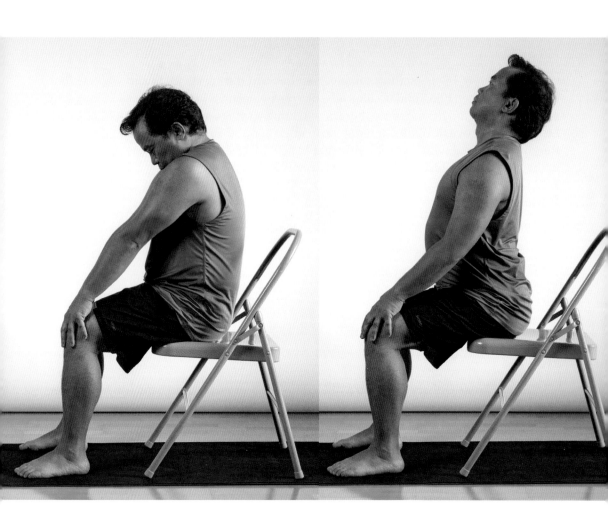

CAT COW IN CHAIR

Marjaryasana Bitilasana

As mentioned, PD reduces flexibility in the spine. This can contribute to increased energy expenditure during ambulation as well as to back and shoulder pain. Cat Cow in Chair is an excellent way to improve mobility of the spine. It is also an effective way to train motor control of the spine, increasing the ability to voluntarily control the position of the spine during movement.

Benefits

- Improves mobility of the spine.
- Opens the lungs for improved breathing.

How To

1. Start seated in a chair, with an upright spine, and feet grounded comfortably on the floor.
2. Relax your hands on your knees or thighs.
3. For Cow, inhale to arch the spine, opening your chest forward and up and drawing the shoulders down your back.
4. For Cat, exhale to round your spine, keeping the hands on the knees or thighs, and drop your chin to your chest. Lift the belly up and in as you round the shoulders and tuck the tailbone slightly.
5. Switch back and forth between Cow and Cat with your inhales and exhales for 5 breath cycles.
6. Return to a neutral spine.

Variations

To challenge yourself, come into Table Top (pages 250-251) on the mat if you are able to perform Cat Cow with the shoulders over the wrists and the hips over the knees.

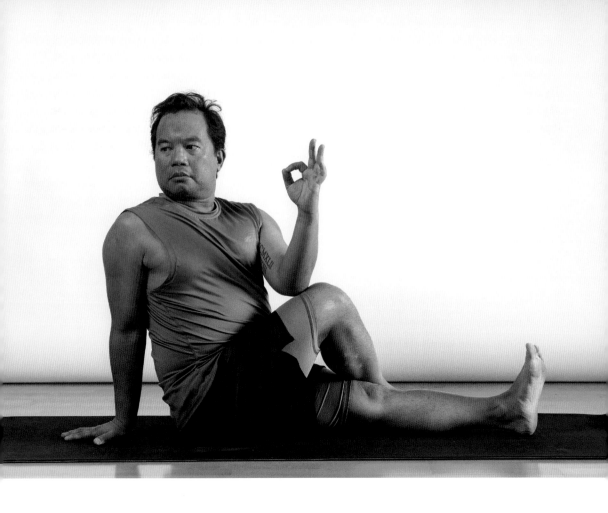

MODIFIED HALF LORD OF THE FISHES

Ardha Matsyendrasana

The most visibly evident symptom of rigidity in the spine is the forward bent presentation, also referred to as stooped posture. Spinal rigidity also decreases the ability to rotate the trunk. This rotational stiffness leads to decreased walking speeds and increased risk of falls. Modified Half Lord of the Fishes can help you regain mobility in spinal rotation, thus freeing up movement in the trunk and improving walking speeds and balance.

Benefits

- Improves spinal rotation.
- Increases hip mobility.
- Stretches the hip flexors.

Precautions

Avoid this pose if you have a current or recently herniated disc.

How To

1. Start in Staff (pages 80-81).
2. Use your hands to lift the right leg and step the right foot to the outside of your left knee.
3. Hug the right knee into your body with your left arm or outer elbow.
4. Place the right hand behind your back to offer stability and leverage for your twist.
5. Make sure both sitting bones remain grounded to the earth; don't let one hip hike up.
6. Inhale to elongate the spine.
7. Exhale, and rotate the torso to the right as you hug the knee in.
8. Continue to inhale and exhale in your twist, elongating your spine with every inhale, and twisting deeper with every exhale.
9. Hold for 5 to 8 breath cycles.
10. To exit the pose, untwist the spine, extend the legs, and switch sides.

Modifications

If one hip wants to lift, sit on blankets or a bolster to lift the hips and even out the pelvis.

Variations

To challenge yourself, bend the bottom leg before you twist.

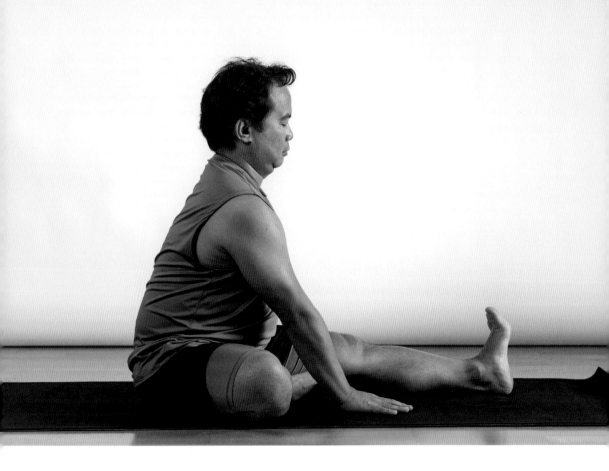

HEAD-TO-KNEE Janu Sirsasana

Another common symptom of PD is bradykinesia, which is slowness of movements. This leads to not utilizing the body's full ROM. Over time, this can result in a loss of muscle flexibility; specifically loss of flexibility in the knee flexor muscles. This often presents as walking with the knees bent, which decreases walking efficiency, diminishes balance, and increases risk of falls. Head-to-Knee is an excellent pose to stretch the knee flexors, improving leg flexibility and thus, walking balance.

Benefits

- Stretches the knee and plantar flexors.
- Increases hip mobility.

Precautions

Avoid this pose if you have a current or recently herniated disc.

How To

1. Start in Staff (pages 80-81).
2. Bend your right knee and place the right foot to the inside of the left thigh.
3. Bring the right knee down to the mat or onto a block.
4. Extend the spine and dorsiflex the left foot (toes up and heel forward).
5. Engage the right leg by pressing the back of the right thigh into the mat.
6. Inhale to lengthen the spine and rotate your torso toward the left foot (you can use your hands on the mat to assist the mild spinal rotation).
7. Exhale to walk your hands toward the left ankle or foot to fold forward at the hips.
8. Make sure that you are not rounding the spine but are maintaining an extended spine with the engagement of the core.
9. Continue to walk the hands forward as much as is comfortable for your forward bend; your hands can rest on the floor, on a strap (see the following modification), or on the shin, ankle, or foot.
10. Hold for 5 to 10 breath cycles.
11. Inhale to sit upright, and switch sides.

Modifications

If you can't reach the floor or the shin (or ankle or foot) comfortably, use a yoga strap around the ball of your foot and hold onto the strap with both hands.

Variations

Place a bolster or blanket on or inside the extended leg to allow your torso to rest on it.

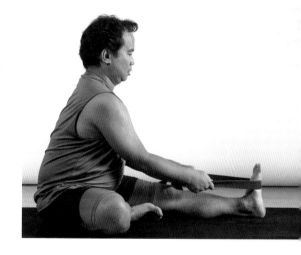

With PD, movements and actions become smaller and slower over time. Therefore, a common practice in treating PD is to utilize large amplitude exercises and learning to Think BIG![16] Performing these exaggerated, big movements retrains the Parkinson's brain with the goal of increasing the size and speed of movements (e.g., standing from a seated position taller and faster).[12] Specifically, research shows that Lee Silverman Voice Treatment (LSVT; exercises that emphasize large amplitude movements) can lead to faster walking with bigger steps and arm swings, better balance, and more ability to twist at the waist.[10] Clinicians also report that LSVT BIG can help people with buttoning their clothes, writing, and other smaller movement (small motor) tasks, as well as large motor movements like dressing, getting up from a seat, and getting into bed.[11]

Poses that include larger amplitude movements also help to improve shoulder strength and ROM.[13] Because of the effects of rigidity and decreased arm swing while walking, those

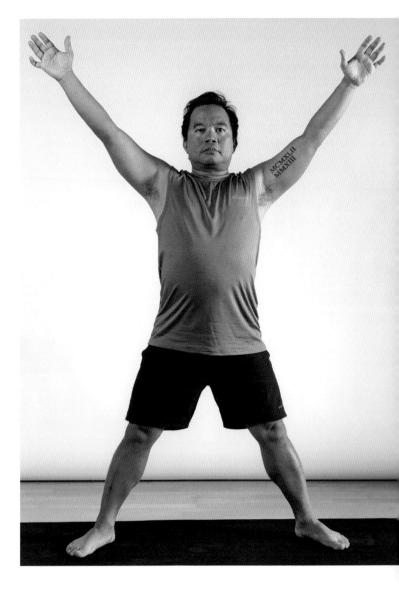

with PD are at an increased risk of developing frozen shoulder (severe tightness of the shoulder joint).[15] The poses in this chapter help to maintain full motion of the shoulders.

You can use these poses in one of two ways. The first way is to practice them traditionally by holding the pose for a few breath cycles; this allows the pose to address balance deficits. The other way is to perform these poses in a repeated fashion to mimic the BIG movements that are often utilized to treat the symptoms of small and slow motions of PD. Additionally, we note that an occasional side effect of PD medications and PD itself is orthostatic hypotension, the decrease in blood pressure during standing.[25] When this occurs, one typically feels dizzy or light-headed. If you are feeling these symptoms, you can modify the poses by performing them in a seated position.

FIVE POINTED STAR Utthita Tadasana

If you were to position your body to take up as much space as possible, you would likely mimic something close to Five Pointed Star. This pose epitomizes a large amplitude movement while strengthening the entire body. The wide stance in the pose helps maintain balance while extending the spine, lifting the chest, and stretching the arms wide.

Benefits

- Strengthens the shoulder abductors.
- Strengthens the knee extensors.
- Strengthens the hip abductors.
- Strengthens the spinal extensors.
- Improves balance.

How To

1. Start in Mountain (pages 216-217), and step or jump the feet wide apart (lengthwise) on the mat.
2. Stretch the arms out to the sides so that the wrists are in line with (over) the ankles.
3. Feet should be pointed toward the corners along the long edge of the mat with the quadriceps and core muscles engaged.
4. Stretch out through your fingertips to engage the arm and upper back muscles.
5. Draw your shoulder blades down your back, relaxing the neck and shoulders.
6. Inhale to extend up through the crown of your head to lengthen the spine.
7. Breathe slowly through your inhales and exhales while you expand outward in every direction with your head, feet, hands, and chest.
8. Hold for 5 to 8 breath cycles, or repeat five times, jumping or walking in and out from Mountain with the legs and arms.
9. To exit the pose, step or jump the feet back together and place the hands in prayer or alongside your body.

Modifications

- Place the hands on the hips.
- Perform in a chair without using the legs and using only the arms.
- Exhaling through the mouth, as in the classic version of this pose, can sometimes cause a bit of dizziness. If so, try exhaling through the nose for a more stable version.

Variations

To challenge yourself, include your voice by making a *Ha* sound as you jump the feet out.

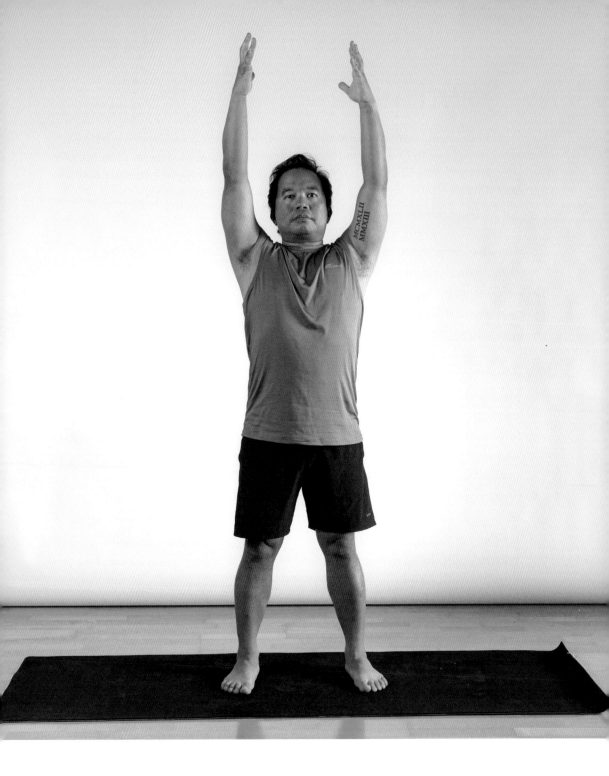

UPWARD SALUTE

Urdhva Hastasana

Any movement requiring the elbows to reach above the shoulders will elicit extension of the thoracic spine. Bringing the arms above the head during Upward Salute improves thoracic extension (and promotes a more upright posture) while also strengthening and stretching the shoulders into flexion (arms up). These features of Upward Salute can help decrease the risk of shoulder pain or injury while also serving as a large amplitude movement.

Benefits

- Strengthens the shoulder flexors.
- Stretches the shoulder extensors.
- Strengthens the knee extensors.
- Improves spinal extension ROM.
- Improves thoracic extension.

How To

1. Start by standing in Mountain (pages 216-217), with the feet directly below the hips and the arms alongside the body.
2. Inhale to reach your arms overhead, biceps next to the ears, and hands facing one another.
3. Relax the shoulder blades down the back as you stretch up through the fingertips and ground the feet down into the floor for stability.
4. Hold for 5 to 8 breath cycles, or repeat five times, coming up and down with your arms and gaze.
5. To exit the pose, release the hands down alongside your body or into Prayer Hands (pages 118-119).

Modifications

If you practice the pose while sitting in a chair, you will still get the benefits of shoulder ROM.

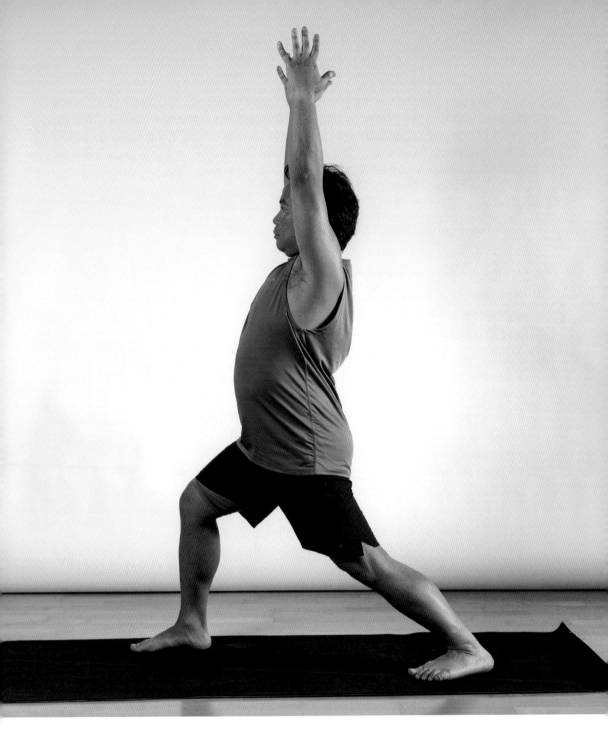

WARRIOR I

Virabhadrasana I

Warrior I provides the same benefits to the spine and shoulders as Upward Salute while also strengthening the legs. Warrior I activates the knee extensor of the front leg and the hip extensors of the back leg, strengthening the base of support (BOS). The goal of this pose is large amplitude, but safety always comes first. The farther apart the feet are placed, the greater challenge is imposed on balance. Initiate this pose by taking a short step and progress into a wider stance over time.

Benefits

- Strengthens the knee extensors.
- Strengthens the knee flexors.
- Strengthens the shoulder flexors.
- Improves spinal extension ROM.
- Strengthens the plantar flexors.
- Strengthens the hip extensors.

How To

1. Starting in Downward-Facing Dog (pages 90-91), step the right foot forward between the hands so that it's placed next to the right thumb, or start from a wide-legged stance on the mat.
2. Spin the left heel down approximately to a 45 degree angle and spin the outer edge of the left foot down so the entire plantar aspect of the foot grounds down.
3. With your right leg bent and thigh parallel to the floor, inhale your arms up to the sky, hands facing each other, fingers pointing up.
4. The back leg remains straight and strong as you anchor the foot to square the hips forward.
5. Lift the lower abdomen up and in as you lengthen the tailbone down.
6. Draw the shoulders down the back, and gaze forward or slightly up between your hands.
7. Hold for 5 to 8 breath cycles, or repeat five times, coming up and down with the arms.
8. To exit the pose, bring the hands down in a swan dive to frame the foot, and return to Downward-Facing Dog or to Mountain (pages 216-217).
9. Repeat on the left side.

Modifications

If this hurts your knee or is too challenging for your balance, shorten your stance and decrease the deep knee bend of the front leg.

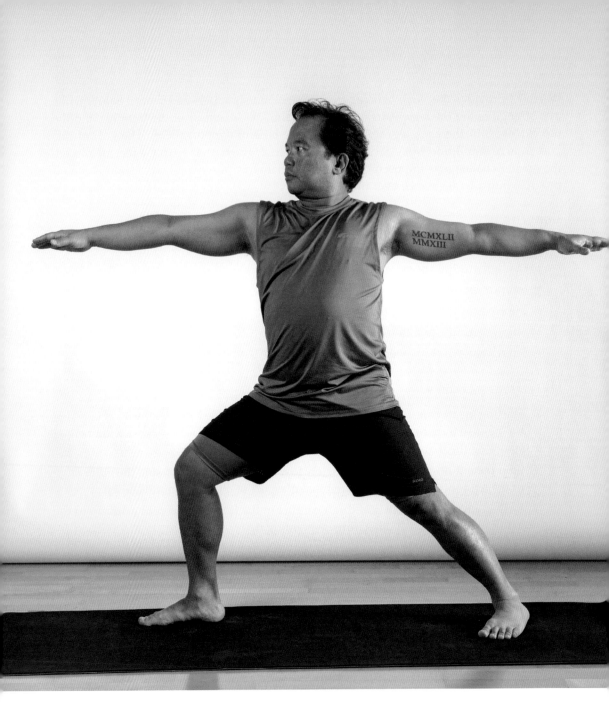

WARRIOR II Virabhadrasana II

There are numerous yoga poses that can be considered large amplitude (one of the main reasons why we are such advocates of yoga for PD). Warrior II is another example of a pose that makes the body big, while strengthening key muscle groups. Weak spinal extensor muscles contribute to the stooped posture that is common with PD. The upright torso and elevation of the arms in Warrior II teaches activation and builds strength in the spinal extensor muscles. Additionally, the opening of the hips laterally (compared to Warrior I) causes further activation of the hip abductors of the front leg, a muscle that is essential for balancing during a single leg stance.

Benefits

- Strengthens the hip abductors.
- Strengthens the hip extensors.
- Strengthens the knee flexors and extensors.
- Strengthen the spinal extensors.
- Strengthens the shoulder flexors.

Precautions

If you have knee issues, be careful not to bend farther than the ankle.

How To

1. Start with your feet wide (3.5 to 4 feet depending on your height) on the mat, right toes in front and pointing forward, and left toes pointing toward the long edge of the mat.
2. Ground all four corners of the feet down, creating a strong base for your legs.
3. As you inhale, extend your arms straight out to the sides, parallel to the floor.
4. Relax the shoulders down and elongate the neck as you gaze over the right fingertips.
5. Bend the right knee with the goal of extending it in line over the right ankle.
6. You can shift the position of your feet to make space.
7. Roll the inner thigh toward the outer hip so you can see the right big toe (it should not be hidden by your right knee). This will maintain alignment of the knee in line with the ankle.
8. Ground the outer edge of your left foot into the floor.
9. Extend the fingertips out with strength and purpose while relaxing the shoulders down your back.
10. Hold for 5 to 8 breath cycles, or move the arms up and down with your breath five times.
11. To exit the pose, place the hands on the hips, straighten the legs, and shift your feet to turn to the other side of the mat, so your left foot is forward.
12. Repeat on the left side.

Variations

To challenge yourself, reach the hands down behind your back and interlace the fingers for a chest stretch and to reverse stooped posture.

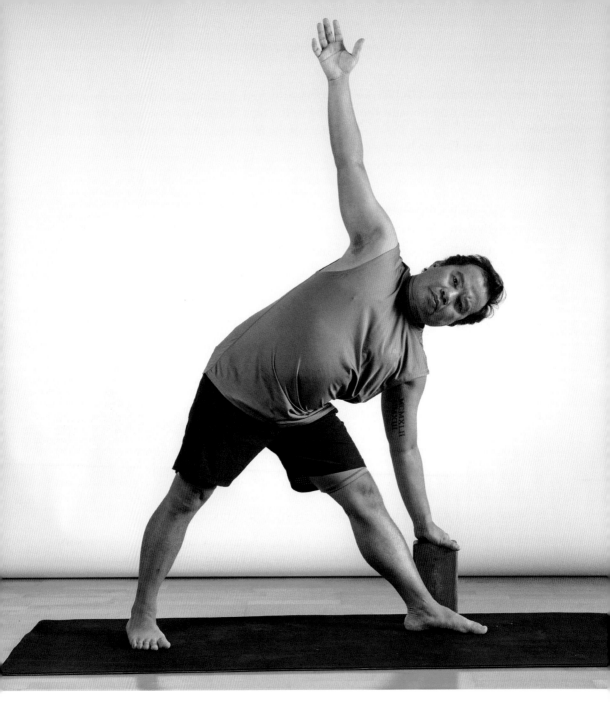

TRIANGLE

Trikonasana

Triangle is part of the large amplitude section because it embodies everything a big move-ment should be: It activates large muscle groups, encourages the body to take up space, and mobilizes the spine. Furthermore, the spinal rotation component of Triangle is an important part of exercise for PD because it improves function and posture by addressing the spinal stiffness so commonly seen in this disease. In Triangle, if your balance feels unsteady, ensure safety by using the bottom arm as additional balance support.

Benefits

- Strengthens the hip abductors.
- Improves spinal rotation.
- Strengthens the shoulder abductors.
- Stabilizes the core.

Precautions

Avoid looking up if you have a neck injury; it's okay to practice this pose with your gaze down toward the floor.

How To

1. Start in Warrior II (pages 212-213), with the left foot forward and the right toes pointing to the long edge of the mat.
2. Keep the arms extended.
3. Straighten the left leg and extend the left fingertips forward, lengthening both sides of your waist.
4. Continue to extend your torso forward in line with your left leg, grounding through the right foot and leg to anchor your movement.
5. Hinge at the left hip, as you rotate the left hand on a block, a chair, or your shin.
6. Stretch your right fingertips up to the sky, expanding your chest and stacking the shoulders.
7. Extend both sides of the waist and rotate the chest to the sky.
8. Your right hip will roll slightly down, which is okay. Make sure that both sides of the torso extend equally long and you are not rounding the right side waist.
9. Try to take some weight off of your left hand so you engage your abdominal muscles to support your spine.
10. Maintain extension of your neck in line with your spine and look up, forward, or down if looking up strains your neck.
11. Hold for 5 breath cycles.
12. To exit the pose, bend the left knee slightly and press firmly into the feet to lift your torso upright again.
13. Switch sides by pivoting your heels or resetting in Downward-Facing Dog (pages 90-91).

Modifications

- For additional support, practice with a wall behind you or a block under your hand.
- Place the hands on blocks or on a chair to protect the back from injury.
- Bend the knee slightly so as not to overstretch the hamstring.

Because of the combined symptoms of rigidity, small and slow movements, and muscle weakness, balance impairments are common in PD. Indeed, falling and the fear of falling lead to significant loss of function and quality of life. Therefore, balance training is a fundamental component of therapy for those with PD to decrease the risk and fear of falling and increase interaction with the community.

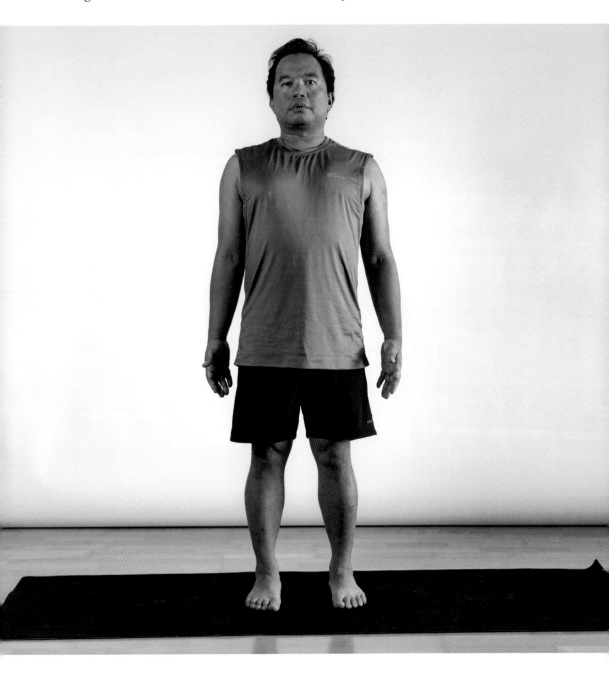

MOUNTAIN Tadasana

Mountain is a great pose to initiate balance and posture training. Mindful standing challenges balance and requires increased muscle activation of the legs and core. This pose is simple enough to allow you to focus on important components of balance in PD: upright posture, equal distribution of weight in the feet, and activation of specific muscle groups, such as the quadriceps and glutes.

Benefits

- Improves balance.
- Improves postural control and awareness.
- Strengthens the hip extensors.
- Strengthens the knee extensors.

How To

1. Start by standing with your feet hip width apart, with a wall behind you or a chair next to you for support if needed.
2. Ground down through all four corners of both feet, lifting the toes, then spreading them wide on the ground.
3. Roll the shoulders down the back and relax your arms alongside your body.
4. Turn the palms slightly forward to open the chest.
5. Engage the quadriceps by lifting your kneecaps while grounding down into your feet.
6. Lift the belly slightly up toward your spine while lengthening the tailbone down toward the heels.
7. Breathe here with the goal of lengthening your spine through the crown of the head, while simultaneously grounding down into your feet.
8. Open your chest, lifting the top of the sternum toward the ceiling. Keep the ribs soft.
9. Relax the jaw and allow the gaze to fall onto the wall or an object in front of you, maintaining an elongated neck.
10. Hold for 8 to 10 breath cycles.

Modifications

Practice in a chair with the feet grounded, arms alongside the body, palms still faced forward, and the crown of the head lifted.

Variations

To challenge yourself, close your eyes, but be sure you have a wall behind you or next to you in case you lose your balance.

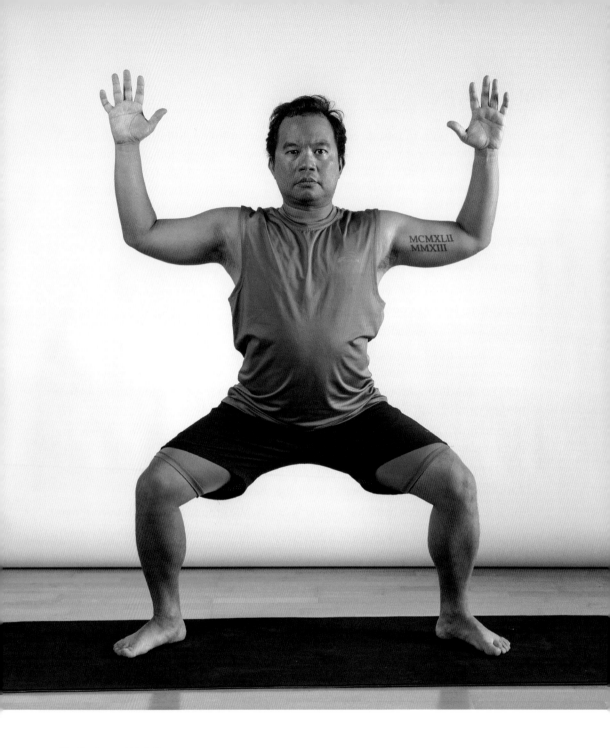

GODDESS

Utkata Konasana

The most difficult aspect of balance in PD is forward and backward control. Because posture and muscle tone are altered, their tendency is to keep COM behind the BOS, leading to a posterior loss of balance, increasing the chance of falls. In Goddess, externally rotating the hips to point the toes away from the midline and focusing on core support forces you to maintain control of forward and backward balance.

Benefits

- Improves balance.
- Stretches the shoulder adductors.
- Stretches the hip adductors.
- Strengthens the hip extensors and abductors.
- Strengthens the knee extensors.

How To

1. Start in Mountain (pages 216-217), and step or jump the feet wide apart on the mat, so that if your arms were outstretched, the ankles would be in line with (over) the ankles.
2. Rotating from the hips, turn the toes out to point to the edges of the mat at 45 degree angles in relation to your midline.
3. Exhale and bend the knees out over the ankles in the same linear plane as the feet.
4. Lower the buttocks down as low as is comfortable, with the goal of eventually lowering them in line with the knees.
5. Stretch the arms out and bend at your elbows so the fingers point up and the palms face forward.
6. Lengthen through your tailbone and engage the core muscles.
7. Hold for 5 to 8 breath cycles, or repeat five times, alternating between straight and bent arms or legs.

Modifications

- Practice the pose in a chair with the feet grounded. Using just your arms, exhale to bring the elbows down and inhale to extend the arms up, repeating several times.
- Bring the arms to Prayer Hands (pages 118-119) at the heart instead of out with bent elbows.

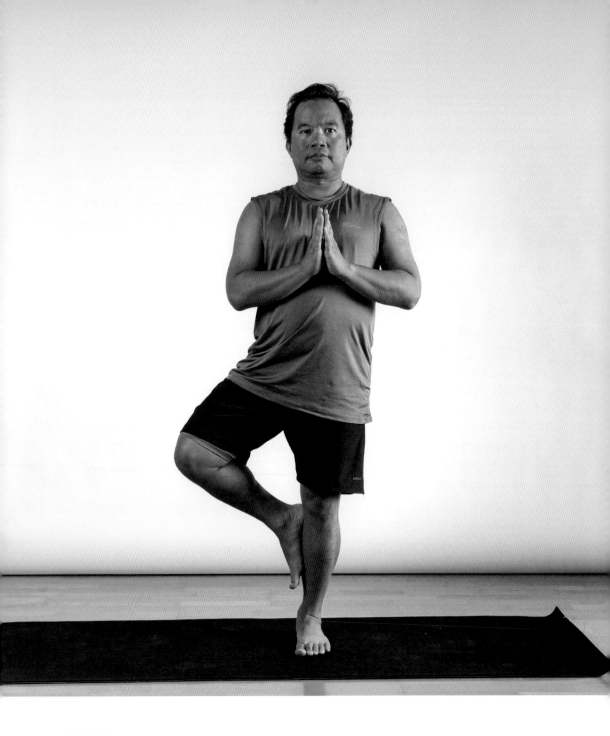

TREE Vrksasana

To improve balance, you must challenge it. Standing on a single leg provides a multidirectional challenge that requires significant lower extremity and core strength. Also, focusing on balance trains you to bring attention to your COM when the BOS is narrowed, thus helping to prevent falls. Depending on the stage of your PD, the traditional version of Tree may be too challenging and should be modified as needed.

Benefits

- Improves balance.
- Strengthens the knee extensors (stance leg).
- Strengthens the hip abductors (stance leg).
- Strengthens the ankle muscles.
- Strengthens the intrinsic foot muscles.

Precautions

Be careful if you have knee instability.

How To

1. Start in Mountain (pages 216-217), with a firm footing on the ground and your gaze focused on an object in front of you.
2. Shift all of your weight to your left leg and bend your right knee up into your chest, catching hold of the knee with your hands.
3. Hold your right ankle with your right hand and place the foot onto your inner calf muscle.
4. Press the left calf back into your right foot so the foot does not overpower the standing leg or cause it to bow out.
5. Reach your arms overhead or keep the hands to prayer at heart center.
6. Lengthen through your tailbone and engage the abdomen as you draw the shoulder blades down the back and open the heart space.
7. Hold for 5 to 10 breath cycles.
8. To exit the pose, step your right foot down and shake it out.
9. Repeat on the other side.

Modifications

- If you have poor balance, try practicing next to a wall or chair. To do so, stand next to a wall at the side of your standing leg. Place your hand on the wall for extra support.
- Keep the toes on the ground with the heel on the ankle if your balance is too challenged with the foot on the calf. Avoid placing the foot on the opposite knee.

Variations

- To add a balance challenge, reach your arms overhead.
- If you feel comfortable and unchallenged with the foot on the calf, you can bring the foot up to the opposite thigh.

Because of factors such as decreased activity levels, small amplitude of movements, and other motor symptoms associated with PD, general weakness is common. Maintaining or improving strength can affect your balance, function, and pain. While the poses just discussed will facilitate improved strength, we will now highlight three muscle groups that, if strengthened, can improve function in PD: hip extensors, knee extensors, and plantar flexors.

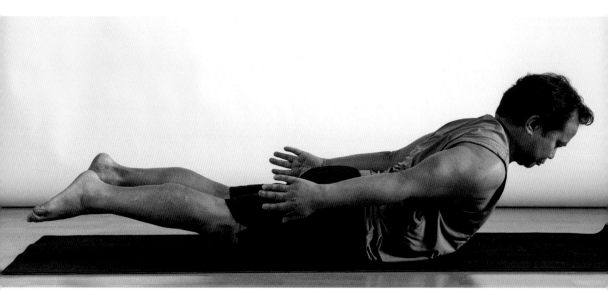

LOCUST Salabhasana

Standing up from a low surface is a functional movement that is commonly difficult for those with PD. This is due to a combination of postural, balance, and strength deficits. The primary therapy to address difficulty standing is to strengthen the hip extensors. Several of the poses already discussed in this chapter will facilitate strengthening of the hip extensors. In particular, Locust allows active isolation of the gluteal muscles and strengthens the postural spinal muscles with the lift of both the legs and chest.

Benefits

- Improves spinal extension.
- Strengthens the hip extensors.

Precautions

Avoid this pose if you are pregnant or if you have severe stenosis of the lumbar spine.

How To

1. Start by lying face down with your forehead on the mat, with hands alongside your body, palms facing the hips.
2. Interlace the fingers as you squeeze the shoulder blades toward each other or keep the hands apart if more comfortable.
3. Inhale, and with the action of dragging your shoulder blades down your back, extend your head, chest, and arms up and back off the mat.
4. Lifting the belly button up and in, start to lift your legs off the mat with the action of reaching the feet behind you and slightly toward each other.
5. Firm and strengthen the legs and buttocks as you extend your arms farther back toward your feet, and your legs higher.
6. Allow the gaze to relax forward or upward, but you can also look down if this is uncomfortable for your neck.
7. You should be balancing on your belly and pelvis.
8. Hold for 5 to 8 breath cycles.
9. Rest by releasing the finger interlace, relaxing the body down, and turning one cheek to the mat.
10. Repeat three more times.

Modifications

- Rest the forehead on the mat to avoid neck strain.
- Place the hands on the ground alongside the body and just lift the legs, *or* keep the legs on the mat and extend the arms only.
- Unlock the hands and extend the arms at your side.

Variations

- *Challenge variations:* Interlace the fingers behind your back and draw the biceps toward each other for increased lift in the chest, *or* reach the arms forward like Superman flying, lifting the hands and feet up and away from the mat.
- *Restorative variation:* Place a bolster under the chest and rest the chest on the bolster. This still allows you to experience spinal extension.

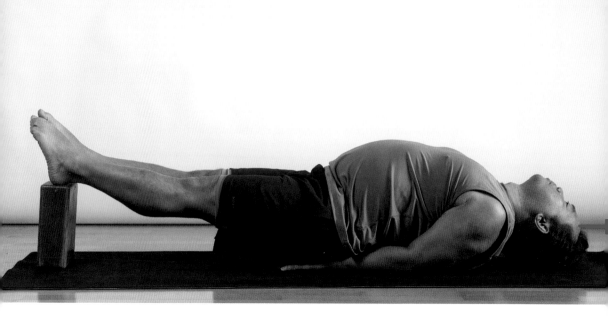

FISH WITH LEGS LIFTED Matsyasana

Increasing knee extensor strength has been shown to improve the quality and efficiency of gait in those with PD. Often the knees remain flexed during the gait cycle (due to small movements). This leads to decreased use of the knee extensors and weakness over time. Many of the poses in the section on large amplitude movements facilitate knee extensor strength. One of the strongest knee extensor muscles (rectus femoris, one of the muscles in the quadriceps muscle group) crosses the hip and knee joint, therefore performing hip flexion and knee extension together with strong activation of this muscle.

A shuffling walking pattern is common in PD. In this pattern, the plantar flexors (calf muscles) are not adequately utilized to push off the ground with the back foot when walking. This greatly reduces stride length and the amount of foot clearance from the ground. It is important to strengthen the plantar flexors while building awareness to their action and purpose. Pointing the toes in Fish With Legs Lifted activates the ankle plantar flexors.

Benefits

- Extends the thoracic spine.
- Strengthens the hip flexors.
- Strengthens the knee extensors.
- Stabilizes the core.

Precautions

Modify this pose by avoiding the neck extension if you have a neck injury.

How To

1. Start by lying on your back on the floor with the knees bent.
2. Lift your hips and slide the hands under the buttocks.
3. Scoot the elbows toward each other to lift the torso and head, creating a kickstand with your elbows.
4. Arch the back, with the chest puffed out, and walk the elbows farther in toward each other.
5. Release the top of your head to the ground. If it does not reach, place a block under the crown of the head.
6. Lift the legs so that they are at a 45 degree angle from the floor, keeping the quadriceps engaged. You can also keep the knees bent to take the strain out of your hips.
7. Point the toes for increased leg strengthening.
8. Hold for 3 to 5 breath cycles.

Modifications

- Keep the legs on the floor and bend the knees with the feet on the floor; you'll still obtain the benefits of the thoracic backbend.
- Rest the feet on blocks for hip flexor support.
- Place a block under your head if your head does not reach the floor behind you.
- If this is too much strain on the back, lift only one leg at a time.

Variations

- *Challenge variation:* Lift the feet off the block to activate and strengthen the core and hip flexor muscles.
- *Restorative variation:* Place a block lengthwise between your shoulder blades and a block flat behind the back of your head.

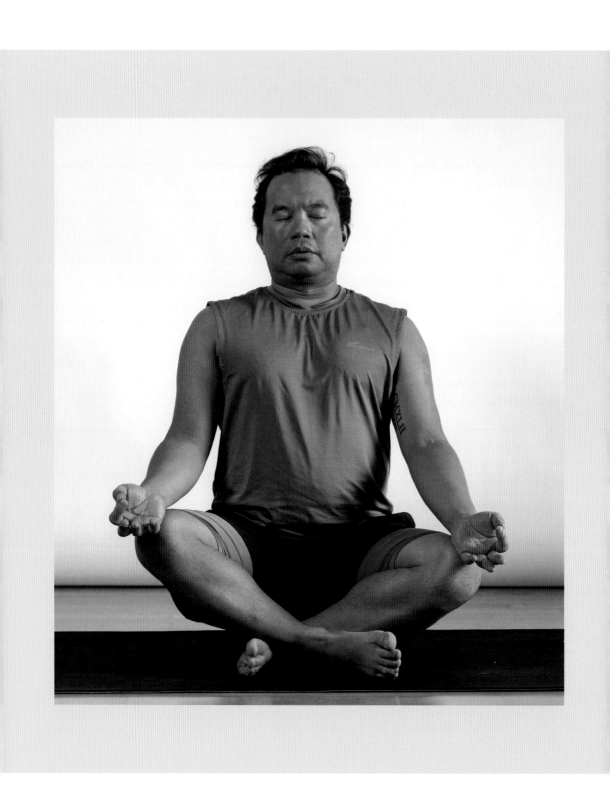

CHANTING

Many of us think of yoga as a set of exercises that enhance flexibility and stamina, with an occasional short meditation thrown in for its calming effects. Thousands of years ago, the rishis, or seers, of India gave us the systems of yoga to bring us into a state of harmony, peace, and ultimately, union with the Divine. Chanting falls under one of the eight limbs of yoga under svadyaya (self-reflection or self-study). But less recognized, chanting is also a form of pranayama (breathing exercise) because each line is chanted on an exhale. Chanting in yoga class is a way to tap into the deeper parts of your being and to connect with your spirit.

Clinically speaking, chanting also helps with breath control for the individual with Parkinson's.[28] Treating a quieted voice has demonstrated improvements in speech among individuals with PD.[22] Training loudness with a focus on specific techniques that improve voice volume has been shown to increase voice amplitude and improve orofacial coordination. Additionally, high-effort voice projection with multiple repetitions also improves voice and facial function.[17] As mentioned earlier, LSVT can also result in improvements in articulation.[26] Part of the neuromuscular pathology of PD involves diaphragmatic weakness, as well as weakness of the accessory respiratory muscles. With chanting in yoga, we increase our ability to exhale deeply, which can enhance phonatory function in PD.

1. Chant *Om* (pronounced A-U-M) with an emphasis on each of the three sounds separately to feel the vibration of each sound distinctly.

2. Start by sitting comfortably on the mat or a chair.

3. Place the backs of the hands on your knees with a focus on lifting the chest and relaxing the shoulders, or bring your hands into Prayer Hands (pages 118-119).

4. Inhale deeply through the nose.

5. As you exhale, open the mouth wide and start to emit the sound *aaaaaaaa* from the depths of your throat. Note that this is not a forceful exhale, but a slow and deliberate emitting of the sound with the goal of loud volume and lengthened exhale.

6. Feel the vibration of the sounds releasing from your entire chest and belly.

7. Transition to the U sound by emitting the sound of *ooooooo* by rounding your lips and concaving the roof of your mouth.

8. Finish with *mmmmmmmm* by closing your lips and feeling the high-frequency vibration in the top of your throat and in your mouth.

9. Use the entire length of the exhale to complete the chant. Spend equal time on each of the three sounds.

10. An important component of chanting *Om* is to allow a moment of silence at the end of the chant.

11. Inhale through your nose with closed lips and repeat again for a total of three or more chants.

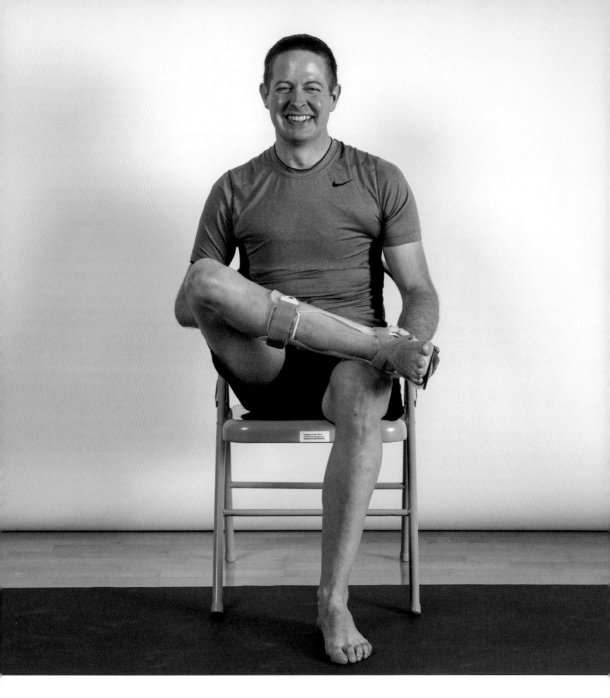

CHAPTER 9

Stroke

A stroke occurs when there is poor or blocked blood flow to a portion of the brain, causing cell damage or death. The result is that the brain does not function properly, with varying levels of severity depending on where the damage occurred and the severity of the damage.[17] A stroke, also known as cerebrovascular accident (CVA), is categorized into two different types:

- *Ischemic:* a blood vessel becomes blocked; tissue that receives blood from this vessel is affected
- *Hemorrhagic:* a blood vessel ruptures, causing bleeding in the brain; due to increased pressure, tissue that receives blood from this vessel as well as surrounding tissue is damaged[3]

Depending on which vessel is compromised, different areas of the brain are affected, influencing the patient's presentation. Hemiparesis, or muscular weakness of the arm and leg on one side of the body, is the most common symptom following a stroke.[4] This side of the body is known as the hemiparetic or affected side. Additional symptoms may include weakness, numbness, slurred speech, or problems with vision.

Strokes are the fourth leading cause of death and the number one cause of disability in older adults in the United States; there are an estimated 6.6 million stroke survivors living in the United States. Approximately 800,000 strokes occur each year in the United States. The prevalence of strokes increases dramatically with age.[4]

Although the most apparent deficit after stroke is typically weakness on the hemiparetic side, there is often significant weakness on what appears to be the strong side.[6] The severity of weakness following a stroke is correlated to a person's independence in performing many functional tasks, including standing, going up and down stairs, and walking.[2] In fact, at three months post-stroke, about 80 percent of people experience difficulty walking.[1]

It is important to note that although symptoms present as weakness or muscle stiffness in the arm, leg, and trunk, there is no direct injury or damage to the musculoskeletal system post-stroke. These symptoms are a direct effect of vascular injury to the brain. However, there are commonly secondary effects of increased weakness, stiffness, and pain that are caused by disuse of the extremities or by moving with compensatory strategies.[5]

Strength training post-stroke has been found to result in improvements in the performance of functional activities.[6] A major goal of post-stroke rehabilitation is to strengthen and stretch muscle to correct posture and asymmetric movement patterns.[5] Yoga can be utilized to achieve this rehabilitative goal, and so much more.

New research suggests that adding yoga to stroke rehabilitation therapy improves the speed and extent of recovery. For example, those who participate in yoga may experience increased flexibility, improved balance, increased strength, a greater range of motion in the neck and hip, and less pain.[17] In addition, because yoga requires intense focus, it enhances neuroplasticity—the ability of the brain's neurons to reorganize, regain function, and form new connections.[19] This enables the brain to correct or adapt to damage caused by a stroke. In stroke patients, yoga has also been found to improve quality of life, reduce fear of falling, and increase independence with daily living activities.[16] Not only does yoga improve balance and flexibility, it has also been shown to result in a stronger and faster gait, longer steps, and increased strength and endurance.[18] In addition, yoga stresses the importance of linking breath to movement, which enhances the overall impact of rehabilitation. Many times, patients hold their breath while exercising, a habit that can negate the benefit of exercise.

GENERAL GUIDELINES

- After a stroke, patients commonly use an ankle or foot brace for balance and stability when standing. If preferred, this brace can be worn during the yoga practice.
- Strengthening all muscle groups is beneficial in those who had a stroke, but emphasis should be placed on the antigravity muscles (hip extensors, knee extensors, and plantar flexors).
- Postural deficits are common. Post-stroke patients typically demonstrate a forward-flexed (bent forward at the waist) posture and may also be leaning toward their hemiparetic side. It is important to strengthen the hip extensors and paraspinal muscles as well as the obliques bilaterally.
- Balance deficits are an ongoing issue after a stroke. It is essential to progressively challenge balance to develop balance and strength. Make modifications to maintain safety while you are working on balance training.
- Using props such as blocks, bolsters, chairs, foam rollers, and more is encouraged.

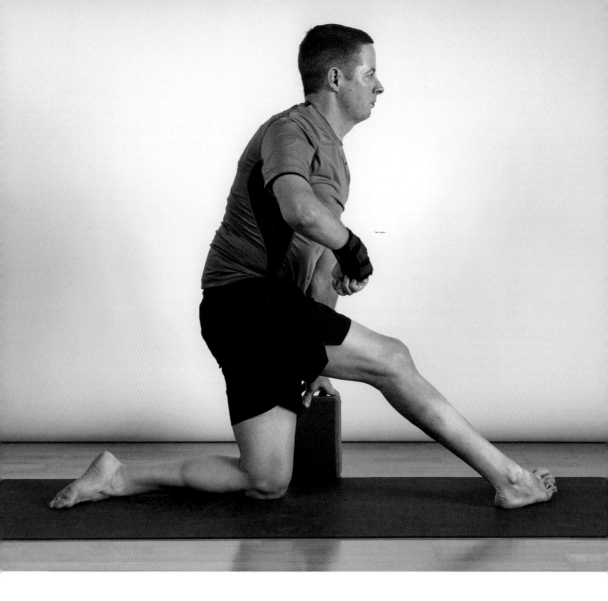

HALF SPLITS

Ardha Hanumanasana

Post-stroke, it is common for muscle weakness to be more prevalent distally than proximally (the ankle is weaker than the hip and the wrist is weaker than the shoulder).[2] Weakness of the plantar flexors (calves) is common in the affected limb and can contribute to several gait deviations. Weakness in this muscle group can lead to a decreased step length (which reduces walking speed), cause hyperextension of the knee (which can cause knee damage), or contribute to the knee staying bent throughout the gait cycle (which can increase the energy required to walk).[8] Half Splits puts the front leg into a nonweight-bearing position in which the ankle can be seen, allowing for visual feedback for the ankle to move into plantar flexion (toes pointed to the ground).

Benefits

- Strengthens the plantar flexors.
- Strengthens the arms and shoulders.
- Strengthens the spinal extensors.
- Stretches the knee flexors.

Precautions

Avoid hyperextending the front knee.

How To

1. Start in Crescent Lunge (pages 238-239), with your right foot forward and your back (left) knee on the ground (use a folded blanket under the knee for cushioning).
2. Steady your hands on blocks, the wall, or a chair to assist your balance.
3. Begin to straighten your front (right) leg by shifting the hips back until they stack over your back knee.
4. Make sure that you feel a stretch, but not strain, in the hamstrings. If you begin to feel strain, maintain a slight bend in the front knee or bring your hands up higher on blocks.
5. Point the toes to ground the ball of the foot down into the mat.
6. Engage your front quadriceps to avoid overextending the knee.
7. Activate the core muscles for balance and breathe here.
8. Hold for 5 to 10 breath cycles.
9. To exit the pose, bend the front knee back into Crescent Lunge and switch sides.

Modifications

Place a block under the front hamstring for more support.

Variations

To challenge yourself, place hands on the mat on either side of your front leg instead of using blocks. If you can maintain your balance, extend your spine long over the front leg, hinging from the hips.

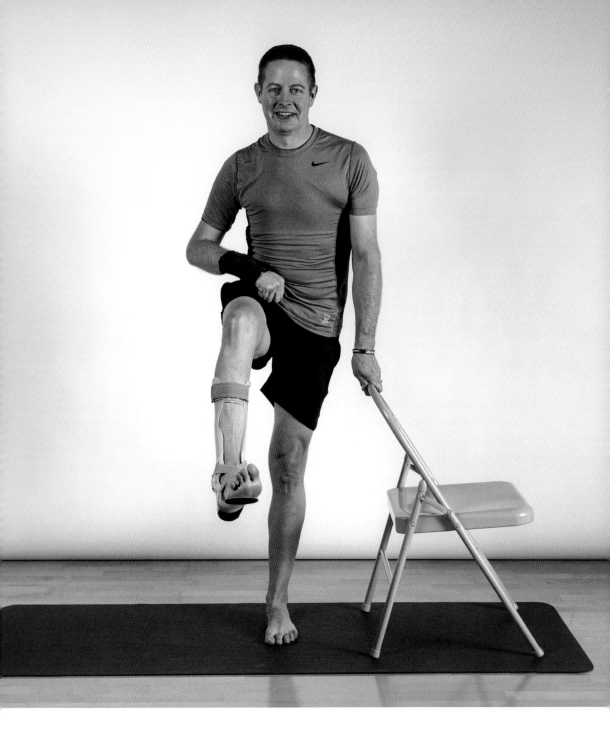

EXTENDED HAND-TO-TOE

Utthita Hasta Padangusthasana

Ankle weakness is common after a stroke, so the hip flexor muscles must be strong to lift the leg to clear the toes when walking (compensating for weak dorsiflexors) and progress the leg forward during gait (to compensate for a lack of push-off due to weak plantar flexors). Hand-to-Toe is highly modifiable and all forms can be utilized to strengthen the hip flexors. Additionally, the dorsiflexors are strengthened by actively flexing the ankle in this pose. When practiced in a modified manner, instead of in traditional Hand-to-Toe, support the thigh with the hand by hooking the hand under the leg. Or if you do not have adequate use of the hand, just lift the corresponding knee up, as pictured.

Benefits

- Strengthens the hip flexors.
- Strengthens the knee extensors.
- Strengthens the dorsiflexors.
- Strengthens the stance hip abductors.

How To

1. Start in Mountain (pages 150-151), with a chair next to your strong leg.
2. Place the strong side hand on the back of a chair next to you.
3. Shift your weight into your strong leg.
4. Bend your weak (hemiparetic) leg up toward your belly. If you'd like, you can scoop up the thigh with your hand.
5. Notice the strength of your standing leg, keep your hand on the chair to maintain your balance, and try to lift the weak side knee higher.
6. Hold for 3 breath cycles and when ready, place the foot back down into Mountain.
7. To exit this pose, sit on the chair to rest.

Modifications

- If you feel unbalanced, you can practice from a seated position, as pictured here.
- You can place the top leg's foot on a chair or an upright block in front of you and practice lifting and relaxing the foot.

Variations

To challenge yourself, try to straighten the raised leg.

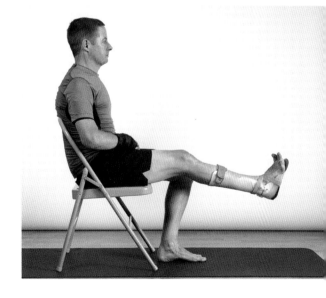

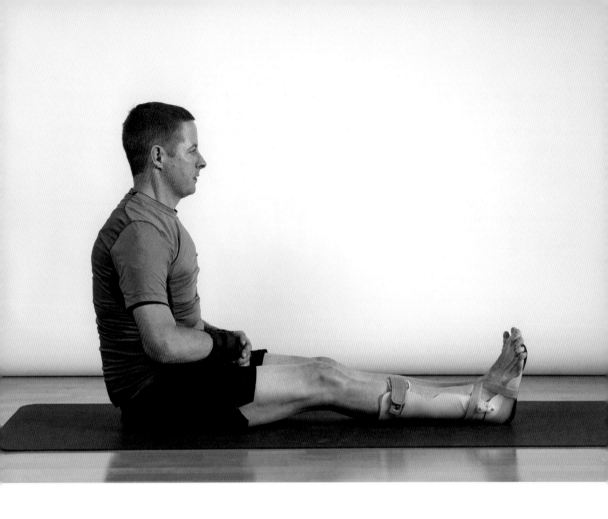

STAFF

Dandasana

Weakness in the knee extensors (quadriceps) increases the risk of the knee buckling, which can lead to a fall; so much so that ankle braces are often used to provide external stability to the knee. Staff activates and strengthens the knee extensors in a stable position in which you receive visual feedback because you see the quadriceps activating and the knees extending.

Benefits

- Strengthens the knee extensors.
- Strengthens the dorsiflexors.
- Strengthens the core.
- Stretches the knee flexors.

How To

1. Start seated with your legs extended in front of you, hands resting beside your hips or in your lap, as pictured.
2. Dorsiflex your feet, extending out through the heels and pointing the toes up and toward your nose.
3. Press the backs of the knees down into the mat as you engage the quadriceps.
4. Roll the shoulders back and engage the belly.
5. Hold for 5 to 10 breath cycles.

Modifications

- Sit facing a wall with your feet flat against the wall to make yourself aware of the dorsiflexion. Press the heels firmly into the wall.
- To emphasize strengthening of the affected side, isolate one leg at a time.
- Wrap a strap around the bottoms of your feet and hold the ends of the strap in your hands to assist with straightening the legs and dorsiflexing the feet.

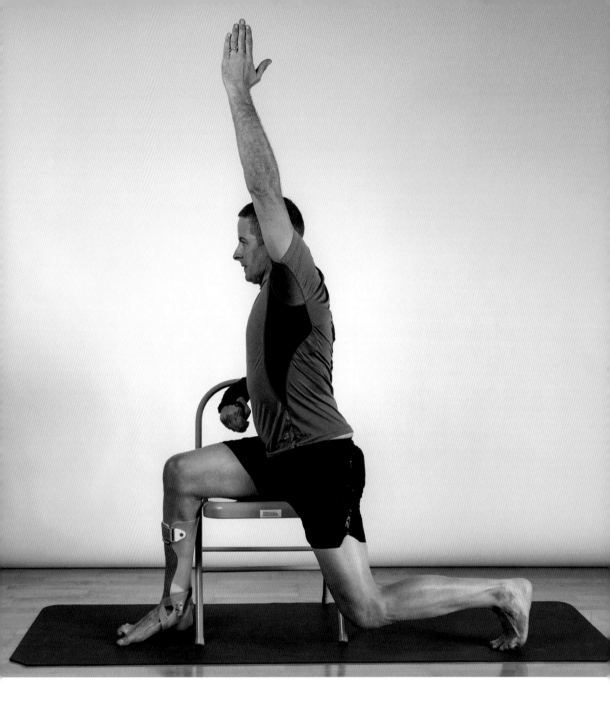

CRESCENT LUNGE

A lunge position is an excellent way to strengthen the knee extensors, decreasing the risk of knee buckling and protecting the knee joint. Because stride length can be adjusted according to ability, Crescent Lunge is an excellent pose to strengthen the knee extensors. Additionally, adductor tightness can create a narrow base of support during standing and walking, contributing to balance deficits. Crescent Lunge addresses this by providing a stretch to the adductors (groin) of the back leg.

Benefits

- Strengthens the knee extensors.
- Strengthens the plantar flexors (back foot).
- Strengthens the hip extensors (back leg).
- Stretches the hip adductors (back leg).

Precautions

Avoid the full expression of this pose if you have severe balance deficits, and instead, utilize the chair as instructed below.

How To

1. Start in Mountain (pages 150-151), with a chair in front of you. Place the weak side hand on the back of the chair and step the weak foot forward over the chair. Use your opposite hand to assist the leg if needed.
2. Rest your front (weak) thigh on the seat of the chair.
3. With the front leg bent and the thigh parallel to the floor, resting on the chair's seat, keep the hand on the chairback, and inhale your arms up to the sky if able. If you do not feel balanced in this, keep your hands on the chair.
4. Try to straighten the back leg as you press back through your left heel. Square the hips forward and attempt to slightly lift your front thigh off of the seat of the chair.
5. Lift the lower abdomen up and in as you lengthen the tailbone down.
6. Draw the shoulders down the back, and gaze forward or slightly up between your hands.
7. Hold for 5 breath cycles.
8. To exit the pose, use your hands on the chair for steadiness and straighten your front leg.
9. Sit on the chair to rest.
10. Repeat with your other (strong) side forward, but do so standing without the front thigh on the seat to strengthen the quadriceps of the front leg. Hold onto a chair for balance as needed.

Modifications

If this hurts your knee, shorten your stance, and reduce the deep knee bend of the front leg.

Variations

To challenge yourself, press down into the feet and try to lift the front thigh off the seat of the chair. Engage the core abdominal muscles.

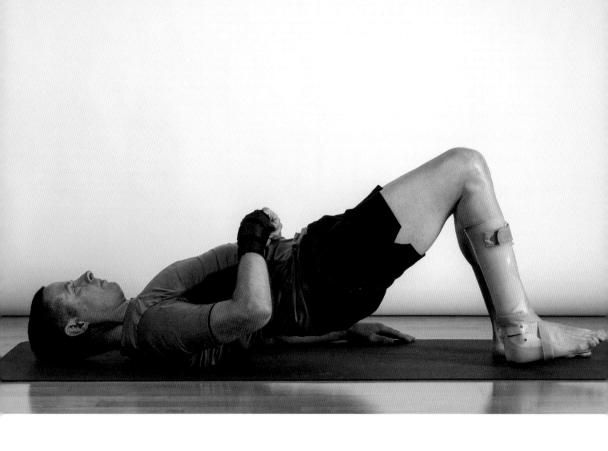

BRIDGE

Setu Bandha Sarvangasana

Strength of the hip extensors is essential for maintaining an upright posture and not bending forward at the waist when standing or walking. Reliance on an assistive device (cane, walker, etc.) and decreased activity level can lead to weakness in the hip extensors. Common in post-stroke, weakness in the hip extensors alters walking posture, which results in a flexed-forward posture at the waist. This abnormal posture increases the risk of knee buckling because the weight of the trunk changes weight-bearing dynamics, pathologically shifting the weight to the front of the knee joint. Bridge improves hip extensor strength and also strengthens the posterior muscles of the trunk and leg to support an upright posture.

Benefits

- Strengthens the hip extensors.
- Strengthens the spinal extensors.
- Strengthens the knee flexors.
- Stretches the hip flexors.

Precautions

Avoid this pose if you have a current or recent cervical spine injury.

Before You Begin

Have a strap or a block handy for modifications.

How To

1. Start by lying on your back with your knees bent, feet flat on the floor, and arms alongside your body with palms facing down.
2. Roll your shoulders underneath you as you begin to lift your hips.
3. Press your feet and shoulders into the mat as you lift your hips.
4. As you rise, walk the feet closer to your buttocks and scoot your shoulders into midline to further elevate the hips and lengthen the tailbone.
5. Knees remain parallel as you engage the inner thighs.
6. Arms remain on the floor, if possible, to support the lift of the hips.
7. Keep your neck neutral by relaxing your chin away from your chest to preserve the natural curve of your cervical spine.
8. Your shoulders, feet, and back of the head support your lift comfortably on the mat because you are using the muscles of your buttocks and back to lengthen your hips.
9. Hold for 5 to 10 breath cycles.
10. To exit the pose, release the hands and slowly roll down your spine.

Modifications

- Place a block between the knees to keep the thighs parallel and in line with the hips.
- Place a block under your hips if the legs cannot support holding the pose.

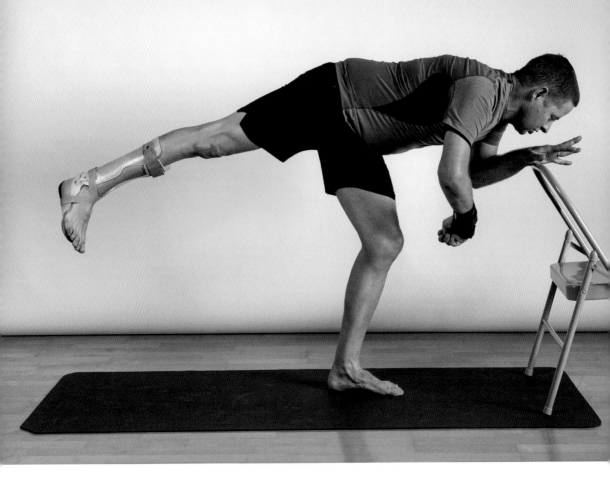

WARRIOR III
Virabhadrasana III

Warrior III is a progression of Bridge in strengthening the hip extensors as well as the knee flexors and spinal extensors. While walking, the hip extensors are used for forward propulsion, therefore hip extensor strength is correlated with faster walking speeds post-stroke.[2] In stroke rehabilitation, gait speed is considered the sixth vital sign; it is correlated with functional mobility, quality of life, and mortality.[13] Post-stroke, to increase stability while walking, the knees tend to stay bent as a compensatory strategy and a co-contraction of both the knee flexors and extensors is often utilized. This can lead to knee flexor tightness. Working to straighten the weak leg as it is elevated in Warrior III can help decrease this knee flexor tightness and improve gait mechanics.

Benefits

- Strengthens the hip extensors.
- Strengthens the spinal extensors.
- Strengthens the dorsiflexors.
- Strengthens and stretches the knee flexors.

Precautions

Perform this pose with the modifications below or with assistive devices (walker, chair, wall, etc.) if you have severe balance deficits.

How To

1. Start in Crescent Lunge (pages 238-239), with the strong foot forward and a chair in front of you.
2. Reach the arms forward and place the hands (or just the strong hand if the weak side arm is contracted) on the back of the chair. If you need to, step your feet forward to reach the chair.
3. Put all your weight onto the strong leg and start to lean the torso forward.
4. Push off of the weak leg, lifting it straight back behind you.
5. Bring the torso and back leg as parallel to the ground as possible, with the goal of creating a T shape with the body.
6. Dorsiflex the lifted foot by pointing the toes to the ground and pressing the heel back in space.
7. Straighten your standing leg by engaging the front quadriceps muscles, but without hyperextending the knee.
8. Internally rotate the back hip so the foot points down to the ground.
9. Continue pressing the standing foot into the ground so as not to collapse into the hip socket, and engage the core muscles.
10. Hold for 3 to 5 breath cycles.
11. To exit the pose, step the lifted foot back into Crescent Lunge or Mountain (pages 150-151).

Modifications

Stand next to a wall, at the side of your strong or standing leg, and place your hand on the wall for extra support.

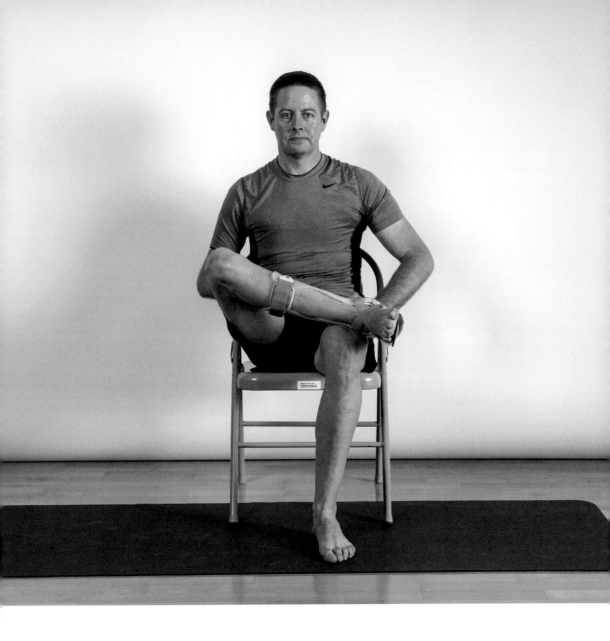

ANKLE-OVER-KNEE

Galavasana

The ankle muscles are commonly affected after a stroke, and typically to a fairly severe degree.[9] Dorsiflexor weakness makes it difficult to lift the toes high enough when stepping forward, creating a risk of catching the foot and tripping. It is common for those who have had a stroke to use a brace to assist in toe clearance. Ankle-Over-Knee allows for active dorsiflexion of the ankle with visual feedback.

Benefits

- Strengthens the ankle dorsiflexors (bent leg).
- Stretches the hip adductors (bent leg).
- Stretches the hip internal rotators (bent leg).
- Strengthens the spinal extensors.

Precautions

Avoid this pose if you have a current or recent knee ligament injury.

How To

1. Sit in a chair with both feet on the floor.
2. Use your hands under the thigh to bring the right leg into your chest.
3. Hook your left hand under the right ankle or foot to rotate the right hip open and place the right foot over the left knee.
4. Use the left hand to dorsiflex the right foot, and the right hand to gently press the right knee down toward the earth.
5. The hands can remain on the foot and knee or come into Prayer Hands (pages 118-119) at the heart.
6. Hold for 3 to 5 breath cycles.
7. To exit the pose, place the hands under the right thigh and ankle again, and rotate the hip back in line with the body as you place the right foot next to the left.
8. Repeat on the left side.

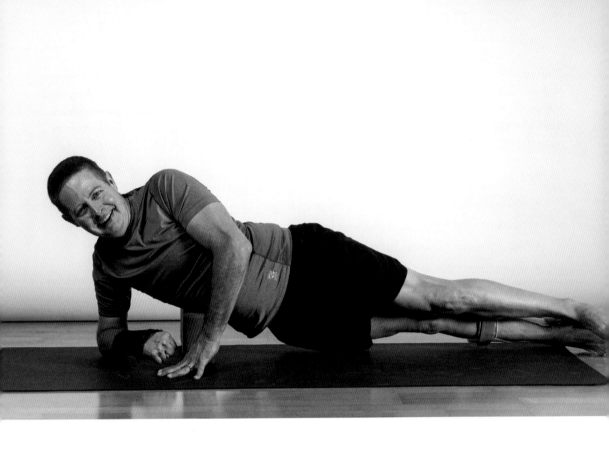

SIDE PLANK

Vasisthasana

Hemiparesis can affect an entire side of your body. While deficits to the arm and leg are most notable, weakness is commonly present in the core muscles as well. Side Plank can help to strengthen the obliques on the affected side. This pose also strengthens the hip abductors, which provide stability while you are standing on one leg. Additionally, this pose involves weight bearing through the affected upper extremity, promoting strength and stabilization.

Benefits

- Strengthens the obliques.
- Strengthens the hip abductors.
- Strengthens the shoulder.
- Strengthens the knee extensors.

How To

1. Start by lying on your weak side.
2. With the assistance of your strong (top) arm on the mat in front of you, come up onto your weak side's forearm.
3. Keeping the strong arm's hand in front of you for balance, press into your weak forearm and lift the hips up and away from the mat. In this move, you will have somewhat rolled onto the front of your shin.
4. Continue to lift up out of the bottom hip so you are balancing on your elbow and bottom foot.
5. Engage the core and lift the outer thighs up to the sky.
6. Hold for 3 to 5 breath cycles.
7. Repeat on the other side.

Modifications

Perform the pose with your back against a wall for support with the legs straight.

Variations

To challenge yourself, come up onto your feet instead of resting on the knee, *or* come up onto your hand instead of resting on the elbow.

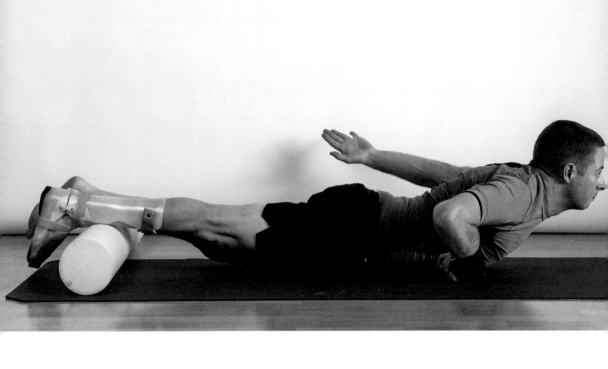

LOCUST Salabhasana

Strengthening the spinal extensors helps you achieve an upright posture and improve walking endurance. Spinal extensor activation decreases with the use of assistive devices and due to increased time spent sitting. Locust provides isolated bilateral spinal extension activation, reminding the body how to activate and utilize this muscle group. Additionally, the unaffected hand can assist the affected arm to straighten behind the back, stretching the affected elbow flexors (biceps). The affected elbow flexors can be tight because the arm often rests with the elbow bent.

Benefits

- Strengthens the spinal extensors.
- Strengthens the hip extensors.
- Stretches the elbow flexors.
- Strengthens the knee extensors.
- Strengthens the ankle plantar flexors.

How To

1. Start by lying face down with your forehead on the mat, hands alongside your hips, palms facing up.
2. Inhale, and with the action of dragging your shoulder blades down your back, extend your head, chest, and arms up and back off the mat.
3. Lifting the belly button up and in, start to lift your legs off the mat with the action of reaching the feet behind you and slightly toward each other. If the legs do not lift, focus on lifting the chest and engaging the belly for optimal spinal extension.
4. Firm and strengthen the legs and buttocks as you extend your arms further back toward your feet, and your legs higher.
5. Allow the gaze to extend forward on the ground or to the space in front of you; you can also look down if that's more comfortable for your neck.
6. You should be balancing on your lower belly and pelvis and engaging the shoulder blades toward midline behind your back.
7. Hold for 5 to 8 breath cycles.
8. Rest by releasing the body down, turning one cheek to the mat, and taking a few breaths.
9. Repeat three more times.

Modifications

- Rest the forehead on the mat during the pose to avoid neck strain.
- Use a foam roller or rolled-up blanket under the hemiparetic ankle to support your legs.

Variations

To challenge yourself, interlace the fingers behind your back and draw the biceps toward each other for increased lift in the chest, *or* reach the arms forward like Superman flying, lifting the arms forward next to your ears and the feet up and away from the mat.

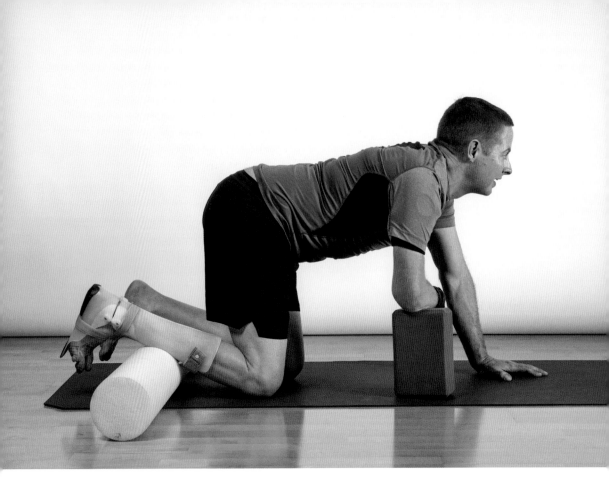

TABLE TOP

Bharmanasana

Weight bearing through the arms brings the head of the humerus (upper arm bone) into close proximity to the socket of the shoulder joint and strengthens the muscles of the shoulder complex. This is important because those who have experienced a stroke may have weakened arms and are at increased risk of shoulder subluxation (partial dislocation). Additionally, weight bearing through the arm activates and strengthens muscles of the elbow and wrist. Table Top allows you to bear weight through the affected arm (and leg) with support from the unaffected extremities. From shifting the weight side to side to lifting an arm or a leg, you can perform several variations of this pose to strengthen the extremities and core.

Benefits

- Strengthens the scapular stabilizers.
- Strengthens the muscles of the shoulder, elbow, and wrist.
- Stretches the wrist and elbow flexors.

Precautions

Avoid this pose if you have a wrist injury.

How To

1. Start in Child's Pose (pages 38-39), with the arms stretched forward. Pull yourself forward on your hands, stacking your hips over the knees and the shoulders over the wrists.
2. Spread the fingers wide, grounding through the thumbs and forefingers.
3. Make sure that the wrist creases are parallel to the front of the mat.
4. Firm the tops of the feet into the mat.
5. Engage the belly button up and in to engage the core abdominal muscles.
6. Relax the shoulders down and elongate the neck by gazing at the front edge of your mat.
7. Knit the ribs in toward midline to firm up the front of the body.
8. Balance your weight evenly between all four limbs.
9. Hold with the core engaged for 5 to 8 breath cycles.

Modifications

- If this hurts your wrists you can come down onto the forearms.
- If you have severe weakness or tightness of an arm, you can still perform the pose on one arm and both legs. Feel free to use a block under the weak arm, as pictured.
- Use a foam roller or rolled-up blanket under the hemiparetic ankle to support your ankles and improve your balance.

Variations

To challenge yourself, lift your weak leg (so the leg still on the ground is your strong leg to maintain balance).

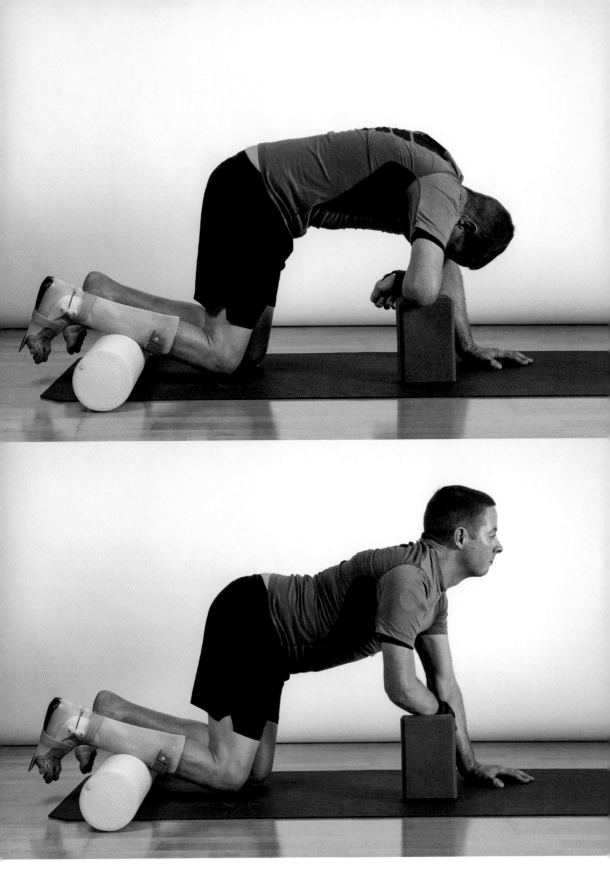

CAT COW

Cat Cow provides all the benefits of Table Top while also improving spine mobility and lumbopelvic control. Because the body is compensating for weakness with compensatory co-contractions, there is generally less movement in the spine during upright activities post-stroke. Cat Cow can help to improve flexion and extension mobility in the spine. Additionally, the active alternation in Cat Cow of the curves of the spine strengthens the core muscles and improves body control.

Benefits

- Improves spinal mobility.
- Strengthens the core.
- Stabilizes the shoulders, elbows, and wrists.
- Stretches the wrist flexors and elbow flexors.

How To

1. Start in Table Top (pages 250-251); be sure your hips are aligned over your knees and your shoulders over your wrists.
2. For Cow, inhale and start to tilt the pelvis as you arch the spine to drop your belly and lift the chest.
3. Press your hands into the mat as you broaden the collarbones and lift the heart to counter the extension of the belly to the floor.
4. For Cat, as you exhale, initiate the spinal movement from the hips to tuck the pelvis underneath you as you start to curve into a rounded spine.
5. In the full expression of Cat, tuck your chin into your chest and tuck your pelvis toward your nose while pressing the hands strongly into the floor.
6. Alternate between Cat and Cow for 5 to 10 breath cycles, inhaling for Cow and exhaling for Cat.

Modifications

- Stand or sit at arm's length from a wall with the hands at the height of your chest, then inhale to lift the chest and arch your back into Cow, then exhale to round your spine into Cat.
- Use a foam roller or rolled-up blanket under the hemiparetic ankle to support your ankles and improve your balance.
- Practice this cycle seated (pages 200-201; see Parkinson's sequence for Cat Cow).
- Place a block under the hemiparetic side to support the arm if that is helpful.

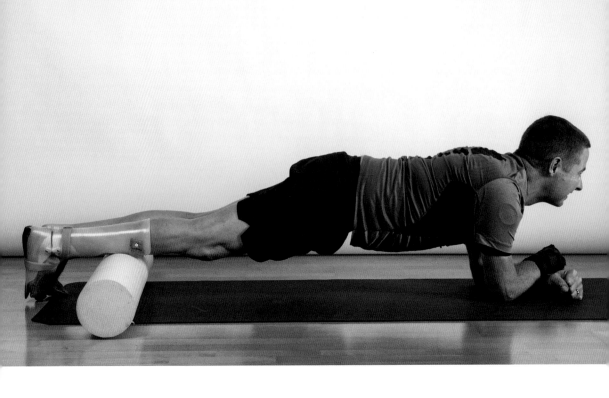

FOREARM PLANK
Phalakasana

Plank strengthens the shoulder complex with an effective isolation of the scapular muscles. These muscles are important for maintaining long-term shoulder mobility and health. Additionally, this pose can be used to strengthen the core muscles, which provide stability during all movements.

Benefits

- Strengthens the shoulder and scapular stabilizers.
- Strengthens the core.
- Strengthens the knee extensors.
- Strengthens the plantar flexors.

How To

1. Start in Table Top (pages 250-251).
2. Walk the elbows down to rest on your forearms, keeping them parallel to one another.
3. Straighten the legs by extending the knees off the floor, pressing back through the heels, and engaging your quadriceps muscles. (Keep the knees down if needed; see the following modification.)
4. Align your body in a straight line from your head and shoulders to your heels.
5. Engage the abdominal muscles in and up, firming your arms in toward midline.
6. Press into the forearms, separating your shoulder blades, drawing your sternum in the direction of your spine, and filling out your thoracic spine.
7. Energize the inner thighs toward each other and up as you press back into your heels and reach forward with your chest, lengthening the spine and neck.
8. Your gaze should rest about two feet in front of the hands on the floor to create a long neck.
9. Be sure the hips do not sag and are in alignment with the chest and legs.
10. Hold for 5 to 8 breath cycles.
11. Come down to rest in Child's Pose (pages 38-39).

Modifications

*   Use a foam roller or rolled-up blanket under the hemiparetic ankle to support your ankles and improve your balance.
*   Place a block under the hips across the width of the hips to support the core. Lift the hips up an inch from the block when ready for more strengthening.
*   Another way to get into the pose is to start in Downward-Facing Dog (pages 90-91), walking the arms down and reaching the chest forward so the hips are in line with the shoulders. You may also start by lying prone and climbing up onto your forearms.
*   *Supported by the knees*: As described, follow the instructions except that in step 3, keep your knees on the ground. Continue engaging the abdominal muscles and hugging the outer arms into midline. Hold for 10 breath cycles and come down to rest in Child's Pose.
*   *Standing:* Face the wall and extend your arms to place your hands on the wall at chest height. Walk the feet back until the hands are at shoulder height and the abdomen engages. You can walk the feet back farther until you feel the upper arm muscles engage. Be sure you are tucking the tailbone so the hips stay in line with the diagonal of the body.

Variations

To challenge yourself, lift one foot off the floor, maintaining neutral position of the hips *or* come up into a full expression of Plank (pages 34-35) with the hands on the mat, aligning the shoulders over the wrists.

THE HOMUNCULUS, MINDFULNESS, AND YOGA NIDRA

Neuroplasticity allows your brain to rewire functions from damaged areas of the brain to new, healthy parts of the brain. A different, healthy area of your brain is capable of picking up the slack. When mobility is affected, for example, new areas of the brain can learn to control the weakened side.[11] After your brain has been damaged by stroke, mood disorders such as anxiety and depression may sometimes prevail.[8] If, instead, you can rewire the brain to participate in a relaxation response via Yoga Nidra, you can use the homunculus and neuroplasticity of the brain to create a whole-hearted, fuller response to the stresses that may arise after a stroke.

The cortical homunculus is a representation of the human body based on a neurological map of the areas of the brain dedicated to processing motor or sensory functions for different parts of the body.[12] Each of the body parts has an existing center in the cerebral gray matter, which researchers have named the *homunculus* or *little man*.[7] Yoga Nidra is a state of consciousness; it is neither sleep nor wakefulness, neither is it concentration nor hypnotism. It can be best defined as an altered state of consciousness.[10] The sequence of rotation of awareness in Yoga Nidra is in accordance with the map in the cerebral gray matter of the brain.[15] When the awareness is rotated in the same sequence again and again, it induces a flow within the neuronal circuit of the homunculus of the brain. This flow brings in a subjective experience of relaxation in the brain. This relaxation response is believed to improve and decrease stress or anxiety, activate the parasympathetic nervous system (the rest and digest portion of the nervous system), and even relieve symptoms of depression.[19]

How To

1. Start by lying in a comfortable position on the mat, palms facing the sky or hands stacked over your heart.
2. Connect to a heartfelt intention or desire during the Yoga Nidra practice.
3. Bring awareness to the breath, not trying to control the breath but resting gentle attention on it.

4. Mentally scan your body. Gradually move your awareness through your body. Sense your jaw, mouth, ears, nose, and eyes. Sense your forehead, scalp, neck, and the inside of your throat. Scan your attention through your left arm and left palm, your right arm and right palm, and then both arms and hands simultaneously. Sense your torso, pelvis, and sacrum. Experience sensation in your left hip, leg, and foot, and then in your right hip, leg, and foot. Sense your entire body as a field of radiant sensation.[14]

5. As you scan the body, notice the sensations that arise. Are you hot or cold? Do you notice aches or tightness? In those places, invite relaxation.

6. Witness your feelings. Do you notice certain emotions that arise during this practice? When you do, touch them lightly with your attention, and let go of them without grasping or following them.

7. After your body scan, allow yourself to rest as long as is comfortable to feel complete relaxation, but without falling asleep.

8. When you are ready, come up to a comfortable seated position to reflect upon the practice.

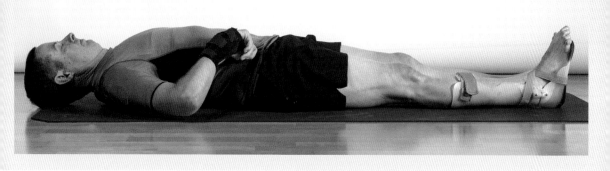

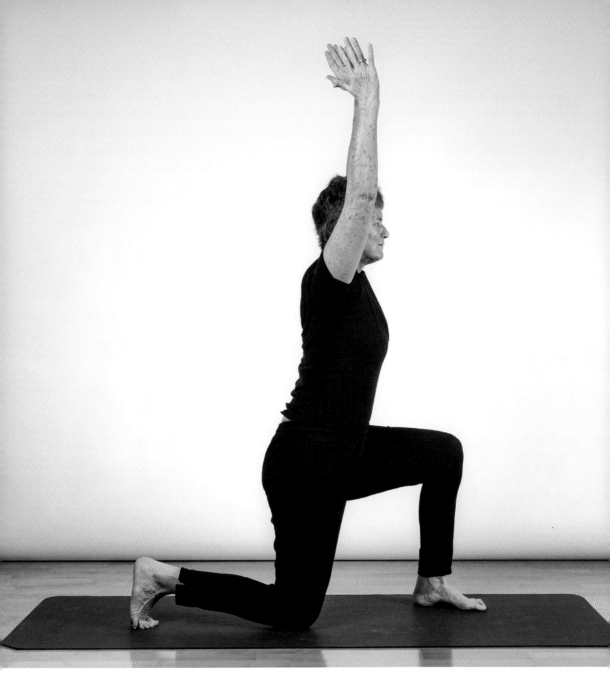

Multiple Sclerosis

Multiple sclerosis (MS) is a chronic neurological disorder in which the body's immune system attacks the brain and the spinal cord, which comprise the central nervous system (CNS). The nerve axons (nerve fibers) in the CNS are wrapped in a fatty substance known as myelin, which acts as an insulator, allowing for effective transmission of signals. In MS, the body's immune system targets and damages myelin in the CNS; this action is known as demyelination. This inflammatory process can also cause damage to the nerve axons themselves, especially in the later stages. Myelin and axonal injury can occur at multiple areas in the CNS, causing impaired nerve conduction and accounting for the wide array of symptoms in MS.[1]

The symptoms of MS are different from patient to patient but commonly include fatigue, spasticity, loss of strength, balance impairments, visual deficits, chronic pain, depression, and cognitive impairment.[3] The onset of the disease typically occurs in young adults aged 20 to 40, and is far more common in females (the ratio of females to males is 3:1).[1] It is estimated that MS affects 400,000 people in the United States and more than 2.5 million people worldwide.[9]

MS has an unpredictable disease course and various patterns of symptom presentation. The most common pattern (80 percent of cases), known as *relapsing-remitting*, is characterized by exacerbations and remissions.[2] Symptoms usually develop over the course of hours to days and then gradually subside over the ensuing weeks to months, though remission may be incomplete. Over time, relapsing-remitting MS may progress to a *secondary-progressive* state, in which there is less symptom resolution between exacerbations.[2]

While current medications for MS are used to ameliorate the severity of exacerbations and reduce the incidence of nerve and myelin damage, there is no cure for MS. Therefore, managing disease progression and symptoms is crucial for maintaining function and quality of life. The National Multiple Sclerosis Society recommends a comprehensive approach for disease management, including exercise and complementary therapies such as yoga.[16]

Although effects on symptom management may vary between individuals, yoga's focus on breath control, strengthening, and flexibility may have therapeutic benefits for patients with MS and improve outcomes such as confidence, mental health, and quality of life. Yoga is a promising method of symptom management for patients with MS.[9]

Pain is a commonly reported symptom for individuals with MS, typically manifesting as back pain, face or eye pain, muscle spasms, pain in the extremities, and headaches.[18] Pain may be a direct symptom of the disease or may arise from secondary causes such as muscle over-contraction. Studies have suggested that participation in a yoga program can lower reports of pain and improve quality of life.[7] MS is a chronic condition and most pain medications are no longer considered appropriate for long-term use; however, alternative pain management strategies such as yoga are beneficial and appropriate.

Mental health is a significant component of quality of life. Up to 50 percent of MS patients experience depression.[8] Increased perceived stress, anxiety, and mental fatigue are also prevalent in individuals with MS.[11] Several studies have explored the effectiveness of nonpharmaceutical approaches to managing mental health in MS. Some of these studies have found that yoga can be an effective tool in lowering levels of depression, anxiety, stress, and fatigue.[8,11,19,20]

Physical symptoms of MS that can be addressed via exercise and yoga include spasticity, balance, and strength. Spasticity, which is present in an estimated 80 percent of MS cases, can cause muscle stiffness, muscle spasms, or cramping.[4] Maintaining muscle flexibility and joint mobility are common treatment goals in patients with MS. Yoga for individuals with MS has been found to significantly improve balance, walking speed, and functional strength.[12,22]

Exercise has multiple benefits, including improving several aspects of physical and mental health for individuals with MS. Yoga is a form of exercise that is regarded as safe and that can be made more accessible for those with MS than many other forms of exercise. In this chapter, we present poses and modifications to address the spasticity, balance deficits, challenges to mental well-being, and strength impairments that are common in MS.

GENERAL GUIDELINES

- People with MS are quick to fatigue. When needed, limit the duration of your practice and incorporate restorative or passive poses.
- A common symptom of MS is poor heat tolerance and overheating, which can exacerbate symptoms. *Hot yoga is contraindicated for those with MS.*
- Make sure you are adequately hydrated before and during practice.
- If you are instructing a class for students with MS, know that slowed cognition and proprioception are prevalent, so in-depth and detailed cueing may be necessary.
- Prioritize poses that target large muscle groups (i.e., quadriceps, hamstrings, glutes).
- Perform poses that require the movement of multiple joints (such as simultaneous hip and knee flexion during Warrior I and Warrior II).
- Urinary incontinence is prevalent for those in the later stages of MS, so we advise practicing near a restroom or incorporating a bathroom break as needed.
- People with MS may have limited range of motion in the legs due to spasticity and decreased activity levels. Poses that focus on flexibility of the lower extremities can be very beneficial.

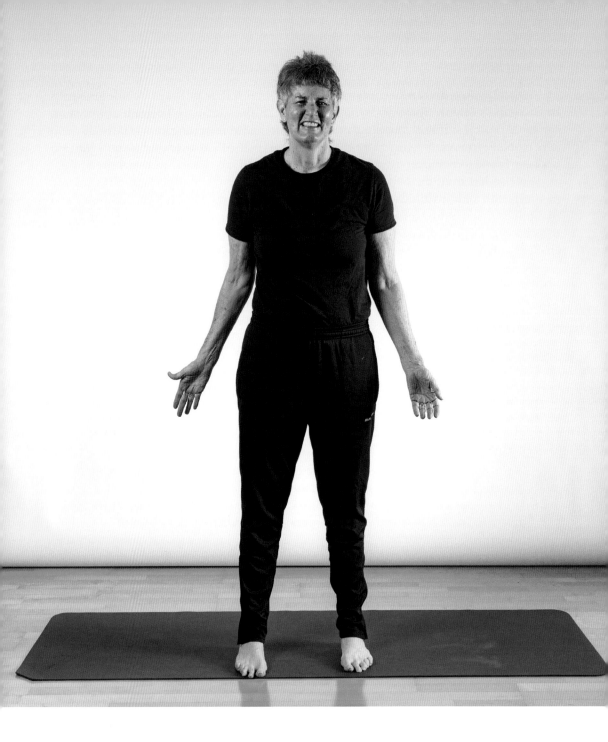

MOUNTAIN   Tadasana

Balance deficits and decreased postural control are common in MS. These impairments contribute to an increased risk of falling. Additional physical aspects that contribute to these impairments include decreased sensation in the legs and an increased sway during quiet stance.[5] Mountain improves postural control by activating the muscles of the legs and core and focusing distribution of weight between both feet.

Benefits

- Improves balance.
- Strengthens the lower extremities.
- Improves posture.

How To

1. Standing with feet hip width apart, ground all four corners of both feet to the mat.
2. Lengthen down through the tailbone, engaging the quadriceps and abdominal muscles.
3. Roll the shoulders down your back, palms facing slightly forward and rotating the inner elbows slightly out.
4. Bring attention to the feet and focus on distributing your weight equally between both feet as you ground them down.
5. Balance the head over the shoulders, drawing the chin slightly back in space.
6. Locate an object or a spot on the wall in front of you to focus your gaze.
7. Hold for 10 or more breath cycles.

Modifications

Practice with a wall behind your back for safety.

Variations

To challenge yourself, try closing your eyes, but if you do so, have a wall behind you for safety.

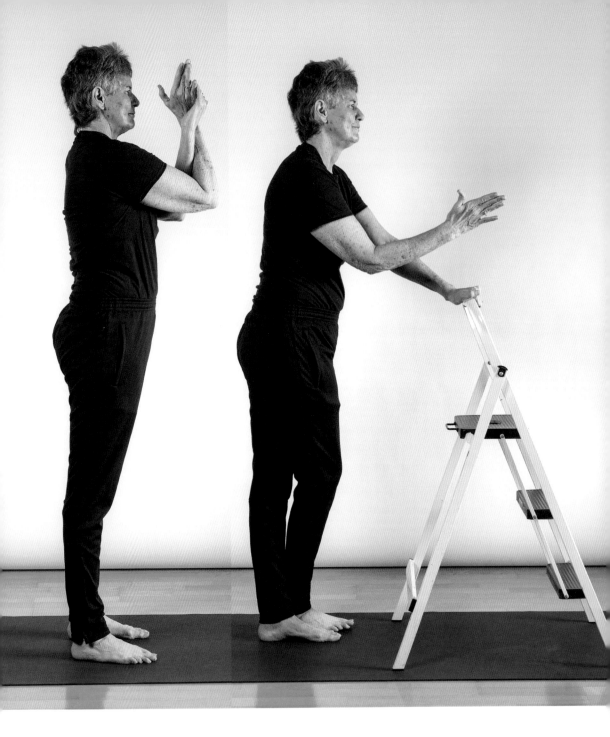

MODIFIED EAGLE

Garudasana

Research suggests that balance-specific training may reduce fall rates and improve balance in people with MS.[6] Any position of single leg standing is considered balance training because it creates a small base of support (the foot) on which you must stabilize the trunk, which is the center of mass. Eagle is highly modifiable, allowing the pose to be used as balance training for people of all abilities.

Benefits

- Improves balance.
- Strengthens the lower extremities.

How To

1. Start in Mountain (pages 262-263).
2. Place your hands on your hips, or hold on to the back of a chair, a stool, or the wall in front of you.
3. Bend your knees very slightly, and shift your weight onto the left foot.
4. Lifting the right leg, cross the right ankle over your left ankle.
5. If possible, balance on your right toes and left foot; if your balance is too precarious like this, cross the ankles with both feet flat on the floor.
6. Hook the right elbow under your left with elbows bent.
7. If you can reach, wrap your arms and hands, and press your palms together (or as close as you can get them).
8. If unable to reach, bring the backs of the hands or forearms to touch, or use a strap.
9. Lift the forearms so that the elbows are as close to the height of your collarbone as possible.
10. Keep your shoulder blades pressing down the back, toward your waist.
11. Square your hips and chest to the front wall.
12. Bend the knees more deeply as you draw your belly up and in.
13. Gaze at the fingertips or at a point in front of you for balance.
14. Hold for 5 to 10 breath cycles, keeping your gaze fixed and soft.
15. Gently unwind your arms and legs and return to Mountain.
16. Repeat on the other side.

Modifications

- You can practice this pose in a chair; refer back to chapter 7, the Seated Eagle pose in a chair (see pages 172-173).
- Perform this pose at whatever level is comfortable. Know that you will likely not be able to wrap your top foot around your standing leg's ankle immediately, but it can be a goal to work toward.
- You can also just practice this pose with the arm and leg movements separately, as pictured here. You will still get the same benefits of balance and scapular stretching.
- You can practice this pose with the wall behind you so that the wall supports your back.

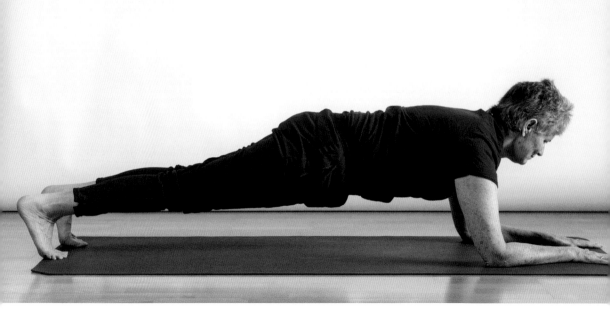

FOREARM PLANK Phalakasana

Decreased postural control is prevalent in MS. Core-strengthening exercises may improve postural control and improve balance. Forearm Plank promotes strength of the core muscles as well as of the legs and arms.

Benefits

- Improves core strength.
- Strengthens the knee extensors.
- Strengthens the hip extensors.
- Strengthens the shoulders.
- Strengthens the ankle plantar flexors.

Precautions

Avoid this pose if you have a current or recent shoulder injury.

How To

1. Start in Downward-Facing Dog (pages 286-287) or lying prone.
2. Walk onto the elbows to rest on your forearms, keeping them parallel to one another.
3. Extend the knees off the floor and engage your quadriceps muscles.
4. Align your body in a straight line from your head and shoulders to your heels.
5. Engage the abdominal muscles in and up, firming your arms in toward midline.
6. Press into the forearms, separating your shoulder blades, drawing your sternum in the direction of your spine, and filling out your thoracic spine.
7. Energize the inner thighs toward each other and up as you press back into your heels and forward with your chest, lengthening the spine and neck.
8. Your gaze should be two feet in front of the hands on the floor for a long neck.
9. Be sure that the hips do not sag and that they are in alignment with the chest and legs.
10. Hold for 5 to 8 breath cycles here and come down to rest in Child's Pose (pages 38-39).

Modifications

- Another way to get into the pose is to start in Table Top (pages 250-251) with the shoulders over the wrists, the core engaged, and first one leg and then the other extended back.
- *On knees:* Start with steps 1 to 5, then lower the knees directly to the floor, without moving your hands and chest. Continue engaging the abdominal muscles and hugging the outer arms into midline. Hold for 10 breaths and come down to rest in Child's Pose.
- *Standing*: Face the wall and extend your arms to place your forearms on the wall at chest height. Walk the feet back until the hands are at shoulder height and the abdomen engages. You can walk the feet back farther until you feel the upper back muscles engage. Be sure you are tucking the tailbone so the hips stay in line with the diagonal of the body.
- For more support, place a block under the hips across the width of the hips, but keep trying to lift the hips up an inch from the block to strengthen the core.

Variations

- To challenge yourself, lift one foot off the floor, maintaining neutral position of the hips, *or* come up into full expression of Plank (pages 34-35) with the hands on the mat, bringing the shoulders over the wrists.
- To challenge yourself, practice Plank on the hands rather than the forearms.

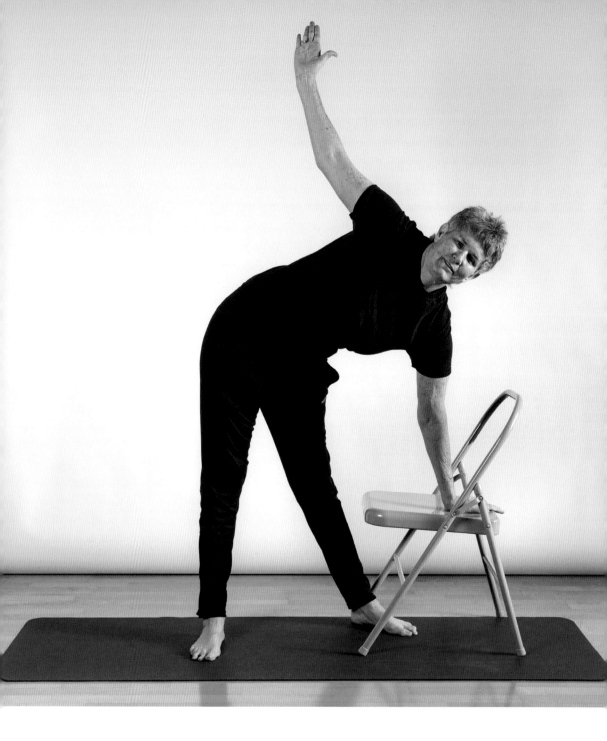

TRIANGLE   Trikonasana

Fatigue and heat sensitivity limit exercise tolerance in people with MS. Therefore, when
you perform strengthening exercises, we recommend emphasizing the use of large muscle
groups and performing multiple-joint exercises to increase the efficiency of exercise.[13] Triangle activates several large muscle groups of the legs and the core and is a quintessential
multijoint exercise.

Benefits

- Strengthens the hip extensors (back leg).
- Strengthens the hip abductors (front leg).
- Strengthens the knee flexors (front leg).
- Strengthens the knee extensors (front leg).
- Strengthens the core.

Precautions

Avoid looking up if you have a neck injury. You can perform this pose with the gaze down toward the floor.

How To

1. Start in Warrior II (pages 272-273), with the left foot forward and a chair or block in front of the foot for the support you will need.
2. Keep the arms extended.
3. Straighten the left leg and extend the left fingertips forward, lengthening both sides of your waist. Rest the left hand on the chair, the block, or your shin for support and balance.
4. Continue to extend your torso forward in line with your left leg, grounding through the right foot and leg to anchor your movement.
5. Hinge at the left hip, as you rotate the left hand on the block, the chair, or your shin.
6. Stretch your right fingertips up to the sky, expanding your chest and stacking the shoulders.
7. Extend both sides of the waist and rotate the chest to the sky.
8. Your right hip will roll slightly down, which is okay. Make sure that both sides of the torso extend equally long and you are not rounding the right side waist.
9. Try to take some weight off of your left hand so you engage your abdominal muscles to support your spine.
10. Maintain extension of your neck in line with your spine and look up, forward, or down if looking up strains your neck.
11. Hold for 5 breath cycles.
12. To exit the pose, bend the left knee slightly and press firmly into the feet to lift your torso upright again.
13. Switch sides by pivoting your heels or resetting in Downward-Facing Dog (pages 286-287).

Modifications

For additional support, practice with a wall behind you and a block under the hand *or* with a chair in front of you, placing your bottom arm on the seat of the chair for support as pictured here.

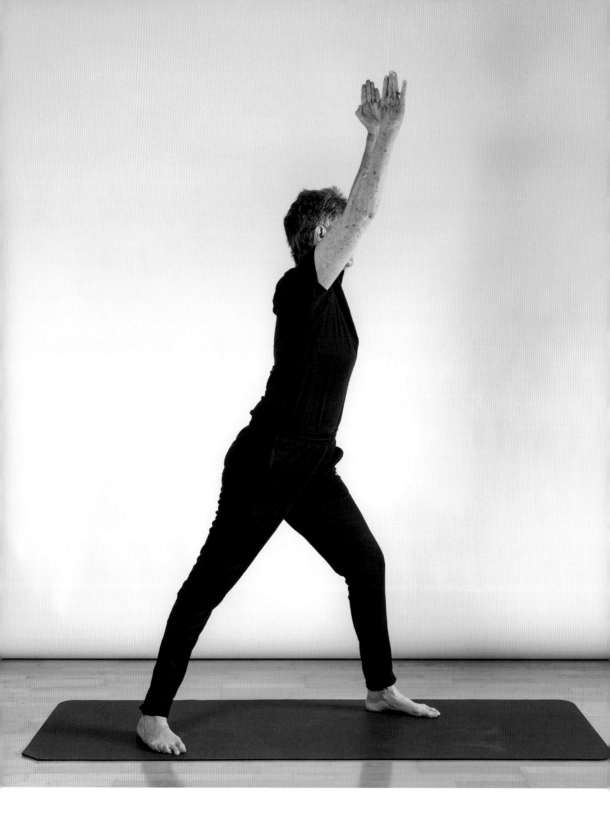

WARRIOR I

Virabhadrasana I

The strength of the knee extensors (quadriceps) is reduced in people with MS. Indeed, greater knee extensor weakness has been correlated with the use of a cane to assist with walking in those with MS.[23] Lunging, as one does during Warrior I, elicits a strong activation of the knee extensors. Additionally, because people with MS tend to walk with a decreased stride length,[23] this pose can be utilized to practice taking a longer step.

Benefits

- Strengthens the knee flexors (front leg) and extensors (back leg).
- Strengthens the hip extensors (back leg) and abductors.
- Stretches the hip flexors.
- Stretches the plantar flexors.

How To

1. Starting in Downward-Facing Dog (pages 286-287), step the left foot forward between the hands so that it's placed next to the left thumb. Alternatively, you can start in a wide-legged stance and turn your body toward the left leg.
2. Spin the right heel down approximately to a 45 degree angle and spin the outer edge of the right foot down so the entire plantar aspect of the foot grounds down.
3. With the left leg bent and the thigh parallel to the floor, inhale your arms up to the sky, hands facing each other, fingers pointing up.
4. The back leg remains straight and strong as you anchor the foot to square the hips forward.
5. Lift the lower abdomen up and in as you lengthen the tailbone down.
6. Draw the shoulders down your back, and gaze forward or slightly up between your hands.
7. Hold for 5 breath cycles.
8. To exit, bring the hands down in a swan dive to frame the foot and return to Downward-Facing Dog or your wide-legged stance.
9. Repeat on the right side.

Modifications

- If this hurts your knee, shorten your stance and decrease the deep knee bend of the front leg.
- Shorten the stance to lessen the challenge to your balance, as pictured here.

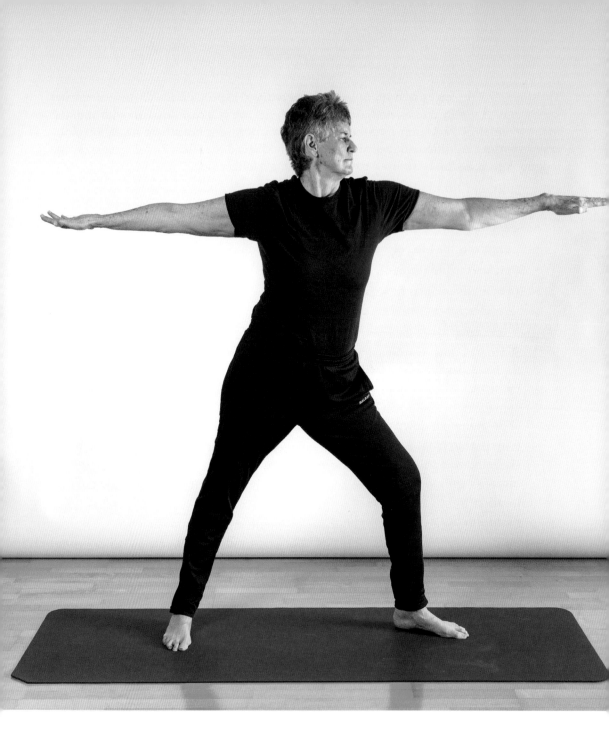

WARRIOR II

Virabhadrasana II

Knee flexor (hamstring) weakness is typical in people with MS. Research suggests that greater knee flexor strength is associated with increased walking speed in MS.[12] In rehabilitation, walking speed is commonly referred to as the sixth vital sign because it is a reflection of overall musculoskeletal and neurologic health.[15] In Warrior II, the knee flexor muscles act to keep the hip and knee in flexion without collapsing under gravity.

Benefits

- Strengthens the knee flexors (front leg).
- Strengthens the knee extensors (back leg).
- Strengthens the hip extensors (both legs).
- Strengthens the hip abductors (both legs).
- Stretches the hip flexors (back leg).

Precautions

If you have knee issues, be careful not to bend the knee so that it extends farther than the ankle.

How To

1. Start with your feet wide (3.5 to 4 feet depending on your height) on the mat, left toes in front and pointing forward, and right foot with toes pointing toward the long edge of the mat.
2. Ground all four corners of the feet down, creating a strong base for your legs.
3. Bend the left knee forward with the goal of extending it in line over the left ankle.
4. You can shift the position of your feet to make space.
5. Roll the inner thigh toward the outer hip so you can see the left big toe (it should not be hidden by your left knee). This will maintain alignment of the knee in line with the ankle.
6. Ground the outer edge of your right foot into the floor.
7. As you inhale, extend your arms straight out to the sides, parallel to the floor.
8. Relax the shoulders down and extend the neck long as you gaze over the left fingertips.
9. Hold for 5 to 8 breath cycles.
10. To exit the pose, place the hands on the hips, straighten the legs, and shift your feet to turn to the other side of the mat, so your right foot is forward.
11. Repeat on the right side.

Modifications

- Decrease the distance between your feet to lessen the challenge to your balance.
- Practice with a wall behind you if you have difficulty with balance in this pose.

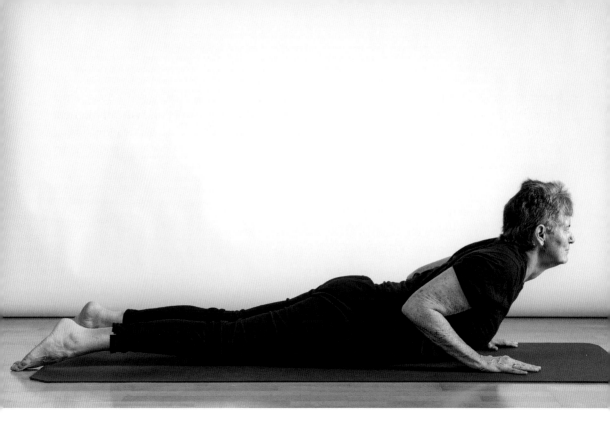

COBRA   Bhujangasana

Cobra is another example of a multijoint-strengthening exercise. This pose activates the functional muscle groups of the spinal extensors and elbow extensors. Additionally, it strengthens the ankle plantar flexors, which are needed to maintain a normal walking speed and can be weak in people with MS.[14]

Benefits

- Strengthens the elbow extensors.
- Strengthens the plantar flexors.
- Strengthens the spinal extensors.
- Stretches the hip flexors.
- Improves spinal extension.

Precautions

Avoid this pose if you are pregnant or if you have a current or recent wrist injury.

How To

1. Start by lying face down with the forehead to the ground, legs extended, and hands directly under the shoulders.
2. Scoop the elbows in toward your body and spread the fingers wide to create a firm foundation with the hands.
3. Press into the hands to lift the chest as you engage the abdominal muscles.
4. Draw the shoulders down your back as you move toward straight arms (it's okay to maintain a bend in your arms for the comfort of your back).
5. Make sure that you continue to engage your abdominal muscles to protect the spine as you lift your heart up and draw the shoulder blades down your back.
6. The head balances comfortably in line with the curve of the spine.
7. The pubic bone rests on the mat, in conjunction with the action of lifting slightly up toward the chest to lengthen the lumbar spine.
8. Hold for 3 to 5 breath cycles.

Modifications

Place a bolster under the belly to take the weight off your arms and shoulders.

Variations

- *Challenge variation:* Walk the hands farther in toward the body to lift the chest higher and move toward a more upright spine. Make sure the shoulders continue to draw down the back and away from the ears, and the abdomen remains engaged.
- *Restorative variation:* Place a bolster under the low belly to support the spine.

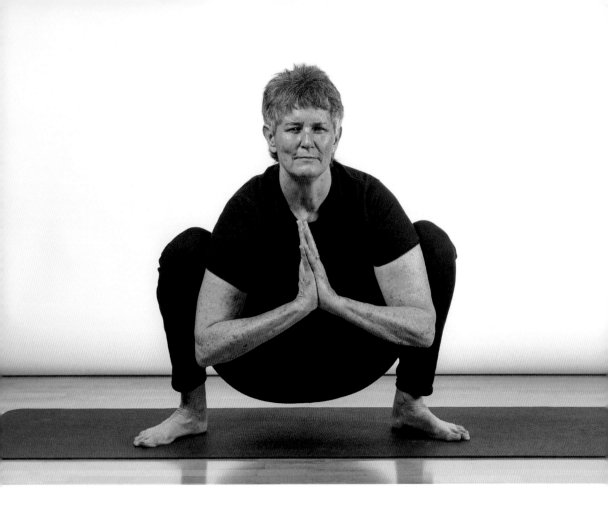

GARLAND Malasana

Urinary incontinence (accidental leakage of urine) is a common symptom of MS.[13] This is often due to decreased control of the urinary sphincter and is associated with weakness in the pelvic floor muscles. Because the pelvic floor works synergistically to respond to the movement of one's inhalation and exhalation, this is an excellent pose to practice activating and strengthening the pelvic floor.

Benefits

- Strengthens the pelvic floor.
- Strengthens the abdominal muscles.
- Improves ankle dorsiflexion.
- Improves wrist extension in Prayer Hands.
- Strengthens the hip adductors.

Precautions

Avoid this pose if you have a recent or current injury to the meniscus of the knee.

How To

1. Stand with your feet slightly farther than hip width apart.
2. Squat down by bending your knees to lower the hips toward the ground.
3. Keep the feet wide enough apart so your feet remain flat on the ground. If the heels rise up, place a rolled-up blanket, a mat, or a wedge under the heels to remain balanced in your feet.
4. Lift the belly button up and in. Draw your palms together in Prayer Hands (pages 118-119). Press the triceps or elbows to the inside of your knees.
5. Engage and lift the pelvic floor up and in, contracting the pelvic floor muscles toward the belly button.
6. Lift the crown of the head up as you also engage the abdomen toward your spine. The hard part will be remembering to breathe; as you clench your pelvic floor and abdomen, you may be tempted to hold your breath. Maintain the contraction while trying to breathe with ease. You'll get the hang of it eventually.
7. Hold for 5 breath cycles.
8. To release, place the hands on the floor and slowly bend forward as you straighten the legs (but keep the knees bent to protect your lower back).

Modifications

- If your heels lift off the floor, place a rolled-up blanket, a mat, or a wedge under the heels.
- Stack blocks under the buttocks and sit on the blocks to support the squat.

Variations

To challenge yourself, step your feet as close together as possible while maintaining the feet flat on the ground.

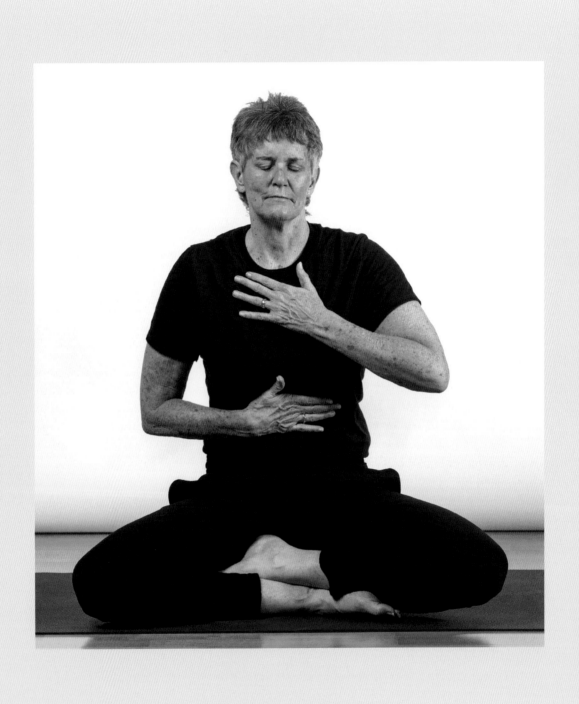

DIAPHRAGMATIC BREATHING

Respiratory muscle weakness can occur during any stage of MS, from mild to moderate disease, and in the end stages of disease.[10] This respiratory muscle weakness can cause impaired ventilation and poor cough reflex, increasing the risk of aspiration and consequent pulmonary disease. Deep diaphragmatic breathing has been shown to improve vital capacity in the lungs, suggesting that breathing exercises might slow down or prevent deterioration of lung function in MS patients.[24] Diaphragmatic breathing is a foundational technique that allows practitioners to exercise the strength of the diaphragm and improve respiratory function. It is also used for relaxation and relief of anxiety and depression. In diaphragmatic breathing, the initial focus of attention is on the expansion of the abdomen, which is why it is sometimes referred to as abdominal or belly breathing.[17]

Here's how to perform diaphragmatic breathing.

1. Start seated on the floor or a chair.
2. Place one hand on the belly and the other on the chest.
3. Feel the belly and chest expand outward on a deep inhalation and notice the expansion of the rib cage with each inhaled breath.
4. Bring attention to the relaxation of the belly and the downward trajectory of the chest as you exhale.
5. Breathe through your nose with the lips gently closed.
6. On your next cycle of breath, inhale on a count of 6 (1-2-3-4-5-6).
7. Transition into your exhale, counting down from 6 (6-5-4-3-2-1).
8. Continue counting; inhale to count up to 6, exhale to count down from 6.
9. Continue for 5 to 10 breath cycles. You can practice for even longer if you want to.
10. The ultimate goal is to integrate diaphragmatic breathing into your physical movements and your yoga practice, and during meditation and relaxation.

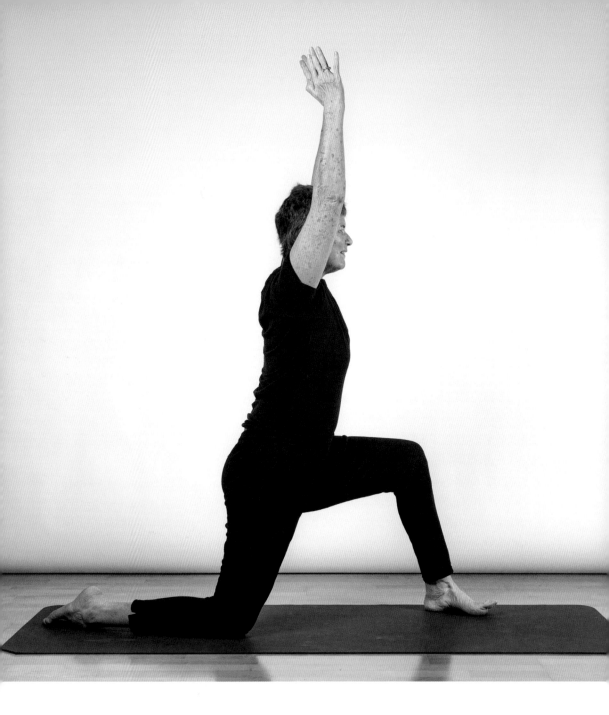

CRESCENT LUNGE

Anjaneyasana

Lower activity levels (increased time spent sitting) and spasticity may contribute to hip flexor tightness. Hip flexor tightness can, in turn, contribute to decreased step length and slower walking speeds. Crescent Lunge allows for an isolated hip flexor stretch of the back leg while using the body's weight to increase the amount of stretch. The hands are available to provide stability if needed.

Benefits

- Stretches the hip flexors (back leg).
- Strengthens the knee extensors (front leg).

How To

1. From Downward-Facing Dog (pages 286-287), raise your left leg up and back to extend the leg.
2. Step the left foot forward in between your hands. If it doesn't make it there with your step, catch the ankle with your hand and assist it forward so it aligns with your hands.
3. Bring your torso upright and bend the front knee.
4. Make sure your knee is above your ankle, not forward of the ankle.
5. Lower the back (right) knee to rest on the ground; you can place a blanket or towel under the knee for cushioning.
6. Extend your arms up with the palms facing each other.
7. Expand your chest to the sky as you draw your arms farther behind your ears, and lift the chest up to deepen the stretch at the front of your right hip.
8. Gaze directly in front of you or slightly up to where the wall meets the ceiling, with the goal of extending the back of your neck.
9. Hold for 5 breath cycles.
10. To exit the pose, release your hands down to the mat to frame the foot and step the left foot back to Downward-Facing Dog.
11. Repeat on the right side.

Modifications

Your hands can be on blocks, on your hips, or in Prayer Hands (pages 118-119), depending on the support you need.

Variations

- *Challenge variation:* Practice with the back knee off the mat for leg strengthening. Note that this tilts the pelvis forward, so you can add a slight bend in the back knee to neutralize the pelvis.
- *Restorative variation:* Place a bolster in front of the back knee and rest the quadriceps on the bolster.

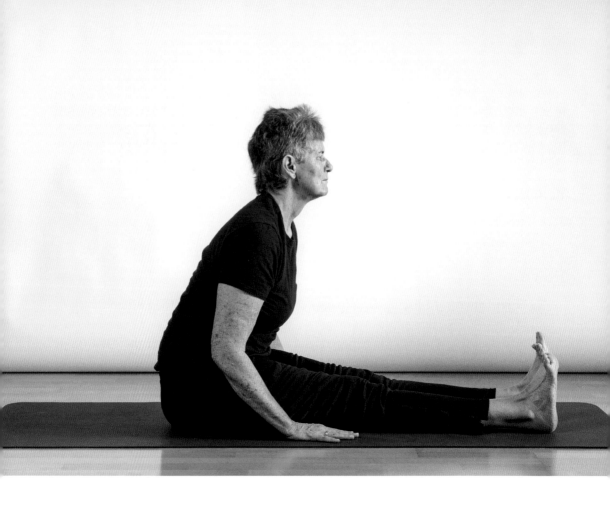

SEATED FORWARD BEND   Paschimottanasana

Tightness in the knee flexors can increase the difficulty of standing from a seated position and decrease the efficiency of walking. The strongest muscle of the knee flexors (biceps femoris) crosses the knee and hip joints. Seated Forward Bend is an ideal pose to lengthen this muscle group because it stretches at both the knee and hip joints.

Benefits

- Stretches the knee flexors.
- Strengthens the knee extensors.
- Stretches the spinal extensors.
- Stretches the ankle dorsiflexors.

Precautions

Avoid this pose if you have a current or recent herniated disc, or if performing it causes tingling, pain, or numbness down the back of one or both legs.

How To

1. From Staff (pages 80-81), inhale to expand your chest and create length in the spine.
2. Engaging the abdominal muscles and quadriceps, bend forward over your straight legs, hinging from the hips as you exhale.
3. Hands rest alongside your legs, with elbows bent to provide support for your spine.
4. Do not round the spine in an attempt to get your forehead closer to your legs; only bend as far as you can while maintaining an extended spine.
5. Engaging the quadriceps, try to straighten your legs and press the backs of the knees toward the floor.
6. With every inhalation, lengthen your spine. With every exhalation, fold deeper into the bend.
7. Maintain length in your neck and keep the abdomen engaged.
8. Hold for 5 breath cycles.

Modifications

- Place a bolster or a folded blanket under your belly to support the spine.
- Separate the feet only as far as you need in order to place a block (on its tall side) between the calves and squeeze the block to engage the legs.
- Place a rolled blanket under the knees to relieve tension in the backs of the knees or hamstrings.

Variations

If you seek to reach your feet, start first with a strap around the feet, and catch hold of one side with each hand.

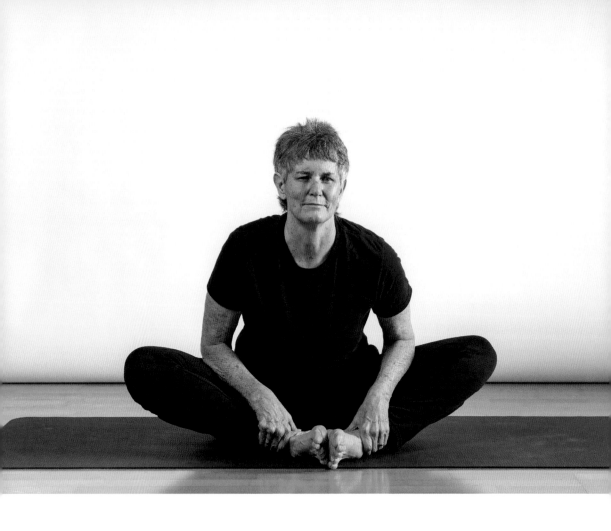

BOUND ANGLE

Baddha Konasana

Spasticity or tightness in the hip adductors (groin) can lead to walking with a scissoring pattern, with one foot directly in front of the other. In advanced forms of MS, hip adductor tightness can create difficulties with lower extremity dressing and hygiene. Bound Angle positions the legs to allow stretching of the hip adductors with the assistance of gravity and the weight of the arms to assist the stretch.

Benefits

- Stretches the hip adductors.
- Strengthens the core.
- Engages the spinal extensors.

How To

1. Start seated on the mat in whatever leg position is comfortable for you.
2. Use the hands to bend the knees into your chest and place the feet flat on the ground.
3. Roll the knees out to the sides, supporting the outer knees with the hands as you bring the bottoms of the feet together to touch.
4. Ground the sitting bones and inhale to lengthen the spine.
5. Hold the feet or ankles with the hands or rest them on your thighs.
6. If your body allows, hinge from your hips to bend forward, maintaining an elongated spine.
7. Hold for 5 to 10 breath cycles.
8. Come up slowly; you can use your hands on your shins or next to you on the ground to help you push up to a straight spine again.

Modifications

- Place blocks under your knees to relieve tension in the hips.
- Bring the feet further away from the pelvis to decrease the flexion in your knees.

Variations

- *Challenge variation:* For a more intense inner thigh stretch, bring the feet closer to the pelvis.
- *Restorative variation:* Position a block on the tall side in front of your feet so you can rest your forehead on the block if you are folding forward.

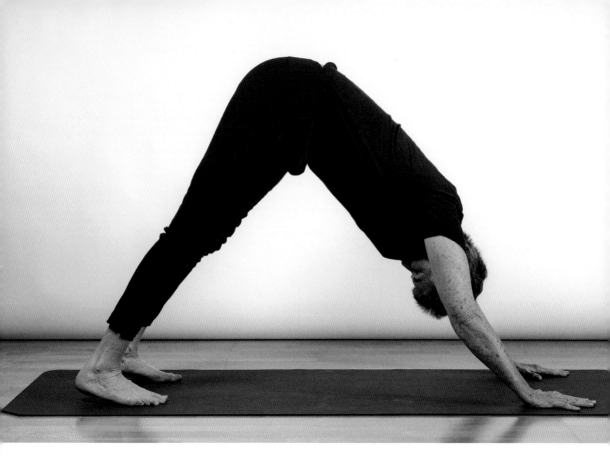

DOWNWARD-FACING DOG   Adho Mukha Svanasana

Spasticity and tightness in the plantar flexors (calves) can contribute to pain in the lower legs and changes in your walking pattern. This, in turn, increases the risk of knee injury. The plantar flexors are some of the strongest muscles of the body and therefore should be stretched while bearing the weight of the body. Downward-Facing Dog provides an excellent position to perform a controlled weight-bearing plantar flexor stretch.

Benefits

- Stretches the plantar flexors.
- Stretches the knee flexors.
- Strengthens the arms.

How To

1. Start in Table Top (pages 250-251), with your hips aligned above your knees and your shoulders above the wrists.
2. Walk the hands forward about half a hand length with the wrist creases parallel to the front of the mat.
3. Tuck the toes, and lift your hips to the sky, creating an upside-down V shape with the body.
4. Drop your chest back toward the shins and maintain a slight bend in the knees to lengthen the lower back and pelvis.
5. Spread the fingers wide and focus on grounding the thumbs and forefingers into the mat as you spiral the upper arms out and the forearms in (elbows should be rolled slightly forward).
6. Press the hands into the mat to create more traction to lift the pelvis up and extend your heels back to lengthen the backs of your legs.
7. Start to straighten your knees, but if you notice that this rounds your low back, keep the knees bent.
8. Lengthen the back of your neck; you can do so by gazing up to the belly or toward the toes.
9. Relax the shoulders down the back and away from the ears.
10. Hold for 5 to 8 breath cycles.
11. To exit the pose, relax your knees back down on the mat and sit your hips back into Child's Pose (pages 38-39).

Modifications

- If this hurts your wrists, you can come down onto the forearms.
- Feel free to pedal the feet by bending first one knee and then the other while you settle into your Downward-Facing Dog.

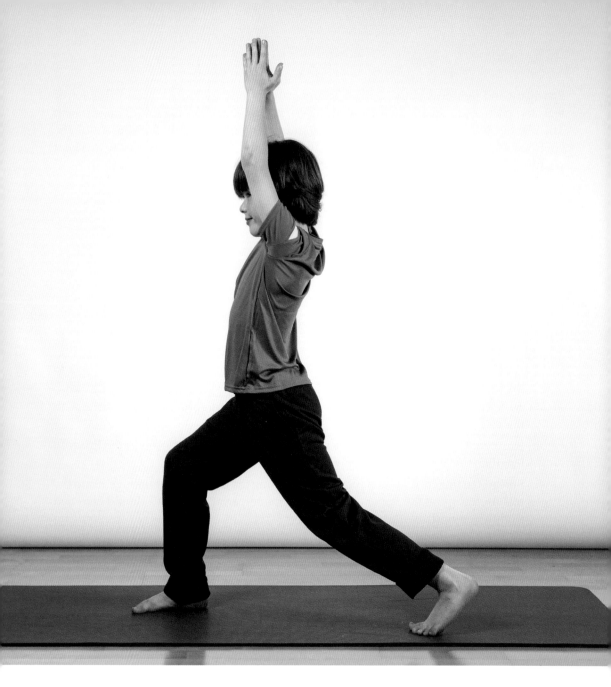

CHAPTER 11
Cerebral Palsy

Cerebral palsy (CP) refers to a group of conditions that involve motor dysfunction affecting muscle tone, posture, or movement. These conditions are due to abnormalities of the developing fetal or infant brain resulting from a variety of causes. Although the disorder itself is not progressive, the clinical presentation may change over time as the central nervous system (CNS) matures. The motor impairment generally results in limitations in functional ability and activity, which can range in severity. Multiple additional symptoms may accompany the primary motor abnormalities, including altered sensation or perception, communication and behavioral difficulties, seizure disorders, and musculoskeletal complications.

CP is characterized by abnormalities of motor activity, tone, and posture. Voluntary movements that should be smooth and coordinated can instead be uncoordinated and limited. Simple actions that are typically performed unconsciously can require significant effort or may not be possible for some patients with CP. In severely affected individuals, an attempted voluntary movement may evoke a primitive reflex, co-contraction of agonist and antagonist muscles, and mass movements (grouped movement of the muscles).[9] For example, attempting to flex one particular joint may involve all segments of a limb, and extension of the fingers may accompany extension of the wrist. In some cases, discrete, isolated movements, such as moving the ankle up and down, may be nearly impossible.

CP is often accompanied by other disorders of cerebral function. Associated abnormalities may affect cognition, vision, hearing, language, cortical sensation, attention, vigilance, and behavior. Some children also have epilepsy, and many have disturbed gastrointestinal function and growth. These dysfunctions may interfere with skilled tasks, regardless of the severity of the motor deficit. In a child with CP, for example, disorders of higher cortical function may interfere with activities of daily living, such as dressing or managing buttons.[7]

Dysfunctions in CP may include, but are not limited to, pain (most common), intellectual disability (50 percent), speech or language disorders, bladder control problems, visual impairments, epilepsy, behavior disorders, hip displacements, sleep disorders, hearing impairments, and gastrostomy tube dependence.[1]

This chapter will focus on how yoga can help those with a specific form of CP, spastic diplegia. In spastic diplegia, spasticity occurs mainly in the legs with little to no involvement in the arms.[6] It is the most common form of CP, accounting for 34 percent of cases.[6] Children with spastic diplegia stand and walk later in life with their feet pointing down and in due to spasticity of the calf muscles. As they age, progressive spasticity of the hip flexors and hamstrings can result in a crouched gait[8] (standing and walking with the knees and hips bent). This crouched gait pattern makes prolonged upright activity difficult. The poses in this chapter will address the muscles that are commonly weak and tight, contributing to the crouched posture.

As we've mentioned, increased muscle tone causes too much muscle tension at rest, impeding the ability to walk, grasp objects, and perform general activities of daily living. Thus, even when the muscle is not being purposely activated, it may still be uncomfortably tense or stiff. This is common in those with spastic CP, causing the extremities to be resistant to movement, and even contorted. Yoga poses that stretch the entire length of a large muscle group may assist in easing high muscle tone and deformations caused by high muscle tone.

Furthermore, the progressive relaxation that accompanies holding yoga poses allows the muscles and tendons to gently stretch, thus providing overall relief in an overactivated musculoskeletal system. With a dedicated yoga practice, over time, the general stress in the body will be reduced, relieving tightness throughout the body's tonic muscles. As the body begins to realign, posture is also improved. One of the great benefits of a yoga practice is a straightening and focus on alignment of the spine. Focus on reducing pressure on the vertebrae and strengthening the core can produce a more limber spine, improving range of motion and relieving muscle tension.

In this chapter, we focus on yoga poses that lengthen the back, stabilize core muscles, and strengthen and stretch the leg muscles that contribute to decreased functional mobility in those with CP.

GENERAL GUIDELINES

- Perform poses that strengthen the extensor muscles of the trunk, hip, and knee to assist in moving out of a crouched posture.
- Individuals with CP often utilize ankle braces while walking; feel free to use these when performing standing or balance poses.
- Consistent core activation should be a focus in every posture.
- It may be helpful for the practitioner to have an assistant to provide balance and stability during a yoga practice.

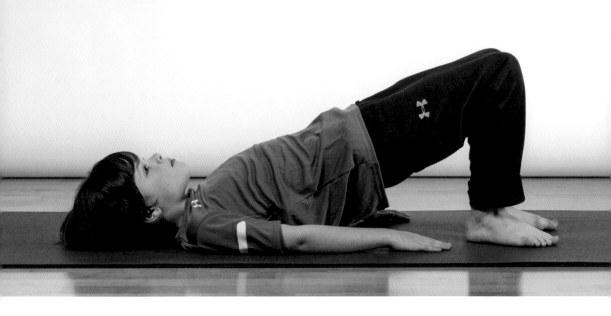

BRIDGE

Setu Bandha Sarvangasana

Bridge is an excellent way to strengthen the posterior leg muscles, which are very functionally important for those with CP. The hip extensors (gluteus maximus) are needed to transfer from a seated to a standing position. Knee flexor (hamstring) strength has been found to be directly correlated with function in CP.[5] The strength of the knee flexors when the knees are bent at various angles coincides with the ease of performing different activities (walking speed and running ability).[5] Bridge can be modified by adjusting the position of the feet to strengthen the knee flexors at different knee joint angles.

Benefits

- Strengthens the hip extensors.
- Strengthens the knee flexors.
- Strengthens the spinal extensors.
- Stretches the hip flexors.

Precautions

Avoid this pose if you have a current or recent neck injury.

Before You Begin

Note that a strap may be needed for modifications.

How To

1. Start by lying on your back with your knees bent, feet flat on the floor, and arms alongside your body with hands facing down.
2. Roll your shoulders underneath you as you begin to lift your hips.
3. Press your feet and shoulders into the mat as you lift your hips higher.
4. As you rise, walk the feet closer toward your buttocks and scoot your shoulders into midline to further elevate the hips and lengthen the tailbone.
5. Keep your knees parallel as you engage the inner thighs.
6. Interlace the fingers underneath you, keep the palms face down on your mat, or hold onto a strap with each hand.
7. Keep your neck neutral by relaxing your chin away from your chest to preserve the natural curve of your cervical spine.
8. Your shoulders, feet, and the back of your head rest comfortably on the mat because you are using the muscles of your buttocks and back to lengthen and lift your hips, not your neck.
9. Hold for 5 to 10 breath cycles.
10. To exit the pose, release the hands if interlaced and slowly roll down your spine.

Modifications

Wrap a strap around the upper thighs to relax the quadriceps and keep the knees in line with the hips to focus on spinal extension.

Variations

- *Challenge variations:* Lift one knee into the belly, *or* for a further challenge, extend that leg straight up.
- *Restorative variation:* Place a block or bolster directly under your sacrum and allow the prop to take the weight of your body. Be sure that you continue to lengthen your neck by resting the head's weight on the back of the head and not on the neck. Lift the chest toward your chin, and your chin slightly up and away from your chest so as not to collapse the neck.

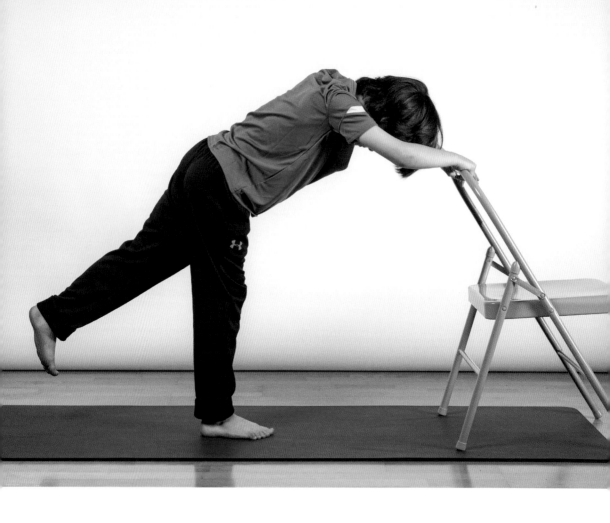

SUPPORTED WARRIOR III Virabhadrasana III

Warrior III is a great progression from Bridge for strengthening the posterior leg muscles. The hip extensors and knee flexors of the stance leg must activate to control the forward motion of the pelvis and trunk. This pose is also an excellent way to strengthen the hip abductor muscles. Using the arms for balance makes the pose accessible for all levels.

Benefits

- Strengthens the hip extensors (standing leg) and abductors (extended leg).
- Strengthens the knee flexors (extended leg) and extensors (standing leg).
- Stretches the knee flexors (standing leg).

Precautions

Avoid this pose if you have a current or recent ankle injury to the standing leg.

How To

1. Start in Crescent Lunge (pages 314-315) with the knee off the ground or Warrior I (pages 296-297) with the right foot forward and a chair in front of you.
2. Reach the arms forward and place the hands on the back of the chair or on a wall. If you need to, step your feet forward so that you can reach the chair.
3. Shift all the weight onto the right leg and start to lean the torso and arms forward.
4. Push off of the left leg, lifting it straight back behind you.
5. Bring the torso and back leg as parallel to the ground as possible, with the goal of creating a T shape with the body.
6. Dorsiflex the foot by pointing the toes to the ground and pressing the heel back behind you.
7. Straighten your standing leg by engaging the front quadriceps muscles, but without hyperextending the knee.
8. Internally rotate the back hip so that the left foot points toward the floor.
9. Continue pressing the standing foot into the ground so as not to collapse into the hip socket and engage the core muscles.
10. Hold for 3 to 5 breath cycles.
11. Exit the pose by stepping the left foot back into Crescent Lunge or Warrior I, then switch sides.

Modifications

Stand next to a wall, at the side of your standing leg. Place your hand on the wall for extra support.

Variations

Start to lift one hand or both away from the chair. Place the hands on the hips, or the arms alongside the torso, instead of in front of you on the chair for extra challenge if you feel secure in your balance.

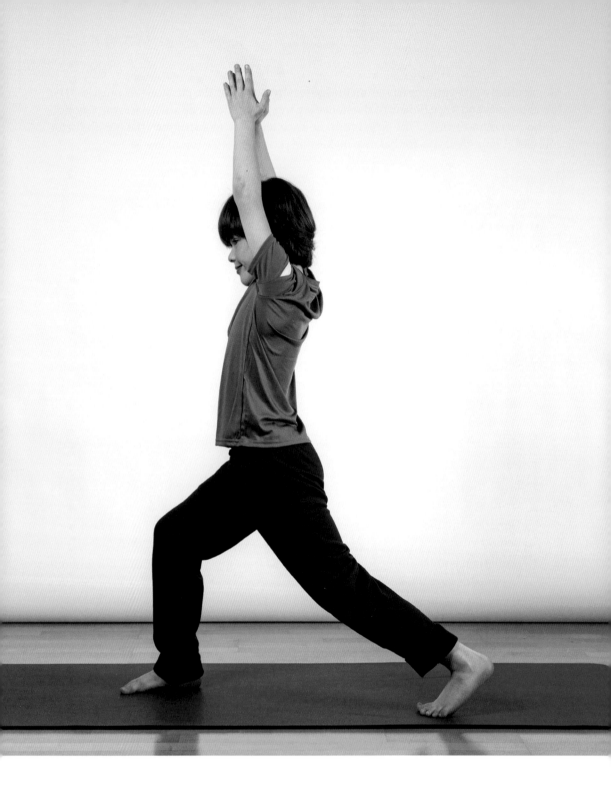

WARRIOR I

Virabhadrasana I

Warrior I promotes strength of the knee extensors (quadriceps). Strength of the knee extensors is emphasized to counteract the characteristic crouched posture common in CP. This pose also strengthens the plantar flexors (calf) of the back leg. Increased plantar flexor strength has been found to improve walking endurance in those with CP.[4]

Benefits

- Strengthens the knee extensors (front leg) and flexors (back leg).
- Strengthens the plantar flexors.
- Strengthens the spinal and hip extensors (back leg).

How To

1. Starting in Downward-Facing Dog (pages 308-309), step the right foot forward between the hands so that it's placed next to the right thumb, or start from a wide-legged stance on the mat.
2. Spin the left heel down approximately to a 45 degree angle and spin the outer edge of the left foot down so the entire plantar aspect of the foot grounds down. If the heel does not reach the ground, it is ok to keep the heel up or place a rolled-up blanket or wedge under the foot.
3. With the right leg bent and the thigh parallel to the floor, inhale your arms up to the sky, hands facing each other, fingers pointing up.
4. The back leg remains straight and strong as you anchor the foot to square the hips forward.
5. Lift the lower abdomen up and in as you lengthen the tailbone down.
6. Draw the shoulders down the back, and gaze forward or slightly up between your hands.
7. Hold for 5 to 8 breath cycles, or repeat five times, coming up and down with the arms.
8. To exit the pose, bring the hands down in a swan dive to frame the foot and return to Downward-Facing Dog, or turn to face the other direction.
9. Repeat on the left side.

Modifications

- If this hurts your knee or is too challenging for your balance, shorten your stance and decrease the deep knee bend of the front leg.
- You can also place your hands on a chair next to or in front of you for balance.

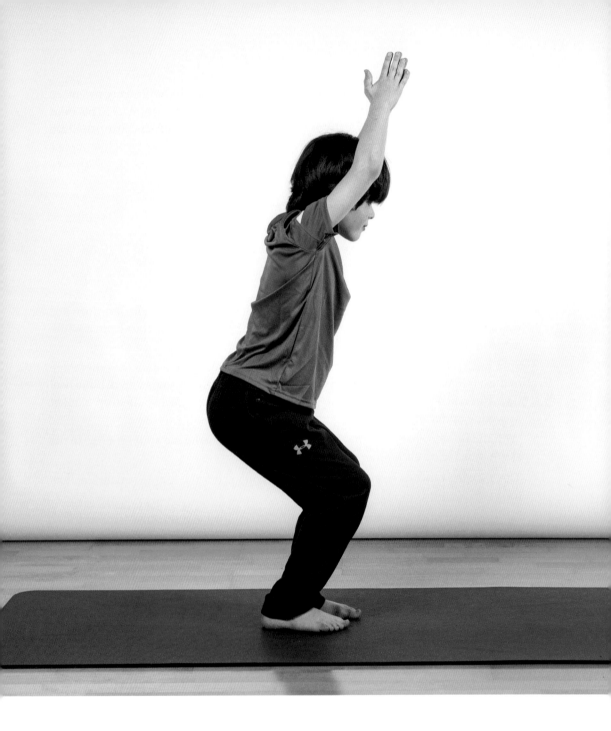

CHAIR

Utkatasana

Knee extensor–strengthening exercises work to facilitate standing without the use of an assistive device (walker or reverse walker). Chair mimics this very functional position while also strengthening the spinal extensor muscles. The key difference between Chair and a crouched posture is that the center of mass (COM) is positioned behind the base of support (the feet), requiring the leg muscles to increase in activation. Chair also improves a crouched posture by focusing on expansion through the chest muscles and strengthening of the upper back muscles.

Benefits

- Strengthens the knee extensors.
- Strengthens the spinal and hip extensors.

How To

1. Start in Mountain (pages 150-151).
2. Bend your knees to sit the hips back, trying to bring your thighs parallel to the floor.
3. Reach your arms overhead alongside your ears and engage your abdomen.
4. Ground through all four corners of the feet.
5. Notice that you are bent at the ankles, knees, and hips.
6. Hold for 5 to 10 breath cycles.
7. To exit the pose, press down into your feet to straighten your legs and stand upright. Relax your arms alongside your body as you come back into Mountain.

Modifications

- Practice with different arm positions, such as Prayer Hands (pages 118-119) at the chest or hands on the hips.
- Place your hands on the back of a chair or a wall in front of you for assistance with balance.

Variations

To challenge yourself, place a block between your knees to engage your inner thighs. Be sure that you still place even weight between your two feet so that you do not collapse into the arches of the feet.

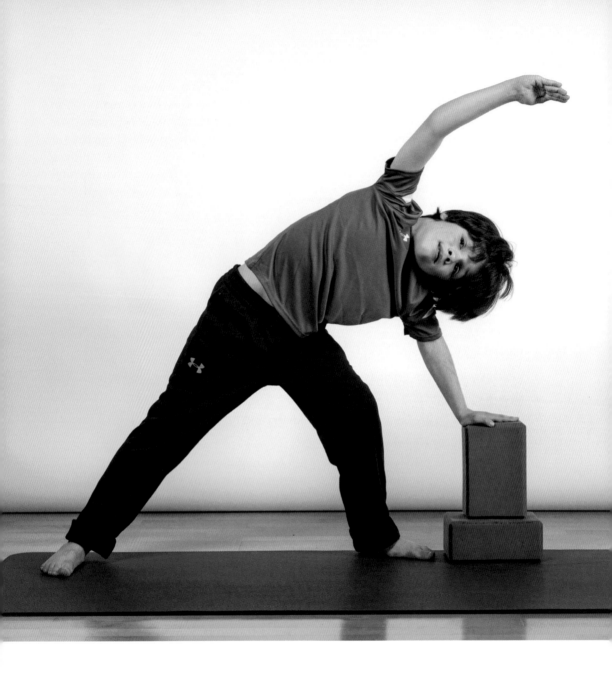

EXTENDED SIDE ANGLE Utthita Parsvakonasana

Scissoring gait is a common gait issue in those with CP.[4] It consists of walking with the feet directly in front of each other or even crossing one another. This is caused by spasticity in the hip adductors (groin) and weakness in the hip abductors. Extended Side Angle stretches the hip adductors while strengthening the hip abductors (especially of the extended leg).

Benefits

- Stretches the hip adductors (both legs).
- Strengthens the hip abductors (both legs).
- Strengthens the obliques.
- Strengthens the plantar flexors.
- Strengthens the knee flexors (back leg) and extensors (front leg).

How To

1. Start in Warrior II (pages 104-105), with the left foot forward.
2. Place the left forearm onto the left thigh, or the left hand to the floor, on a chair, or on a block outside your foot.
3. Extend the right arm over the right ear to feel the extension in your right side body. The palm faces down to the ground with the fingers extending out in front of you.
4. Extend both sides of the waist to reach out and over the front thigh.
5. Engage the abdomen to protect the spine and side body.
6. Your gaze can be to your right hand, the ground, or straight forward, depending on which is most comfortable for your neck.
7. Hold for 5 breath cycles.
8. To exit the pose, turn the torso to the mat to frame the left foot with your hands, and step back to Downward-Facing Dog (pages 308-309) before switching sides.

Modifications

You can perform this pose with a chair under the front thigh for support.

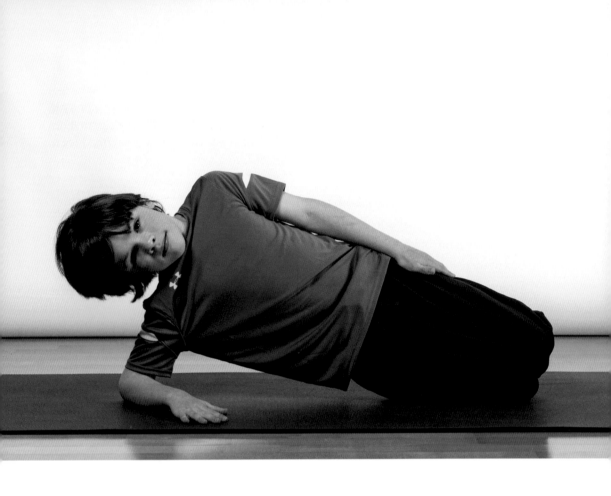

SIDE PLANK

Vasisthasana

To keep the pelvis elevated against gravity, Side Plank elicits a very strong contraction of the hip abductors. Hip abductor strength has been found to be correlated to increased walking speed and the ability to climb stairs in those with CP.[2] This is likely because both of these tasks require single leg standing time during which the hip abductors must act to stabilize the pelvis. Side Plank also strengthens all the muscles of the shoulder joint. This is important because use of walkers and wheelchairs in those with CP increases the risk of shoulder pain or injury.[11]

Benefits

- Strengthens the hip abductors (bottom leg).
- Strengthens the shoulder muscles (bottom arm, or both if top arm is lifted).
- Strengthens the obliques.
- Strengthens the knee extensors if this pose is performed with the legs straight.

Precautions

Avoid this pose if you have a shoulder injury.

How To

1. From Forearm Plank (pages 100-101), rotate onto the right forearm, positioning it so it is parallel to the front of the mat.
2. Roll to the outer edge of your right foot or knees if your legs remain bent, as pictured, stacking your left thigh over the right.
3. Press the hips up and away from the mat, engaging the core and right inner thigh up into the left leg.
4. Lift the left fingertips to the sky or keep the arm alongside the body, as pictured.
5. Press the right forearm down into the mat as you stack the shoulders and lift the hips further away from the mat.
6. Gaze forward or up to the left hand.
7. Hold for 3 to 5 breath cycles.
8. Repeat on the other side.

Modifications

As noted above, if balancing with the legs straight is too challenging, keep the knees bent and shins on the mat.

Variations

To challenge yourself, come up on the hand instead of resting on the elbow, *or* for even more challenge, lift the top leg so the foot comes in line with the hip.

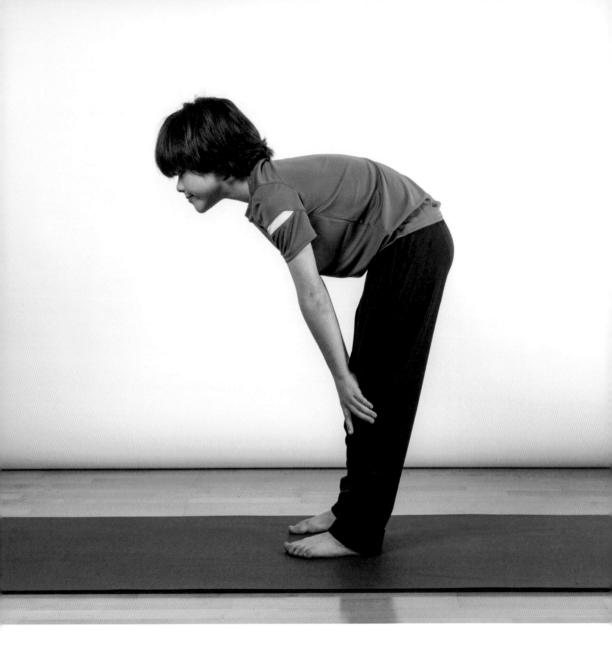

HALF STANDING FORWARD BEND

Ardha Uttanasana

In the characteristic crouched posture, individuals with CP demonstrate a pronounced lumbar lordosis (swayback). This is caused by tightness in the hip flexors, resulting in an anteriorly tilted pelvis. Due to this tendency of swayback, spinal extensor weakness is common.[11] Half Standing Forward Bend allows you to focus on strengthening the spinal extensors in an extremely accessible way.

Benefits

- Strengthens the spinal extensors.
- Stretches the knee flexors.

How To

1. Start in a Standing Forward Bend (see figure D on page 108), feet hip width apart and knees slightly bent.
2. Place the hands on the shins or quadriceps, on blocks, or on a chair, and inhale to extend the chest forward.
3. Engage the abdominal muscles up and in as you begin to straighten your legs, pressing the hips back to extend the chest forward.
4. Be sure your lower back feels supported as you spread the collarbones apart.
5. Hold for 1 to 5 breath cycles.
6. To exit the pose, fold forward over bent legs, relaxing your head toward the ground.

Modifications

You can perform this pose in front of a wall, placing your hands on the wall for support.

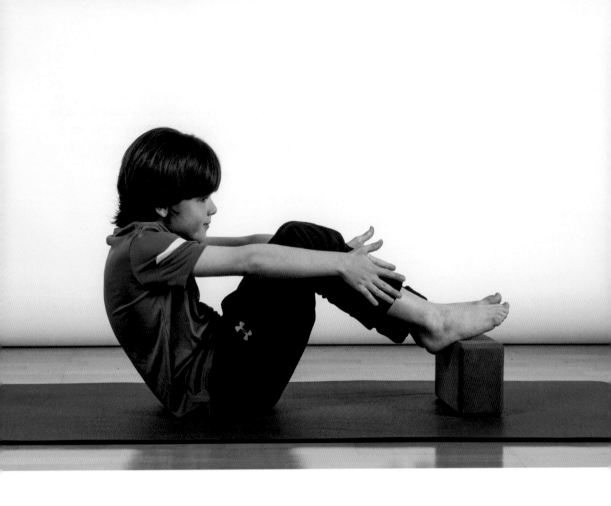

MODIFIED BOAT Navasana

Decreased postural control is one of the primary dysfunctions associated with CP.[2] Therefore, core strengthening is a goal of exercise for those with CP. Boat requires a co-contraction of the abdominal and spinal extensor muscles, offering dual benefits for core strength. Additionally, Boat facilitates strengthening of the hip flexors. Strength of this muscle group is associated with improved walking speeds and stair-climbing in CP.

Benefits

- Strengthens the abdominal muscles.
- Strengthens the spinal extensors.
- Strengthens the hip flexors.

How To

1. Start seated with your knees bent and feet flat on the floor.
2. Place your hands behind your knees and start to lean back with the chest lifted, noticing the core activation that is starting to take place.
3. Draw the belly button up and in as you begin to lift the feet off the mat.
4. Engage your abdomen and lift the chest, drawing the shoulders back.
5. Let go of the legs and extend your arms forward alongside your knees with your palms facing your legs.
6. Be sure the neck remains comfortable by keeping the chest lifted.
7. Your torso, pelvis, and upper legs will be in a V shape with the hips as the fulcrum.
8. Feet should be neutral, not flexed.
9. Hold for 3 to 5 breath cycles.

Modifications

Place the feet on blocks for additional support, with the goal of eventually lifting the feet off the blocks. Try lifting one foot at a time to improve core strength.

Variations

To challenge yourself, straighten the legs or bring the arms overhead.

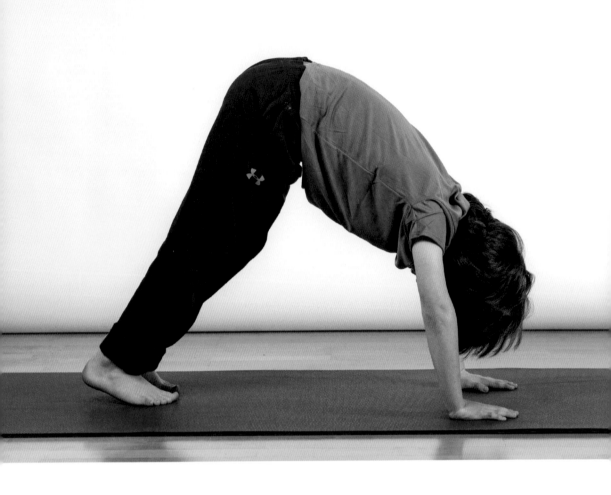

DOWNWARD-FACING DOG Adho Mukha Svanasana

Another gait deviation sometimes found in CP is called toe walking. In this pattern, leg weakness and ankle plantar flexor tightness cause compensatory walking on the balls of the feet with the heels elevated. Downward-Facing Dog provides an excellent position to perform a controlled weight-bearing stretch to the plantar flexors and decrease the toe walking gait pattern.

Benefits

- Stretches the knee and plantar flexors.
- Strengthens the spinal extensors.
- Strengthens the arms.

How To

1. Start in Table Top (pages 250-251), with your hips aligned above your knees and shoulders above the wrists.
2. Walk the hands forward about half a hand length with the wrist creases parallel to the front of the mat.
3. Tuck the toes and lift your hips to the sky, creating an upside-down V shape with the body.
4. Drop your chest back toward the shins and maintain a slight bend in the knees to lengthen the lower back and pelvis.
5. Spread the fingers wide and focus on grounding the thumbs and forefingers into the mat as you spiral the upper arms out and the forearms in (elbows should be rolled slightly forward).
6. Press the hands into the mat to create more traction to lift the pelvis up and extend your heels back to lengthen the backs of your legs and ankles. Focus on pressing the heels back to attain this stretch.
7. Start to straighten your knees, but if you notice that this rounds your low back, keep the knees bent.
8. Lengthen the back of your neck; you can do so by gazing up to the belly or toward the toes.
9. Relax the shoulders down the back and away from the ears.
10. Hold for 5 to 8 breath cycles.
11. To exit, relax your knees back down on the mat and sit your hips back into Child's Pose (pages 38-39).

Modifications

- If this hurts the wrists, you can come down onto the forearms.
- You can pedal the feet by bending one knee and then the other while you settle into your Downward-Facing Dog.
- Practice against a wall by facing the wall, placing the hands at shoulder height, and walking the feet back. This allows both the spine to lengthen and the hamstrings to stretch, but without bringing the head below the heart.

Variations

- *Challenge variation:* Lift one leg at a time.
- *Restorative variation:* Place a bolster under the crown of the head for further support.

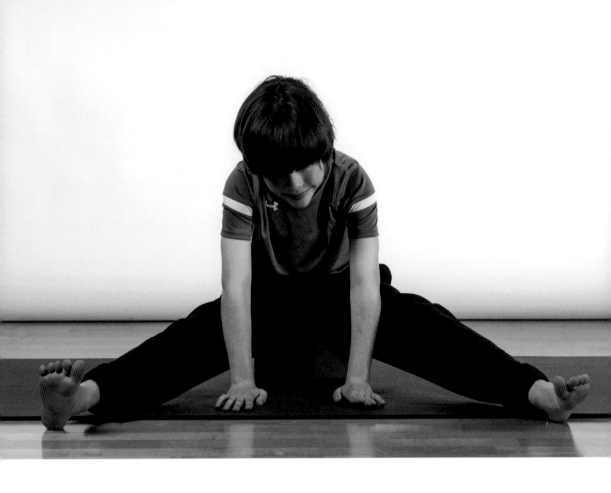

WIDE-ANGLE SEATED FORWARD BEND

Upavistha Konasana

As mentioned, hip adductor tightness or spasticity is common in those with CP. Thus, emphasis on flexibility training of the hip adductor muscles can greatly improve function and gait. Wide-Angle Seated Forward Bend provides a beneficial stretch to the hip adductors as well as to the knee flexor muscles.

Benefits

- Stretches the hip adductors.
- Stretches the knee flexors.

How To

1. Start seated in a comfortable position.
2. Extend your legs wide apart, enough so that you feel a stretch in the inner thighs (adductors).
3. Place your hands in front of you and extend the spine long.
4. Dorsiflex the feet, rolling the inner thighs out and behind you, toes and knees pointed up.
5. Press out through the heels to extend the knees toward straight.
6. Hinging from the hips, start to walk your hands forward so the torso comes forward between the legs.
7. Maintain a long spine and make sure that the toes remain pointed upward as you continue bending forward; do not let the spine round.
8. Bend as far as is comfortable for you, then hold for 5 to 10 breath cycles.
9. To exit the pose, walk the hands back until your spine is upright again. Place the hands under the knees to bend the knees back into a comfortable seated position.

Variations

- Place a block in front of you to rest your head.
- Place a bolster or a stack of blankets lengthwise in front of you to rest your torso down.
- Sit up on a block to take the strain away from your lower back and assist the spinal extension, as pictured.

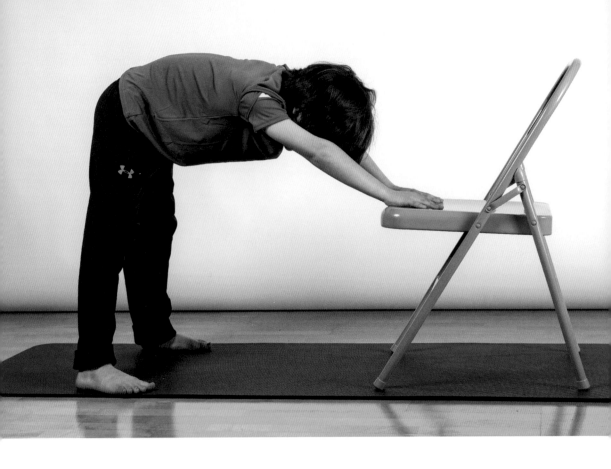

MODIFIED WIDE-LEGGED STANDING FORWARD BEND
Prasarita Padottanasana

This pose can be used as an alternative or a progression for stretching the hip adductors and knee flexors in Wide-Angle Seated Forward Bend. Furthermore, bringing your trunk (the COM) in front of the feet while they are in contact with the ground can elicit a stretch to the plantar flexors.

Benefits

- Stretches the hip adductors.
- Stretches the knee flexors.
- Stretches the plantar flexors.

Precautions

- Make sure that your balance is safe; if needed, bend forward with the arms on the seat of a chair.
- If it is uncomfortable to bring your head below your heart, just bend halfway.

How To

1. Start in Mountain (pages 150-151), with a chair or the wall in front of you for support.
2. With hands on your hips, step your feet wide apart (about 3 to 4 feet); the width should be measured so that if you were to extend the arms out to the sides, your ankles would align below your wrists.
3. Point the toes forward so that the feet are parallel to one another.
4. With hands on the hips or resting your hands on the wall or chair in front of you, engage the upper legs as you ground down through all four corners of both feet.
5. Inhale to lift the chest and extend the spine.
6. Hinging from the hips, exhale to bend forward as far as is comfortable for you. Again, rest the hands on the wall or chair in front of you if needed.
7. If you have the flexibility to bend forward over the legs, rest your hands on blocks, on your shins, or on the floor.
8. Make sure you maintain a lengthened, not rounded, spine as you bend forward.
9. Keep the neck relaxed.
10. Hold for 5 to 10 breath cycles.
11. To exit the pose, walk the hands up the wall, or place your hands on the hips again. Inhale to rise into an upright position and step your feet together. Be sure to come up slowly; you might feel light-headed when you first come up so refrain from any quick movements out of the pose.

Modifications

- Just bend halfway if it is not comfortable to position your head below your heart.
- You can use the back of a chair if you do not want to use the wall.
- You can use blocks in front of you to rest your hands on if you do not want to use the wall or a chair.

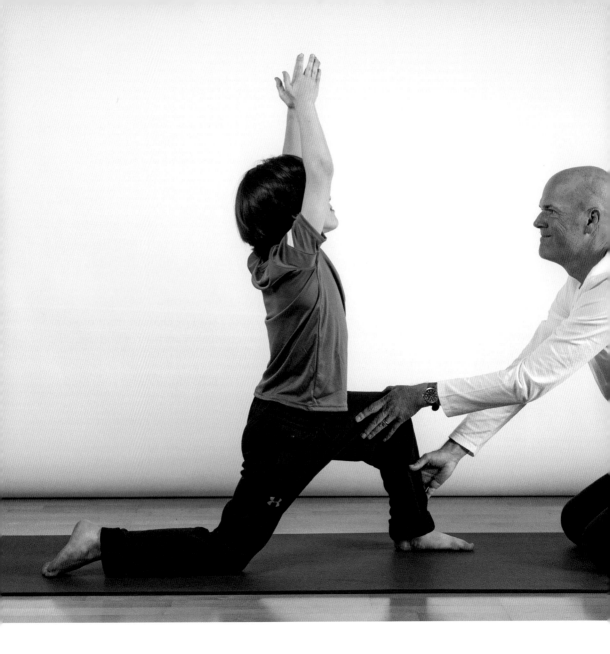

CRESCENT LUNGE Anjaneyasana

Spasticity or tightness in the hip flexors contributes to the characteristic crouched posture of CP. The tight hip flexors pull the pelvis forward into an anterior pelvic tilt, bringing the trunk forward with it, creating the characteristically hunched and crouched posture of CP. Crescent Lunge allows for an isolated hip flexor stretch of the back leg while using the body weight to increase the stretch, reversing tightened hip flexors. Place the hands on blocks or the wall to provide stability if needed.

Benefits

- Stretches the hip flexors (back leg).
- Strengthens the knee extensors (front leg).
- Strengthens the spinal extensors.

How To

1. From Downward-Facing Dog (pages 308-309), raise your left leg up and back to extend the leg.
2. Step the left foot forward in between your hands. If you can't make it there with your step, catch the ankle with your hand and assist it forward so it aligns with your hands.
3. Bring your torso upright and bend the front knee.
4. Make sure your knee is above your ankle, not forward of the ankle.
5. Lower the back (right) knee to rest on the ground; you can place a folded blanket or towel under the knee for cushioning.
6. Extend your arms up with the palms facing each other.
7. Expand your chest to the sky as you draw your arms further behind your ears and lift the chest up to deepen the stretch at the front of your right hip.
8. Gaze directly in front of you or slightly up to where the wall meets the ceiling, with the goal of extending the back of your neck.
9. Hold for 5 breath cycles.
10. To exit the pose, release your hands down to the mat to frame the foot and step the left foot back to Downward-Facing Dog.
11. Repeat on the right side.

Modifications

- Your hands can be on blocks, on your hips, or in Prayer Hands (pages 118-119), depending on the support you need.
- If balance is difficult here, start with your front leg alongside the wall to help maintain balance or enlist an assistant to stabilize the knee, as pictured here.

Variations

- *Challenge variation:* Perform the pose with the back knee off the mat for leg strengthening. Note that this tilts the pelvis forward, so you can add a slight bend in the back knee to neutralize the pelvis.
- *Restorative variation:* Place a bolster in front of the back knee and rest the quadriceps on the bolster.

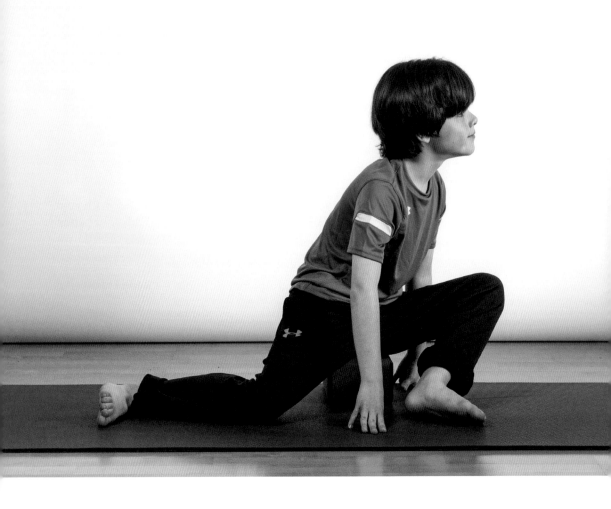

PIGEON Eka Pada Rajakapotasana

Pigeon is another pose that provides stretch to the hip flexor muscles (in the back leg). Additionally, this pose provides a stretch to the hip adductors of the front leg. The flexibility of these muscles is integral to walking, particularly in individuals with spastic CP who default into a crouched posture.

Benefits

- Stretches the hip flexors (back leg) and adductors (front leg).
- Strengthens the spinal extensors.
- Strengthens the elbow extensors.

Precautions

Avoid this pose if you have certain knee injuries that cause pain when weight is placed on the lateral aspect of the front knee.

Before You Begin

Have a block handy to put under the front hip.

How To

1. Start in Downward-Facing Dog (pages 308-309).
2. Shift halfway forward with your hips and bend your left knee while rotating your hip out so that your left ankle slides behind your right wrist.
3. Your left lateral shin will relax onto the floor and the left knee will rest lateral to the alignment of the hip.
4. Rest your hip on a block to try to square your hips forward.
5. Extend your right leg back with a straight knee, hip rotated slightly inward, and right upper thigh resting on the floor. Don't worry if your hip does not rotate inward; you will get there with practice.
6. With the hands supporting you, settle into the hip stretch; walk the hands back alongside the hips, or place the hands on blocks next to the hips.
7. The torso lifts up and the lower back lengthens with core engagement.
8. If this feels uncomfortable, scoot your left foot closer to your body.
9. Hold for 3 to 5 breath cycles.
10. To exit the pose, tuck the right toes under to straighten the leg, press into the hands to lift the left leg up and back again into Downward-Facing Dog.
11. Switch to the right side.

Modifications

Place a block or a folded blanket under the front hip to support your pelvis and achieve a leveling of the hips.

Variations

- *Challenge variations:* Bend your back knee and use the same-side hand to hold the foot or ankle to deeply stretch the quadriceps and the hip flexor, *or* practice without a block under the front hip.
- To make the pose even more challenging, walk the foot closer to the right wrist, to bring the left shin parallel to the front of the mat.
- *Restorative variations:* From the upright position, walk the hands forward to lie over the front leg, *or* rest your forehead on stacked hands, a folded blanket, or a block. You can also place a folded blanket under the back knee for cushioning.

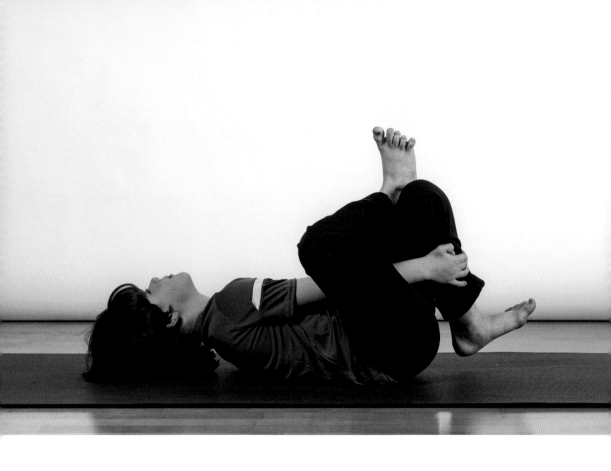

RECLINING PIGEON   Supta Eka Pada Rajakapotasana

Reclining Pigeon provides stretch to the hip flexor muscles for the bent leg, and also stretches the hamstrings of the opposite leg and the low back. It also provides protection for the knee for those with sensitive knee joints or if you find upright Pigeon uncomfortable.

Benefits

- Stretches the glutes and hip flexors of the bent leg.
- Stretches the low back.

How To

1. Lying on your back, bend the knees and place the feet on the floor, walking them under the knees, hip width apart.
2. Bend the right knee into the chest and place your right ankle above your left knee, creating a figure 4 with your legs.
3. Draw your left knee in to your chest and thread your right arm through the triangle created by your ankle and knee.
4. Interlace your fingers around the left shin or the back of your left thigh and draw your knees close to your chest.
5. Your head and shoulders should be resting on the ground. If they need to come off the floor to catch hold of the shin or thigh, you can use a strap to draw your legs in to the body.
6. Bonus: You can push your right knee away with your right arm while simultaneously drawing the left knee in for increased stretch.
7. Relax your sacrum, head, and shoulders on the ground while you draw the knees in.
8. Hold for 5 to 10 breath cycles.
9. To exit the pose, uncross and extend the legs.
10. Switch sides.

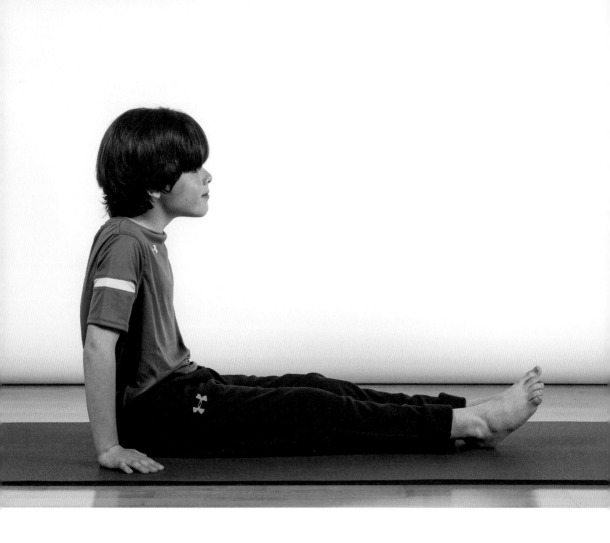

STAFF

Dandasana

Knee flexor tightness or spasticity has a significant functional impact on those with CP, so much so that some patients require hamstring lengthening surgery.[6] Knee flexor tightness and the consequent bent knees severely limit gait efficiency. Staff straightens the knees in a nonweight-bearing position, allowing for gentle stretching of the knee flexors. A yoga strap across the bottoms of the feet can also be used to stretch the plantar flexors.

Benefits

- Stretches the knee and plantar flexors.
- Strengthens the spinal extensors.
- Strengthens the knee extensors.

How To

1. Start seated with your legs extended in front of you, hands resting beside your hips with the palms facing down and fingers spread wide.
2. Dorsiflex your feet, extending out through the heels and pointing the toes up and toward the sky.
3. Press the backs of the knees down into the mat as you engage the quadriceps.
4. Roll the shoulders back and engage the belly.
5. Hold for 5 to 10 breath cycles.

Modifications

Sit facing a wall with your feet flat against the wall for awareness in dorsiflexion. Press the heels firmly into the wall.

Glossary

Chapter 1

Acquired disability — A disability that has developed during an individual's lifetime.

Adaptive yoga — Yoga postures adapted to all types of disabilities and bodies with the goal of improving function and quality of life.

Assistive device — A device used by people with disabilities to increase the ease of performing activities of daily living.

Base of support (BOS) — The area underneath a person that includes every point of contact the person makes with a supporting surface. These points of contact may be body parts, crutches, or a chair.

Center of mass (COM) — The point of the body at which its mass is most concentrated; this is the point around which the force of gravity acts.

Closed chain exercise — An exercise in which the hand or foot is fixed in space and cannot move.

Congenital disability — A condition present at birth, regardless of origin, which causes a decrease in function.

Meditation — A practice whereby an individual uses a technique (such as mindfulness, or focusing the mind on a particular object, single word, or activity) to train attention and awareness and to achieve a mentally clear and emotionally calm and stable state.

Mindfulness — A mental state achieved by focusing awareness on the present moment while calmly acknowledging and accepting one's feelings, thoughts, and bodily sensations, used as a therapeutic technique.

Nervous system — The complex collection of nerves and specialized cells known as neurons that transmit signals between different parts of the body.

Open chain exercise — An exercise in which the hand or foot is free to move.

Physical disability — A limitation of an individual's physical functioning, mobility, dexterity, or stamina.

Pose — In the context of yoga, a body position encompassed within the study and principles of hatha yoga.

Pranayama — The practice of breath control and breathing exercises in yoga.

PWD — Person(s) (or people) with disabilities (or disability).

Rehabilitation — The restoration of a person's health or normal life through training and therapy after injury or illness.

Relaxation response — The opposite of the body's stress response; a natural method of engaging the parasympathetic nervous system to reverse the effects of stress.

Yoga asana — A body position encompassed within the study and principles of hatha yoga.

Chapter 2

Antagonist muscle — Produces an opposing joint force to the muscles that are causing joint movement. These muscles aid in controlling and slowing down motion.

Core stability — A person's ability to use the postural muscles to control the position and movement of the spine and pelvis.

Core strength — The strength of the postural muscles.

Locomotion — Movement from one place to another.

Muscle activation — The contraction or engagement of a muscle.

Muscle control — The use of the nervous system to perform intentional, directed movement.

Muscle fibers — The individual contractile units within a muscle; a single muscle cell. Large bundles of muscle fibers form muscles.

Muscle flexibility — The ability of a muscle to increase in length and therefore allow movement in a joint or a series of joints.

Muscle groups — Muscles that are located close to one another and produce the same joint movements.

Musculoskeletal system — Provides form, support, stability, and movement to the body. It is made up of the bones of the skeleton, muscles, cartilage, tendons, ligaments, joints, and other connective tissue that supports and binds tissues and organs together.

Object manipulation — Interaction with objects in the environment, typically performed by using the hands to grasp and use an object for specific functional tasks.

Postural muscles — Found deep in the body, particularly in the pelvis, abdomen, and back. They include all the muscles of the spine, from the lower back up to the base of the neck.

Stabilization — The process of being made unlikely to move.

Chapter 3

Acute low back pain — Pain located in the low back that has been present for less than eight weeks.

Chronic low back pain — Pain located in the low back that has been present for longer than three months.

Cognitive behavioral therapy — A common type of talk therapy (psychotherapy) that focuses on challenging and changing unhelpful cognitive distortions and behaviors, improving emotional regulation, and developing coping strategies that target solving current problems.

Core activation — Contraction or activation of the postural muscles.

Extension — The action of bending backward.

Flexion — The action of bending forward.

Mindfulness-based stress reduction (MBSR) — A mindfulness training program to assist people with stress, anxiety, depression, and pain.

Physical therapy — A branch of rehabilitative health that uses specific exercise and equipment to help people with injuries regain or improve physical ability.

Radiculopathy—A condition due to a compressed nerve in the spine that can cause pain, numbness, tingling, or weakness along the course of the nerve. When this occurs in the low back, symptoms are felt in the legs.

Rotation—The action of twisting.

Spinal extension–based exercise—An exercise that incorporates moving the spine backwards, creating an arch.

Spinal loading—The application of force to the bones or joints of the spine.

Spinal stress—Excessive force on the bones or joints of the spine; may cause pain or injury over time.

Spinal traction—A form of decompression therapy for the spine that relieves pressure.

Subacute low back pain—Pain located in the low back that has been present between eight weeks and three months.

Trunk exercise—An exercise of the area of the body between the waist and the neck, excluding the arms.

Chapter 4

Degeneration—The process of being worn down or deteriorating.

Dorsiflexion—The action of raising the foot upward toward the lower leg.

End range position—The position of a joint or body part when it is moved as far as it can in that direction.

Full weight-bearing exercise—An exercise in which the limb being used is supporting the body's full weight.

Joint capsule—The tissue surrounding a joint, providing passive stability to the joint.

Joint cartilage—The smooth tissue that covers the ends of bones where they come together to form joints.

Joint impairment—A mobility deficit occurring at a joint, most commonly manifesting as stiffness or weakness.

Joint mobility—How much a joint can move.

Knee extensor activation—Contraction of the muscles that elicits extension of the knee joint.

Load—An external force acting on a muscle, bone, or joint.

Nonweight-bearing exercise—An exercise in which the limb being used has no weight placed on it.

Osteoarthritis—The wearing down of the protective cartilage at the end of bones where joints are formed. Occurs gradually and worsens over time.

Partial weight-bearing exercise—An exercise in which the limb being used is supporting between 30 and 50 percent of the body weight.

Proprioception—Perception or awareness of the position and movement of the body.

Range of motion (ROM)—The amount of movement possible around a joint or body part.

Stability — The state of resistance to change.

Surface area — The total area that the surface of an object occupies.

Chapter 5

Active pose — A pose that, once achieved, requires significant effort to maintain.

Biofeedback — The process of gaining greater awareness of many physiological functions of the body. This is achieved via performing a task while receiving visible or audible information in direct feedback regarding the performance of that specific task.

Contractures — Permanent shortening and hardening of muscles, tendons, or other tissue, often leading to deformity and rigidity of joints.

Dynamic exercise — An exercise that incorporates specific joints or whole-body movement.

High-intensity exercise — An exercise that requires significant effort and results in a significant increase in heart rate between short recovery periods.

Inflammatory markers — Proteins (biomarkers) released into the bloodstream during inflammation.

Joint erosion — Damage to bone caused by destruction of the cartilage and bone barrier.

Joint motion — The available motion of a joint.

Muscle atrophy — The wasting away or loss of muscle tissue, typically caused by lack of physical activity.

Passive pose — A pose that, once achieved, requires little work to maintain, such as Child's Pose.

Polyarthritis — The presence of arthritis in several joints.

Resultant disability — A disability that results directly from disease or injury.

Rheumatoid arthritis — A symmetric, inflammatory, peripheral polyarthritis of unknown origin, causing chronic inflammation that most commonly affects the lining of joints. It typically leads to deformity through the stretching of tendons and ligaments and destruction of joints through the erosion of cartilage and bone.

Rheumatoid nodule — A firm, palpable lump that develops under the skin. This symptom is unique to rheumatoid arthritis and usually occurs near joints affected by the condition.

Chapter 6

Assistive device — A device people with disabilities use to increase the ease of performing activities of daily living.

Community ambulation — Locomotion outside the home that allows people to interact with their environment, such as visits to the bank, pharmacy, and grocery store.

Gait abnormality — A deviation from typical walking. Problems in the nervous or musculoskeletal system manifest as gait abnormalities.

Gait pattern — The unique way an individual walks.

Gait training—A type of physical therapy that has the goal of improving an individual's ability to walk.

Intact (or sound) limb—A limb that has not undergone amputation.

Peripheral vascular disease (PVD)—A condition in which fatty deposits and calcium build up in the walls of the blood vessels, reducing blood flow to the limbs, which results in pain in the affected muscles.

Prosthetic device—A device that replaces a missing body part.

Prosthetic training—The process of learning to regain function and mobility with the use of a prosthetic device.

Residual limb—The portion of a limb that remains after an amputation.

Vascular disease—Any abnormal condition of the blood vessels.

Chapter 7

Compensatory movement—Movement used to achieve functional motor skills when a normal movement pattern is not available.

Complete paralysis—The inability to feel or contract the affected muscle groups at all.

Joint contracture—A condition of shortening and hardening of muscles, tendons, or other tissue, often leading to deformity and rigidity of the affected joints.

Muscle spasticity—A condition in which muscles stiffen or tighten, preventing normal fluid movement. The muscles remain contracted and resist being stretched, thus inhibiting free-flowing movement.

Neuropathic pain—Pain caused by damage or disease affecting the nervous system, typically manifesting as burning, tingling, stabbing electric shock, or pins-and-needles sensations.

Partial paralysis—Weakness or loss of sensation in a muscle or group of muscles, but without total loss of function.

Passive joint movement—The motion of a joint performed through no effort of the muscles or joints involved.

Sensory deprivation—The reduction or removal of stimuli from an area of the body.

Spinal cord—A long, thin, tubular structure made up of nervous tissue, which extends from the base of the brain to the lumbar region of the vertebral column. It carries the incoming and outgoing messages between the brain and the rest of the body.

Tone abnormality—The resistance to passive stretching of a muscle.

Voluntary muscle activation—The intentional contraction of a muscle.

Chapter 8

Akinesia—A decreased ability to move muscles voluntarily.

BIG movements—A therapy program for patients with Parkinson's disease with the goal of reducing the symptoms of pathologically small, slow movements by the repeated performance of big, whole-body movements.

Gait disturbance — A deviation from typical walking.

Isokinetic contractions — Contractions that allow muscles to exert maximum force at a constant speed within a joint's range of motion. The benefits vary by the speed at which they are performed. Low-velocity exercises increase muscle strength while high-velocity exercises assist in recovery of muscle endurance following an injury.

Kyphosis — An exaggerated, hunched rounding of the upper back.

Large amplitude pose — A yoga pose selected for the big size of its movements.

Lee Silverman Voice Treatment (LSVT) — A program designed to increase vocal intensity in patients with Parkinson's disease.

Motor task function — Movements and actions of the muscles that serve specific functions.

Rigidity — Stiff or inflexible muscles. Rigidity is one of the primary motor dysfunctions of Parkinson's disease.

Chapter 9

Asymmetric movement pattern — When the movement of one side of the body is significantly different from that of the other side of the body.

Cerebrovascular accident (CVA) — The medical term for a stroke, it describes damage occurring to the brain when its blood supply is interrupted, resulting in the impairment of brain function in the corresponding area of the brain.

Hemiparesis — Muscle weakness on one side of the body that decreases function and movement of the arms, legs, and facial muscles on that side.

Neuroplasticity — The ability of the brain to change and adapt, forming new connections or finding alternative pathways to optimize neural networks.

Postural deficit — An impairment in the ability to obtain or maintain an upright position.

Chapter 10

Axon — A long, slender projection of a nerve cell that conducts electrical impulses from the nucleus of the nerve to the nerve ending to allow it to communicate with other nerve cells, muscles, or glands.

Central nervous system (CNS) — Consists of the brain and spinal cord; controls most of the body's functions.

Demyelination — Damage to the myelin, resulting in neurological problems.

Myelin — An insulating sheath that covers nerve fibers, increasing the speed at which nerve impulses are conducted.

Relapsing-remitting — A form of MS in which patients have episodes of worsening symptoms (relapse) and periods of stability between episodes (remission).

Secondary-progressive — A form of MS in which symptoms steadily worsen with no periods of remission (improvement of symptoms).

Chapter 11

Agonist muscle — A muscle that causes a movement to occur by being activated.

Gastronomy tube — A tube inserted through the abdomen to deliver nutrition directly into the stomach. This is done in instances where an individual has difficulty swallowing.

Mass movement — Movement that occurs across multiple joints, using multiple muscle groups.

Spastic diplegia — A form of CP that manifests as high and constant tightness in the muscles of the lower extremities.

References

Preface

1. Desikachar, K. *The Yoga of the Yogi: The Legacy of T. Krishnamacharya*. New York: Macmillan, 2011.

Chapter 1

1. Büssing, A., T. Ostermann, R. Lüdtke, and A. Michalsen. Effects of yoga interventions on pain and pain-associated disability: A meta-analysis. *J Pain* 13, no. 1 (2012): 1-9.

2. Chou, R., A. Qaseem, V. Snow, et al. Clinical Efficacy Assessment Subcommittee of the American College of Physicians; American College of Physicians; American Pain Society low back pain guidelines panel diagnosis and treatment of low back pain: A joint clinical practice guideline from the American College of Physicians and the American Pain Society. *Ann Intern Med* 147, no. 7 (2007): 478-91.

3. Cohen, E.T., D. Kietrys, S.G. Fogerite, M. Silva, K. Logan, D.A. Barone, et al. Feasibility and impact of an 8-week integrative yoga program in people with moderate multiple sclerosis-related disability: A pilot study. *Int J MS Care* 19, no. 1 (2017): 30-39.

4. Curtis, K., S.L. Hitzig, G. Bechsgaard, C. Stoliker, C. Alton, N. Saunders, et al. Evaluation of a specialized yoga program for persons with a spinal cord injury: A pilot randomized controlled trial. *J Pain Res* 10 (2017): 999-1017.

5. Desveaux, L., A. Lee, R. Goldstein, and D. Brooks. Yoga in the management of chronic disease: A systematic review and meta-analysis. *Med Care* 53, no. 7 (2015): 653-61.

6. Field, T. Yoga research review. *Complement Ther Clin Pract* 24 (2016): 145-61.

7. Imai, A., K. Kaneoka, Y. Okubo, I. Shiina, M. Tatsumura, S. Izumi, and H. Shiraki. Trunk muscle activity during lumbar stabilization exercises on both a stable and unstable surface. *J Orthop Sport Phys* 40, no. 6 (2010): 369-75. https://doi.org/10.2519/jospt.2010.3211.

8. Justice, L.C., C. Brems, and C. Jacova. Exploring strategies to enhance self-efficacy about starting a yoga practice. *Ann Yoga Phys Ther* 1 (2016): 1-7.

9. Krahn, G.L., D.K. Walker, and R. Correa-De-Araujo. Persons with disabilities as an unrecognized health disparity population. *Am J Public Health* 105, Suppl 2 (2015): S198-206.

10. Kwon, Y.J., S.J. Park, J. Jefferson, and K. Kim. The effect of open and closed kinetic chain exercises on dynamic balance ability of normal healthy adults. *J Phys Ther Sci* 25, no. 6 (2013): 671-74. https://doi.org/10.1589/jpts.25.671.

11. Nagi, S. "Some Conceptual Issues in Disability and Rehabilitation." In M.B. Sussman, ed., *Sociology and Rehabilitation*. Washington, DC: American Sociological Association, 1965.

12. Ostelo, R.W., M.W. van Tulder, J.W. Vlaeyen, S.J. Linton, S.J. Morley, and W.J. Assendelft. Behavioural treatment for chronic low-back pain. *Cochrane Database Syst* 1 (2005).

13. Rimmer, J.H., et al. Rationale and design of a scale-up project evaluating responsiveness to home exercise and lifestyle tele-health (super-health) in people with physical/mobility disabilities: A type 1 hybrid design

effectiveness trial. *BMJ Open* 9, no. 3 (2019): e023538.

14. Schmid, A.A., K.K. Miller, M. Van Puymbroeck, and N. Schalk. Feasibility and results of a case study of yoga to improve physical functioning in people with chronic traumatic brain injury. *Disabil Rehabil* 38, no. 9 (2016): 914-20.

15. Sharpe, P.A., S. Wilcox, D.E. Schoffman, B. Hutto, and A. Ortaglia. Association of complementary and alternative medicine use with symptoms and physical functional performance among adults with arthritis. *Disabil Health J* 9, no. 1 (2016): 37-45.

16. Thomas, E.V., J. Warren-Findlow, and J.B. Webb. Yoga is for every (able) body: A content analysis of disability themes within mainstream yoga media. *Int J Yoga* 12, no. 1 (2019): 68.

17. Verbrugge, L.M., and A.M. Jette. The disablement process. *Soc Sci Med* 38, no. 1 (1994): 1-4.

18. World Health Organization. World Report on Disability. Geneva, Switzerland: World Health Organization (2011).

Chapter 2

1. Panjabi, M.M. The stabilizing system of the spine: Part II. Neutral zone and instability hypothesis. *J Spinal Disord* 5, no. 4 (1992): 390-97. https://doi.org/10.1097/00002517-199212000-00002.

Chapter 3

1. Bergquist-Ullman, M., and U. Larsson. Acute low back pain in industry. A controlled prospective study with special reference to therapy and confounding factors. *Acta Orthop Scand* 170 (1977): 1-117.

2. Bevevino, A., D. Kang, S. Pangarkar, F. Sandbrink, and C. Aberle. United States Department of Veterans Affairs,

Department of Defense. Clinical Practice Guideline for Diagnosis and Treatment of Low Back Pain. September 2017.

3. Chou, R., R. Deyo, J. Friedly, et al. AHRQ Comparative Effectiveness Reviews. Noninvasive Treatments for Low Back Pain. Rockville, MD: Agency for Healthcare Research and Quality (US), 2016.

4. Demirel A., M. Oz, Y. Ozel, H. Cetin, and O. Ulger. Stabilization exercise versus yoga exercise in non-specific low back pain: Pain, disability, quality of life, performance: a randomized controlled trial. *Complement Ther Clin Pract* 35 (2019): 102-08. http://doi:10.1016/j.ctcp.2019.02.004.

5. Dieleman, J.L., R. Baral, M. Birger, et al. US spending on personal health care and public health, 1996-2013. *JAMA* 316, no. 24 (2016): 2627-46.

6. George, S.Z. Fear: A factor to consider in musculoskeletal rehabilitation. *J Orthop Sports Phys Ther* 35, no. 5 (2006): 264-66. http://dx.doi.org/10.2519/jospt.2006.0106.

7. Kuo, C.S., H.T. Hu, R.M. Lin, K.Y. Huang, P.C. Lin, Z.C. Zhong, and M.L. Hseih. Biomechanical analysis of the lumbar spine on facet joint force and intradiscal pressure: A finite element study. *BMC Musculoskelet Disord* 11, no. 1 (2010). https://doi.org/10.1186/1471-2474-11-151.

8. Long, L., A. Huntley, and E. Ernst. Which complementary and alternative therapies benefit which conditions? A survey of the opinions of 223 professional organizations. *Complement Ther Med* 9, no. 3 (2001): 178-85.

9. Patil, N.J., R. Nagaratna, P. Tekur, P.V. Manohar, H. Bhargav, and D. Patil. A randomized trial comparing effect of yoga and exercises on quality of life in among nursing population. *Int J Yoga* 11, no. 3 (2018): 208-14.

10. Phimphasak, C., M. Swangnetr, R. Puntumetakul, U. Chatchawan, and R. Boucaut. Effects of seated lumbar extension postures on spinal height and lumbar range of motion during prolonged sitting. *Ergonomics* 59, no. 1 (2015): 112-20. https://doi.org/10.1080/00140139.2015.1052570.

11. Pincus T., A.K. Burton, S. Vogel, and A.P. Field. A systematic review of psychological factors as predictors of chronicity/disability in prospective cohorts of low back pain. *Spine* 27, no. 5 (2002): E109-20.

12. Steenstra, I.A., J.H. Verbeek, M.W. Heymans, and P.M. Bongers. Prognostic factors for duration of sick leave in patients sick listed with acute low back pain: a systematic review of the literature. *Occup Environ Med* 62, no. 12 (2005): 851-60. http://dx.doi.org/10.1136/oem.2004.015842.

13. Thelin, A., S. Holmberg, and N. Thelin. Functioning in neck and low back pain from a 12-year perspective: A prospective population-based study. *J Rehabil Med* 40, no. 7 (2008): 555-61. http://dx.doi.org/10.2340/16501977-0205.

Chapter 4

1. Ackland, D.C., M. Denton, A.G. Schache, M.G. Pandy, and K.M. Crossley. Hip abductor muscle volumes are smaller in individuals affected by patellofemoral joint osteoarthritis. *Osteoarthritis Cartilage* 27, no. 2 (2019): 266-72. https://doi.org/10.1016/j.joca.2018.09.013.

2. Bannuru, R.R., M.C. Osani, E.C. Vaysbrot, N.K. Arden, K. Bennell, S.M.A. Bierma-Zeinstra, V.B. Kraus, et al. OARSI guidelines for the non-surgical management of knee, hip, and polyarticular osteoarthritis. *Osteoarthritis Cartilage* 27, no. 11 (2019). https://doi.org/10.1016/j.joca.2019.06.011.

3. Bolgla, L.A., and T.L. Uhl. Electromyographic analysis of hip rehabilitation exercises in a group of healthy subjects. *J Orthop Sports Phys Ther* 35, no. 8 (2005). https://doi.org/10.2519/jospt.2005.2066.

4. Calatayud, J., S. Borreani, J. Martin, F. Martin, J. Flandez, and J.C. Colado. Core muscle activity in a series of balance exercises with different stability conditions. *Gait Posture* 42, no. 2 (2015): 186-92. https://doi.org/10.1016/j.gaitpost.2015.05.008.

5. Cibulka, M.T., N.J. Bloom, K.R. Enseki, C.W. MacDonald, J. Woehrle, C.M. McDonough, et al. Hip and mobility deficits — hip osteoarthritis. *J Orthop Sports Phys Ther* 47, no. 6 (2017): A1-A37. https://doi.org/10.2519/jospt.2017.0301.

6. De l'Escalopier, N., P. Anract, and D. Biau. Surgical treatments for osteoarthritis. *Ann Phys Rehabil Med* 59, no. 3 (2016): 227-33.

7. Dunlop, D.D., S.L. Hughes, P. Edelman, R.M. Singer, and R.W. Chang. Impact of joint impairment on disability-specific domains at four years. *J Clin Epidemiol* 51, no. 12 (1998): 1253-61.

8. Edd, S.N., J. Favre, K. Blazek, P. Omoumi, J.L. Asay, and T.P. Andriacchi. Altered gait mechanics and elevated serum pro-inflammatory cytokines in asymptomatic patients with MRI evidence of knee cartilage loss. *Osteoarthritis Cartilage* 25, no. 6 (2017): 899-906. https://doi.org/10.1016/j.joca.2016.12.029.

9. Ekstrom, R.A., R.A. Donatelli, and K.C. Carp. Electromyographic analysis of core trunk, hip, and thigh muscles during 9 rehabilitation exercises. *Journal of Orthopaedic & Sports Physical Therapy* 37, no. 12 (2007): 754-62. https://doi.org/10.2519/jospt.2007.2471.

10. Foucher, K.C., and M.A. Wimmer. Contralateral hip and knee gait biomechanics are unchanged by total

hip replacement for unilateral hip osteoarthritis. *Gait Posture* 35, no. 1 (2012): 61-65. https://doi.org/10.1016/j.gaitpost.2011.08.006.

11. Goh, S.-L., M.S.M. Persson, J. Stocks, Y. Hou, N.J. Welton, J. Lin, M.C. Hall, M. Doherty, and W. Zhang. Relative efficacy of different exercises for pain, function, performance and quality of life in knee and hip osteoarthritis: Systematic review and network meta-analysis. *Sports Med* 49, no. 5 (2019). https://doi.org/10.1007/s40279-019-01082-0.

12. Hafer, J.F., J.A. Kent, and K.A. Boyer. Physical activity and age-related biomechanical risk factors for knee osteoarthritis. *Gait Posture* 70 (2019): 24-29.

13. Hart, J.M., B. Pietrosimone, J. Hertel, and C.D. Ingersoll. Quadriceps activation following knee injuries: A systematic review. *J Athl Train* 45, no. 1 (2010): 87-97. https://doi.org/10.4085/1062-6050-45.1.87.

14. Kampshoff, P., K. Van Doormaal, and V. Meerhoff. KNGF guideline for physical therapy in patients with osteoarthritis of the hip and knee. *Supplement to the Dutch Journal of Physical Therapy* 120, no. 1 (2010).

15. Kim, C., M.C. Nevitt, J. Niu, et al. Association of hip pain with radiographic evidence of hip osteoarthritis: diagnostic test study. *BMJ* (2015): 351. https://doi.org/10.1136/bmj.h5983.

16. Loureiro, A., M. Constantinou, L.E. Diamond, B. Beck, and R. Barrett. Individuals with mild-to-moderate hip osteoarthritis have lower limb muscle strength and volume deficits. *BMC Musculoskelet Dis* 19, no. 1 (2018). https://doi.org/10.1186/s12891-018-2230-4.

17. Neelapala, Y.V., M.B. Raghava, and P. Shah. Hip muscle strengthening for knee osteoarthritis. *J Geriatr Phys Ther* 43, no.

18. Pua, Y.-H., T.V. Wrigley, S.M. Cowan, and K.L. Bennell. Hip flexion range of motion and physical function in hip osteoarthritis: Mediating effects of hip extensor strength and pain. *Arthritis Rheum* 61, no. 5 (2009): 633-40. https://doi.org/10.1002/art.24509.

19. Steinhilber, B., G. Haupt, R. Miller, P. Janssen, and I. Krauss. Exercise therapy in patients with hip osteoarthritis: Effect on hip muscle strength and safety aspects of exercise—Results of a randomized controlled trial. *Mod Rheumatol* 27, no. 3 (2016): 493-502. https://doi.org/10.1080/14397595.2016.1213940.

20. Suetta, C., P. Aagaard, S.P. Magnusson, L.L. Andersen, S. Sipila, A. Rosted, et al. Muscle size, neuromuscular activation, and rapid force characteristics in elderly men and women: Effects of unilateral long-term disuse due to hip osteoarthritis. *J Appl Physiol* 102, no. 3 (2007): 942-48.

21. Tateuchi, H., H. Akiyama, K. Goto, K. So, Y. Kuroda, and N. Ichihashi. Gait- and posture-related factors associated with changes in hip pain and physical function in patients with secondary hip osteoarthritis: A prospective cohort study. *Arch Phys Med Rehabil* 100, no. 11 (2019). https://doi.org/10.1016/j.apmr.2019.04.006.

22. Wang, Y., S. Lu, R. Wang, P. Jiang, F. Rao, B. Wang, Y. Zhu, Y. Hu, and J. Zhu. Integrative effect of yoga practice in patients with knee arthritis. *Medicine (Baltimore)* 97, no. 31 (2018). https://doi.org/10.1097/md.0000000000011742.

23. Wyndow, N., N.J. Collins, B. Vicenzino, K. Tucker, and K.M. Crossley. Foot and ankle characteristics and dynamic knee valgus in individuals with patellofemoral osteoarthritis. *J Foot Ankle Res* 11, no. 65 (2018). https://doi.org/10.1186/s13047-018-0310-1.

Chapter 5

1. Astin, J.A., W. Beckner, K. Soeken, M.C. Hochberg, and B. Berman. Psychological interventions for rheumatoid arthritis: A meta-analysis of randomized controlled trials. *Arthritis Rheum* 47, no. 3 (2002): 291-302.

2. Badsha, H., C. Leibman, A. Mofti, and K.O. Kong. The benefits of yoga for rheumatoid arthritis: Results of a preliminary, structured 8-week program. *Rheumatol Int* 29, no. 12 (2009): 1417-21.

3. Bartlett, S.J., H. Steffany, C.M. Moonaz, S. Bernatsky, and C.O. Bingham. Yoga in rheumatic diseases. *Curr Rheumatol Rep* 15, no. 12 (2013): 387.

4. Burmester, G.R., and J.E. Pope. Novel treatment strategies in rheumatoid arthritis. *Lancet* 389, no. 10086 (2017): 2338-48.

5. Combe, B. Early rheumatoid arthritis: Strategies for prevention and management. *Best Pract Res Clin Rheumatol* 21, no. 1 (2007): 27-42.

6. Evans, S., M. Moieni, R. Taub, S.K. Subramanian, J.C. Tsao, B. Sternlieb, and L.K. Zeltzer. Iyengar yoga for young adults with rheumatoid arthritis: Results from a mixed-methods pilot study. *J Pain Symptom Manage* 39, no. 5 (2010): 904-13.

7. Firestein, G.S. Evolving concepts of rheumatoid arthritis. *Nature* 423, no. 6937 (2003): 356.

8. Hurkmans, E., F.J. van der Giesen, T.P. Vliet Vlieland, et al. Dynamic exercise programs (aerobic capacity and/or muscle strength training) in patients with rheumatoid arthritis. *Cochrane Database Syst Rev* 4 (2009).

9. Kavuncu, V., and D. Evcik. Physiotherapy in rheumatoid arthritis. *MedGenMed* 6, no. 2 (2004): 3.

10. Kay, J., and K.S. Upchurch. ACR/EULAR 2010 rheumatoid arthritis classification criteria. *Rheumatology (Oxford)* 51 (2012), Issue suppl 6: vi5-9.

11. Kumar, K. Complete the course of sleep through yoga nidra. *Nature Wealth* 7 (2008).

12. Lorig, K., and J. Fries. *The arthritis helpbook: A tested self-management program for coping with arthritis and fibromyalgia.* Boston: Da Capo Press, 2009.

13. Metsios, G.S., and A. Lemmey. Exercise as medicine in rheumatoid arthritis: Effects on function, body composition, and cardiovascular disease risk. *J Clin Exerc Physiol* 4, no. 1 (2015): 14-22.

14. Mishra, B. The effect of yoga nidra in the management of rheumatoid arthritis. *Anc Sci Life* 32, Suppl 1 (2012): S118.

15. Munneke, M., Z. de Jong, A.H. Zwinderman, H.K. Ronday, D. van Schaardenburg, B.A. Dijkmans, H.M. Kroon, T.P. Vliet Vlieland, and J.M. Hazes. Effect of a high-intensity weight-bearing exercise program on radiologic damage progression of the large joints in subgroups of patients with rheumatoid arthritis. *Arthritis Rheum* 53, no. 3 (2005): 410-17.

16. Pradhan, E.K., M. Baumgarten, P. Langenberg, B. Handwerger, A.K. Gilpin, T. Magyari, M.C. Hochberg, and B.M. Berman. Effect of mindfulness-based stress reduction in rheumatoid arthritis patients. *Arthr Rheum* 57, no. 7 (2007): 1134-42.

17. Salmon, V.E., S. Hewlett, N.E. Walsh, J.R. Kirwan, and F. Cramp. Physical activity interventions for fatigue in rheumatoid arthritis: A systematic review. *Phys Ther Rev* 22, no. 1-2 (2017): 12-22.

18. Stack, R.J., L.H. van Tuyl, M. Sloots, L.A. van de Stadt, W. Hoogland, B. Maat, et al. Symptom complexes in patients with seropositive arthralgia and in patients newly diagnosed with rheumatoid arthritis: A qualitative exploration of

symptom development. *Rheumatology (Oxford)* 53, no. 9 (2014): 1646-53.

19. Stenström, C.H. Therapeutic exercise in rheumatoid arthritis. *Arthr Rheum* 7, no. 4 (1994): 190-97.

20. Van den Ende, C.H., T.P. Vliet Vlieland, M. Munneke, and J.M. Hazes. Dynamic exercise therapy in rheumatoid arthritis: A systematic review. *Br J Rheumatol* 37, no. 6 (1998): 677-87.

21. Verhoeven, F., N. Tordi, C. Prati, C. Demougeot, F. Mougin, and D. Wendling. Physical activity in patients with rheumatoid arthritis. *Joint Bone Spine* 83, no. 3 (2016): 265-70.

22. Wang, M.Y., S.S.Y. Yu, R. Hashish, S.D. Samarawickrame, L. Kazadi, G.A. Greendale, and G. Salem. The biomechanical demands of standing yoga poses in seniors: The Yoga Empowers Seniors Study (YESS). *BMC Complement Altern Med* 13, no. 8 (2013).

23. Ward, L., G.J. Treharne, and S. Stebbings. The suitability of yoga as a potential therapeutic intervention for rheumatoid arthritis: A focus group approach. *Musculoskeletal Care* 9, no. 4 (2011): 211-21.

24. Young, A., J. Dixey, N. Cox, P. Davies, J. Devlin, P. Emery, S. Gallivan, et al. How does functional disability in early rheumatoid arthritis (RA) affect patients and their lives? Results of 5 years of follow-up in 732 patients from the Early RA Study (ERAS). *Rheumatology (Oxford)* 39, no. 6 (2000): 603-11.

Chapter 6

1. Chui, K.C., Y. Sheng-Che, J. Milagros, and M.M. Lusardi. *Orthotics and Prosthetics in Rehabilitation*. Philadelphia: Saunders, 2019.

2. Dillingham, T.R., L.E. Pezzin, and E.J. Mackenzie. Limb amputation and limb deficiency. *Southern Med J* 95, no. 8 (2002): 875-83. https://doi.org/10.1097/00007611-200295080-00019.

3. Gallagher, P., M.-A. O'Donovan, A. Doyle, and D. Desmond. Environmental barriers, activity limitations and participation restrictions experienced by people with major limb amputation. *Prosthet Orthot Int* 35, no. 3 (2011): 278-84. https://doi.org/10.1177/0309364611407108.

4. Isakov, E., H. Burger, J. Krajnik, M. Gregoric, and C. Marincek. Knee muscle activity during ambulation of trans-tibial amputees. *J Rehabil Med* 33, no. 5 (2001): 196-99. https://doi.org/10.1080/165019701750419572.

5. Miller, W.C., and A.B. Deathe. A prospective study examining balance confidence among individuals with lower limb amputation. *Disabil Rehabil* 26, no. 14-15 (2004): 875-81. https://doi.org/10.1080/09638280410001708887.

6. Miller, W.C., M. Speechley, and B. Deathe. The prevalence and risk factors of falling and fear of falling among lower extremity amputees. *Arch Phys Med Rehabil* 82, no. 8 (2001): 1031-37. https://doi.org/10.1053/apmr.2001.24295.

7. Moura, V.L., K.R. Faurot, S.A. Gaylord, J.D. Mann, M. Sill, C. Lynch, and M.Y. Lee. Mind-body interventions for treatment of phantom limb pain in persons with amputation. *Am J Phys Med Rehab* 91, no. 8 (2012): 701-14. https://doi.org/10.1097/phm.0b013e3182466034.

8. Nadollek, H., S. Brauer, and R. Isles. Outcomes after trans-tibial amputation: The relationship between quiet stance ability, strength of hip abductor muscles and gait. *Physiother Res Int* 7, no. 4 (2002): 203-14. https://doi.org/10.1002/pri.260.

9. Renzi, R., N. Unwin, R. Jubelirer, and L. Haag. An international comparison of lower extremity amputation rates. *Ann Vasc Surg* 20, no. 3 (2006): 346-50. https://doi.org/10.1007/s10016-006-9044-9.

10. Schoppen, T., A. Boonstra, J.W. Groothoff, J. de Vries, L.N. Goeken, and W.H. Eisma. Physical, mental, and social predictors of functional outcome in unilateral lower-limb amputees. *Arch Phys Med Rehabil* 84, no. 6 (2003): 803-11. https://doi.org/10.1016/s0003-9993(02)04952-3.

11. Vanicek, N., S. Strike, L. McNaughton, and R. Polman. Gait patterns in transtibial amputee fallers vs. non-fallers: Biomechanical differences during level walking. *Gait Posture* 29, no. 3 (2009): 415-20. https://doi.org/10.1016/j.gaitpost.2008.10.062.

12. van Velzen, J.M., C.A. van Bennekom, W. Polomski, J.R. Slootman, L.H. van der Woude, and H. Houdijk. Physical capacity and walking ability after lower limb amputation: A systematic review. *Clin Rehabil* 20, no. 11 (2006): 999-1016. https://doi.org/10.1177/0269215506070700.

13. Wilken, J.M., and R. Marin. Gait analysis and training of people with limb loss. https://pdfs.semanticscholar.org/805d/0c8e2974f45beb3ee5219cc2709c1eb95eb2.pdf.

14. Wong, C.K., et al. Exercise programs to improve gait performance in people with lower limb amputation: A systematic review. *Prosthet Orthot Int* 40, no. 1 (2014): 8-17. https://doi:10.1177/0309364614546926.

Chapter 7

1. Beninato, M., K.S. Okane, and P.E. Sullivan. Relationship between motor FIM and muscle strength in lower cervical-level spinal cord injuries. *Spinal Cord* 42, no. 9 (2004): 533-40. https://doi.org/10.1038/sj.sc.3101635.

2. Boninger, M.L. Preservation of upper limb function following spinal cord injury: A clinical practice guideline for health-care professionals. *J Spinal Cord Med* 28, no. 5 (2005): 434-70. https://doi.org/10.1080/10790268.2005.11753844.

3. Durán, F.S., L. Lugo, L. Ramírez, and E. Eusse. Effects of an exercise program on the rehabilitation of patients with spinal cord injury. *Arch Phys Med Rehabil* 82, no. 10 (2001): 1349-54. https://doi.org/10.1053/apmr.2001.26066.

4. Fawcett, J.W., A. Curt, J.D. Steeves, W.P. Coleman, M.H. Tuszynski, D. Lammertse, P.F. Bartlett, et al. Guidelines for the conduct of clinical trials for spinal cord injury as developed by the ICCP panel: Spontaneous recovery after spinal cord injury and statistical power needed for therapeutic clinical trials. *Spinal Cord* 45, no. 3 (2006): 190-205. https://doi.org/10.1038/sj.sc.3102007.

5. Frownfelter, D.L., and E.W. Dean. *Cardiovascular and Pulmonary Physical Therapy: Evidence to Practice*. St. Louis, MO: Mosby, 2012.

6. Frye, S.K., P. Richley Geigle, H.S. York, and W.M. Sweatman. Functional passive range of motion of individuals with chronic cervical spinal cord injury. *J Spinal Cord Med* 42, no. 22 (2019): 1-7. https://doi.org/10.1080/10790268.2019.1622239.

7. Fujiwara, T., Y. Hara, K. Akaboshi, and N. Chino. Relationship between shoulder muscle strength and functional independence measure (FIM) score among c6 tetraplegics. *Spinal Cord* 37, no. 1 (1999): 58-61. https://doi.org/10.1038/sj.sc.3100715.

8. Jackson, A.B., and M.L. Sipski. Invited review shoulder pain in chronic spinal cord injury, Part 1: Epidemiology, etiology, and pathomechanics. *J Spinal Cord Med* 28, no. 2 (2005): 81-91. http://doi.org/10.1080/10790268.2005.11753803.

9. National Spinal Cord Injury Statistical Center, Facts and Figures at a Glance. Birmingham, AL: University of Alabama at Birmingham, 2018.

10. Nawoczenski, D.A., J.M. Ritter-Soronen, C.M. Wilson, B.A. Howe, and P.M. Ludewig. Clinical trial of exercise for shoulder pain in chronic spinal injury. *Phys Ther* 86, no. 12 (2006): 1604-18. https://doi.org/10.2522/ptj.20060001.

11. Somers, M.F. *Spinal Cord Injury Functional Rehabilitation*. Boston: Pearson Education International, 2010.

Chapter 8

1. Abe, K., Y. Uchida, and M. Notani. Camptocormia in Parkinson's disease. *Parkinson's Dis* (2010): 1-5. https://doi.org/10.4061/2010/267640.

2. Allen, N.E., A.K. Schwarzel, and C.G. Canning. Recurrent falls in Parkinson's disease: A systematic review. *Parkinson's Dis* (2013).

3. Amara, A.W., and A.A. Memon. Effects of exercise on non-motor symptoms in Parkinson's disease. *Clin Ther* 40, no. 1 (2018): 8-15.

4. Bega, D., et al. Yoga versus resistance training in mild to moderate severity Parkinson's disease: A 12-week pilot study. *J Yoga Phys Ther* 6 (2016): 222.

5. Birtwell, K., L. Dubrow-Marshall, R. Dubrow-Marshall, et al. A mixed methods evaluation of a Mindfulness-Based Stress Reduction course for people with Parkinson's disease. *Complement Ther Clin Pract* 29 (2017): 220.

6. Boulgarides, L.K., E. Barakatt, and B. Coleman-Salgado. Measuring the effect of an eight-week adaptive yoga program on the physical and psychological status of individuals with Parkinson's disease. A pilot study. *Int J Yoga Ther* 24 (2014): 31-41.

7. Colgrove, Y.S., et al. Effect of yoga on motor function in people with Parkinson's disease: A randomized, controlled pilot study. *J Yoga Phys Ther* 2 (2012): 112.

8. Comella, C.L., G.T. Stebbins, N. Brown-Toms, and C.G. Goetz. Physical therapy and Parkinson's disease: A controlled clinical trial. *Neurology* 44 (1994): 376.

9. Cummings, J.L. Depression and Parkinson's disease: A review. *American J Psychiatry* 149, no. 4 (1992): 443.

10. Ebersbach, G., et al. Amplitude-oriented exercise in Parkinson's disease: A randomized study comparing LSVT-BIG and a short training protocol. *J Neural Transm (Vienna)* 122, no. 2 (2015): 253-56.

11. Fox, C.M., et al. The science and practice of LSVT/LOUD: Neural plasticity-principled approach to treating individuals with Parkinson disease and other neurological disorders. *Sem Speech Lang* 27, no. 4 (2006): 283-99.

12. Fox, C., et al. LSVT LOUD and LSVT BIG: Behavioral treatment programs for speech and body movement in Parkinson disease. *Parkinson's Dis* (2012). https://doi.org/10.1155/2012/391946.

13. Janssens, J., et al. Application of LSVT BIG intervention to address gait, balance, bed mobility, and dexterity in people with Parkinson disease: a case series. *Phys Ther* 94, no. 7 (2014): 1014-23.

14. Kwok, J.Y.Y., J.C.Y. Kwan, M. Auyeung, et al. Effects of mindfulness yoga vs stretching and resistance training exercises on anxiety and depression for people with Parkinson disease: A randomized clinical trial. *JAMA Neurol* 76, no. 7 (2019): 755.

15. Lakke, J.P.W.F. Axial apraxia in Parkinson's disease. *J Neurol Sci* 69, no. 1-2 (1985): 37-46.

16. LSVT BIG treatment. n.d. Accessed October 2019. www.lsvtglobal.com/LSVTBig.

17. McHenry, M. The effect of increased vocal effort on estimated velopharyngeal orifice area. *Am J Speech Lang Pat* 6, no. 4 (1997): 55-61.

18. Ni, M., et al. Comparative effect of power training and high-speed yoga on motor function in older patients with Parkinson disease. *Arch Phys Med Rehabil* 97, no. 3 (2016): 345-54.e15.

19. Ni, M., K. Mooney, and J.F. Signorile. Controlled pilot study of the effects of power yoga in Parkinson's disease. *Complement Ther Med* 25 (2016): 126-31.

20. Parkinson, J. *An Essay on the Shaking Palsy.* London: Sherwood, Neely, and Jones, 1817.

21. Ramig, L.O., S. Countryman, C. O'Brien, M. Hoehn, and L. Thompson. Intensive speech treatment for patients with Parkinson disease: Short and long-term comparison of two techniques. *Neurology* 47, no. 6 (1996): 1496-1504.

22. Ramig, L.O., et al. Intensive voice treatment (LSVT) for patients with Parkinson's disease: A 2 year follow up. *J Neurol Neurosurg Psychiatry* 71, no. 4 (2001): 493-98.

23. Roland, K.P. Applications of yoga in Parkinson's disease: A systematic literature review. *Res Rev Parkinson* 4 (2014): 1-8.

24. Roland, K.P. Yoga for Parkinson's: What the research says. (2015). www.michaeljfox.org/news/yoga-parkinsons-what-research-says.

25. Senard, J.M., et al. Prevalence of orthostatic hypotension in Parkinson's disease. *J Neur Neurosurg Psychiatry* 63, no. 5 (1997): 584-89.

26. Smith, A., L. Goffman, H.N. Zelaznik, G. Ying, and C. McGillem. Spatiotemporal stability and patterning of speech movement sequences. *Exp Brain Res* 104, no. 3 (1995): 493-501.

27. Spindler, B. Yoga therapy and Parkinson's disease. Accessed October 2019. https://yogainternational.com/article/view/yoga-therapy-and-parkinsons-disease.

28. Tanner, M., L. Rammage, and L. Liu. Does singing and vocal strengthening improve vocal ability in people with Parkinson's disease? *Arts Health* 8, no. 3 (2016): 199-212.

29. Vandenberg, B.E., J. Advocat, C. Hassed, et al. Mindfulness-based lifestyle programs for the self-management of Parkinson's disease in Australia. *Health Promot Int* (2019) 34, no. 4: 668.

30. Van Den Eeden, S.K., C.M. Tanner, A.L. Bernstein, et al. Incidence of Parkinson's disease: Variation by age, gender, and race/ethnicity. *Am J Epidemiol* 157, no. 11 (2003): 1015.

Chapter 9

1. Algurén, B., Å. Lundgren-Nilsson, and K.S. Sunnerhagen. Functioning of stroke survivors—A validation of the ICF core set for stroke in Sweden. *Disabil Rehabil* 32, no. 7 (2009): 551-59. https://doi.org/10.3109/09638280903186335.

2. Andrews, A.W., and R.W. Bohannon. Distribution of muscle strength impairments following stroke. *Clin Rehabil* 14, no. 1 (2000): 79-87. https://doi.org/10.1191/026921500673950113.

3. Ay, H., K.L. Furie, A. Singhal, et al. An evidence-based causative classification system for acute ischemic stroke. *Ann Neurol* 58, no. 5 (2005): 688.

4. Benjamin, E.J., et al. Heart disease and stroke statistics-2018 update: A report from the American Heart Association. *Circulation* 137, no. 12 (2018): e67.

5. Beyaert, C., R. Vasa, and G.E. Frykberg. Gait post-stroke: Pathophysiology and rehabilitation strategies. *Neurophysiol Clin* 45, no. 4-5 (2015): 335-55. https://doi.org/10.1016/j.neucli.2015.09.005.

6. Bohannon, R.W. Muscle strength and muscle training after stroke. *J Rehabil Med* 39, no. 1 (2007): 14-20. https://doi.org/10.2340/16501977-0018.

7. Catani, M. A little man of some importance. *Brain* 140, no. 11 (2017): 3055-61.

8. D'Anci, K.E., et al. Treatments for poststroke motor deficits and mood disorders: A systematic review for the 2019 US Department of Veterans Affairs and US Department of Defense guidelines for stroke rehabilitation. *Ann Intern Med* 171, no. 12 (2019): 906-15.

9. Dragert, K., and E.P. Zehr. High-intensity unilateral dorsiflexor resistance training results in bilateral neuromuscular plasticity after stroke. *Exp Brain Res* 225, no. 1 (2012): 93-104. https://doi.org/10.1007/s00221-012-3351-x.

10. Kumar, K. Yoga nidra and its impact on students' well being. *Yoga-Mimasa* 36, no. 1 (2004): 31-35.

11. Lusk, J. *Yoga Nidra for Complete Relaxation and Stress Relief.* Oakland, CA: New Harbinger Publications, 2015.

12. Marieb, E., and K. Hoehn. *Human Anatomy and Physiology.* 7th ed. San Francisco: Pearson Benjamin Cummings, 2007.

13. Middleton, A., S.L. Fritz, and M. Lusardi. Walking speed: The functional vital sign. *J Aging Phys Act* 23, no. 2 (2015): 314-22. https://doi.org/10.1123/japa.2013-0236.

14. Miller, R. 2013. 10 steps of yoga nidra. Updated April 5, 2017. www.yogajournal.com/meditation/10-steps-of-yoga-nidra.

15. Saraswati, S.S., et al. *Yoga nidra.* Bihar School of Yoga, 1984.

16. Schmid, A.A., et al. Poststroke balance improves with yoga: A pilot study. *Stroke* 43, no. 9 (2012): 2402-07.

17. Schmid, A.A., et al. Yoga leads to multiple physical improvements after stroke, a pilot study. *Complement Ther Med* 22, no. 6 (2014): 994-1000.

18. Song, H.-S., and J.-Y. Kim. The effects of yoga exercise on balance and gait velocity in stroke patient. *Journal of the Korea Academia-Industrial cooperation Society* 14, no. 1 (2013): 294-300.

19. Tolahunase, M.R., et al. Yoga- and meditation-based lifestyle intervention increases neuroplasticity and reduces severity of major depressive disorder: A randomized controlled trial. *Restor Neurol Neurosci* 36, no. 3 (2018): 423-42.

Chapter 10

1. Amatya, B., F. Khan, and M. Galea. Rehabilitation for people with multiple sclerosis: An overview of Cochrane Reviews. *Cochrane Database Syst Rev* (2019). https://doi.org/10.1002/14651858.cd012732.pub2.

2. Amatya, B., L. La Mantia, M. Demetrios, and F. Khan. Non-pharmacological interventions for spasticity in multiple sclerosis. *Cochrane Database Syst Rev* (2012). https://doi.org/10.1002/14651858.cd009974.

3. Beer, S., F. Khan, and J. Kesselring. Rehabilitation interventions in multiple sclerosis: An overview. *J Neurol* 259, no. 9 (2012): 1994-2008. https://doi.org/10.1007/s00415-012-6577-4.

4. Bethoux, F., and M.A. Willis. "Spasticity Management in Multiple Sclerosis." In R.J. Fox, A.D. Rae-Grant, and F. Bethoux, eds., *Multiple Sclerosis and Related Disorders.* New York: Springer, 2018. https://doi.org/10.1891/9780826125941.0030.

5. Cameron, M.H., and S. Lord. Postural control in multiple sclerosis: Implications for fall prevention. *Curr Neurol Neurosci Rep* 10, no. 5 (2010): 407-12. https://doi.org/10.1007/s11910-010-0128-0.

6. Cattaneo, D., J. Jonsdottir, M. Zocchi, and A. Regola. Effects of balance exercises on people with multiple sclerosis: A pilot study. *Clin Rehabil* 21, no. 9 (2007): 771-81. https://doi.org/10.1177/0269215507077602.

7. Doulatabad, S.N., K. Nooreyan, A.N. Doulatabad, and Z.M. Noubandegani. The effects of pranayama, hatha and raja yoga on physical pain and the quality of life of women with multiple sclerosis. *Afr J Tradit Complement Altern Med* 10, no. 1

(2012). https://doi.org/10.4314/ajtcam. v10i1.

8. Feinstein, A., N. Rector, and R. Motl. Exercising away the blues: Can it help multiple sclerosis-related depression? *Mult Scler J* 19, no. 14 (2013): 1815-19. https://doi. org/10.1177/1352458513508837.

9. Frank, R., and J. Larimore. Yoga as a method of symptom management in multiple sclerosis. *Front Neurosci* 9 (2015). https://doi.org/10.3389/ fnins.2015.00133.

10. Gosselink, R., L. Kovacs, P. Ketelaer, H. Carton, and M. Decramer. Respiratory muscle weakness and respiratory muscle training in severely disabled multiple sclerosis patients. *Arch Phys Med Rehabil* 81, no. 6 (2000): 747-51.

11. Grossman, P. Effects of a cognitive-behavioural mindfulness intervention upon quality of life, depression and fatigue among multiple sclerosis (MS) patients. http://isrctn.org/ (2013). https://doi.org/10.1186/isrctn21643919.

12. Guner, S., and F. Inanici. Yoga therapy and ambulatory multiple sclerosis assessment of gait analysis parameters, fatigue and balance. *J Bodyw Mov Ther* 19, no. 1 (2015): 72-81. https://doi. org/10.1016/j.jbmt.2014.04.004.

13. Halabchi, F., Z. Alizadeh, M.A. Sahraian, and M. Abolhasani. Exercise prescription for patients with multiple sclerosis: Potential benefits and practical recommendations. *BMC Neurol* 17, no. 1 (2017). https://doi.org/10.1186/s12883-017-0960-9.

14. Jørgensen, M.L.K., U. Dalgas, I. Wens, and L.G. Hvid. Muscle strength and power in persons with multiple sclerosis — A systematic review and meta-analysis. *J Neurol Sci* 376 (2017): 225-41. https://doi. org/10.1016/j.jns.2017.03.022.

15. Middleton, A., S.L. Fritz, and M. Lusardi. Walking speed: The functional vital sign. *J Aging Phys Act* 23, no. 2 (2015): 314-22.

16. National Multiple Sclerosis Society. Living well with MS. Accessed December 3, 2019. https://www.nationalmssociety. org/living-well-with-MS.

17. Novotny, S., and L. Kravitz. The science of breathing. *IDEA Fitness Journal* 4, no. 2 (2007, February): 36-43.

18. O'Connor, A.B., S.R. Schwid, D.N. Herrmann, J.D. Markman, and R.H. Dworkin. Pain associated with multiple sclerosis: Systematic review and proposed classification. *Pain* 137, no. 1 (2008): 96-111. https://doi.org/10.1016/j. pain.2007.08.024.

19. Oken, B.S., S. Kishiyama, D. Zajdel, D. Bourdette, J. Carlsen, M. Haas, C. Hugos, D.F. Kraemer, J. Lawrence, and M. Mass. Randomized controlled trial of yoga and exercise in multiple sclerosis. *Neurology* 62, no. 11 (2004): 2058-64. https://doi. org/10.1212/01.wnl.0000129534.88602.5c.

20. Pritchard, M., P. Elison-Bowers, and B. Birdsall. Impact of Integrative Restoration (IRest) meditation on perceived stress levels in multiple sclerosis and cancer outpatients. *PsycEXTRA Dataset*, 2009. https://doi.org/10.1037/e741342011-166.

21. Ronai, P., T. Lafontaine, and L. Bollinger. Exercise guidelines for persons with multiple sclerosis. *Strength Cond J* 33, no. 1 (2011): 30-33. https://doi.org/10.1519/ ssc.0b013e3181fd0b2e.

22. Salgado, B.C., M. Jones, S. Ilgun, G. McCord, and M. Loper-Powers. Effects of a 4-month Ananda Program on physical and mental health outcomes for persons with multiple sclerosis. *Int J Yoga Therap* 23 (2013): 27-38.

23. Thoumie, P., D. Lamotte, S. Cantalloube, M. Faucher, and G. Amarenco. Motor determinants of gait in 100 ambulatory

patients with multiple sclerosis. *Mult Scler J* 11, no. 4 (2005): 485-91. https://doi.org/10.1191/1352458505ms1176oa.

24. Westerdahl, E., et al. Deep breathing exercises with positive expiratory pressure in patients with multiple sclerosis—A randomized controlled trial. *Clin Respir J* 10, no. 6 (2016): 698-706.

Chapter 11

1. Ashwal, S., et al. Practice parameter: Diagnostic assessment of the child with cerebral palsy: Report of the Quality Standards Subcommittee of the American Academy of Neurology and the Practice Committee of the Child Neurology Society. *Neurology* 62, no. 6 (2004): 851-63.

2. Dallmeijer, A.J., E.A. Rameckers, H. Houdijk, S. De Groot, V.A. Scholtes, and J.G. Becher. Isometric muscle strength and mobility capacity in children with cerebral palsy. *Disabil Rehabil* 39, no. 2 (2015): 135-42. https://doi.org/10.3109/09638288.2015.1095950.

3. Dewar, R., S. Love, and L.M. Johnston. Exercise interventions improve postural control in children with cerebral palsy: A systematic review. *Dev Med Child Neurol* 57, no. 6 (2014): 504-20. https://doi.org/10.1111/dmcn.12660.

4. Ferland, C., C. Lepage, H. Moffet, and D.B. Maltais. Relationships between lower limb muscle strength and locomotor capacity in children and adolescents with cerebral palsy who walk independently. *Phys Occup Ther Pediatr* 32, no. 3 (2011): 320-32. https://doi.org/10.3109/01942638.2011.631102.

5. Hong, W.H., H.C. Chen, I.H. Shen, C.Y. Chen, C.L. Chen, and C.Y. Chung. Knee muscle strength at varying angular velocities and associations with gross motor function in ambulatory children with cerebral palsy. *Res Dev Disabil*

33, no. 6 (2012): 2308-16. https://doi.org/10.1016/j.ridd.2012.07.010.

6. Huntsman, R., E. Lemire, J. Norton, A. Dzus, P. Blakley, and S. Hasal. The differential diagnosis of spastic diplegia. *Arch Dis Child* 100, no. 5 (2014): 500-04. https://doi.org/10.1136/archdischild-2014-307443.

7. Novak, I., et al. Clinical prognostic messages from a systematic review on cerebral palsy. *Pediatrics* 130, no. 5 (2012): e1285-e1312.

8. Rodda, J., and H.K. Graham. Classification of gait patterns in spastic hemiplegia and spastic diplegia: A basis for a management algorithm. *Eur J Neurol* l8, no. s5 (2001): 98-108. https://doi.org/10.1046/j.1468-1331.2001.00042.x.

9. Rosenbaum, P., Paneth, N., Leviton, A., et al. A report: The definition and classification of cerebral palsy April 2006 [published correction appears in Dev Med Child Neurol. 2007 Jun;49(6):480]. *Dev Med Child Neurol Suppl.* 109 (2007): 8-14.

10. Selber, P.R.P., and H.K. Graham. Pelvic tilt changes after hamstring lengthening in children with cerebral palsy. *J Pediatr Orthop* 39, no. 5 (2019). https://doi.org/10.1097/bpo.0000000000001422.

11. Wright, M., and L. Wallman. "Cerebral Palsy." In S. Campbell, R. Palisano, and M. Orlin, eds., *Physical Therapy for Children*, 4th ed., 577-627. St. Louis, MO: Elsevier Saunders, 2012.

About the Authors

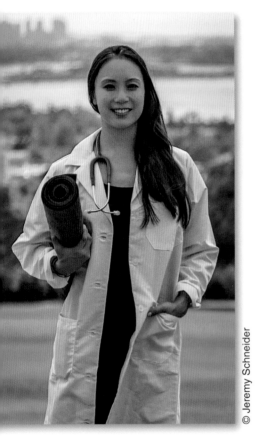

© Jeremy Schneider

Ingrid Yang, MD, JD, E-RYT 500, C-IAYT, is a deeply knowledgeable, creative, and inspiring yoga therapist, teacher, and physician. She earned her doctorate of medicine from Rush Medical College in Chicago, Illinois. She then received postgraduate residency training at Northwestern's Feinberg School of Medicine, where she specialized in physical medicine and rehabilitation, completing a year of inpatient rehabilitation medicine training. Dr. Yang subsequently completed an internal medicine residency at Scripps Green Hospital in San Diego, California. She was awarded her juris doctorate at Duke University School of Law and received her bachelor of arts in economics at Barnard College in New York City. Her first book, *Hatha Yoga Asanas: A Pocket Guide to Personal Practice*, was published by Human Kinetics in 2011. Dr. Yang leads teacher trainings, workshops, and retreats all over the world. She seeks to integrate her background in allopathic medicine with the ancient teachings of the centuries-old yoga traditions. Her teaching is seeded deeply in dharmic philosophies and an expert grasp of movement kinesiology. Her special focus on the physiology of healing through breath work, meditation, and mind–body connection brings a unique and joyful perspective to the practice and study of yoga. Prior to her current work, Dr. Yang was an intellectual property attorney; founded and owned Blue Point Yoga Center in Durham, North Carolina; and entertained audiences as a jazz singer in Australia.

Kyle Fahey, DPT, PT, is a doctor of physical therapy and senior physical therapist at the Shirley Ryan AbilityLab in Chicago, Illinois, the world's largest and top-ranked acute rehabilitation hospital. As a graduate of Northwestern University's doctor of physical therapy program, Dr. Fahey is an expert in biomechanics and rehabilitation for those with severe disabilities in all levels of rehab. He develops programs for his patients to regain and preserve strength, endurance, and balance following debilitating injury or illness. In 2017, Dr. Fahey was made Shirley Ryan's pain management physical therapy director and specialist. In this role, he formulates 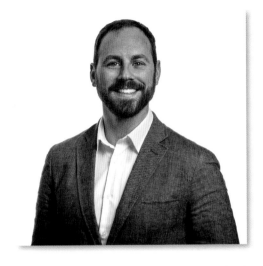 pain-specific interventions and consultations to individuals with a wide variety of medical diagnoses throughout the hospital. He is the founder and creator of a weekly wheelchair yoga program for the hospital and seamlessly integrates adaptive yoga into his treatments. Dr. Fahey is also the chairman of the Telehealth and Technology in Practice Committee of the Illinois Physical Therapy Association and serves as an active member of the American Physical Therapy Association. As a leader in the physical therapy telehealth initiative, he strives to improve access to physical therapy care and believes that everyone can benefit from rehab.

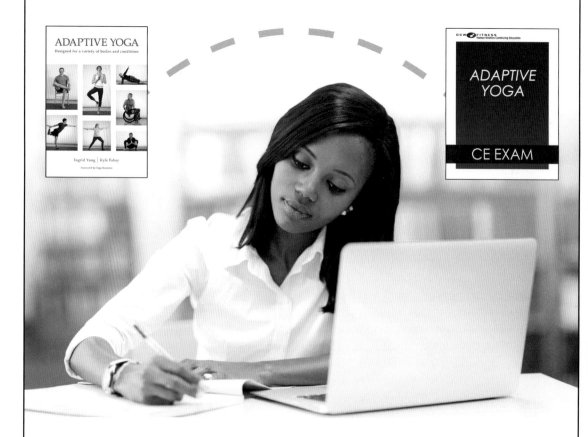
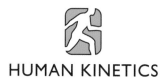